Horizons in Medicine

······ *number* 13

Edited by

Stephanie Amiel MD FRCP

RD Lawrence Professor of Diabetic Medicine
Department of Diabetes, Endocrinology and Internal Medicine,
Guy's, King's and St Thomas' School of Medicine, London

Royal College of
Physicians of London

Publisher's Acknowledgements

The Royal College of Physicians is pleased to acknowledge generous support towards the cost of production of this book from:

Pfizer Pharmaceuticals Group

GlaxoSmithKline Medical Fellowship

Cover illustrations

Front cover: Mucosa-associated *Escherichia coli* obtained from Crohn's disease tissue, demonstrating their ability to invade intestinal cells. From: Rhodes J. Advances in inflammatory bowel disease.

Back cover (top): An extracellular plaque consisting of a core of amyloid peptide surrounded by neuritic change, revealed by silver staining in Alzheimer disease brain. From: Lovestone S. Alzheimer's disease: from palliation to modification.

Back cover (bottom): Hepatic and splenic AA amyloid deposits in a patient with rheumatoid arthritis. From: Hawkins P. Amyloidosis.

Royal College of Physicians of London
11 St Andrews Place, London NW1 4LE

Registered Charity No. 210508

Copyright © 2002 Royal College of Physicians of London
ISBN 1 86016 154 5

Typeset by Dan-Set Graphics, Telford, Shropshire
Printed in Great Britain by The Lavenham Press Ltd, Sudbury, Suffolk

British Library Cataloguing in Publication Data
A catalogue record of this book is available from the British Library

Editor's preface

I wanted 'my' Advanced Medicine Conference to be the best ever. It was not, of course, as these annual conferences are of a uniformly high standard and always both enjoyable and enlightening, but I think it was of a standard comparable to the rest and – in retrospect – I enjoyed it enormously. I think the audience did too.

When I set out to create the programme, I was aware that the aim of the conference was to present advanced science as it applies to current clinical practice. The challenge was the greater as 2000 was also the first year of the 'General Medicine for Specialists' conferences, designed to present state-of-the-art clinical practice to Fellows and Members – a nice distinction, as of course the Advanced Medicine Conference audience is composed of clinicians, and they want to hear information that is exciting but also relevant to their practice.

I quickly realised that I could not compile an appropriate programme single-handed. This is the era of the specialist and, while I could provide many 'names' in my own field (diabetes), my last personal exposure to oncology, for example, was in my registrar post in 1981. I had no doubt that the specialty – and its exponents – had moved on since then! I am extraordinarily grateful to the speakers, chairmen and colleagues who helped me to compile innovative programmes in their field: Professor David Kerr of Birmingham, Professors Gulam Mufti and Simon Wessley and Drs John Costello, Hugh Cairns and Martyn Thomas of King's College Hospital, Professor Ian Gilmore of Liverpool, and Professor Sir George Alberti, occasionally of Newcastle. Without their advice and help, the glittering array of speakers might have shone a little less brilliantly. I am also grateful to the organiser of last year's conference, Peter Weissberg, who was my role model throughout. It is a reflection of the quality of both the conference and the speakers that the audience also contributed significantly to its success, enlivening the programme during discussions.

The speakers not only delivered highly professional and topical presentations but they also generously provided manuscripts over which they took at least as much trouble. The subsequent publication is presented here and reflects the excitement and utility of the conference itself. As with others in the series, *Horizons in Medicine 13* relates current research to current practice in a range of specialist areas of interest to the generalist, and features a series of discussions on 'hot topics' of the year 2001. This year, for the first time, the *Horizons* series is being recognised officially as a 'Continuing Professional Development' reading text, but I hope it will appeal to clinicians at every stage of their careers. I can certify from experience that reading this volume and attending these conferences can alter clinical practice. I used some of the evidence to treat a patient with a highly effective treatment extracted from a chapter I had edited the previous week!

The conference and this publication would not have the reputation they deserve were it not for the highly professional attentions of the College staff. I cannot sign off without specifically thanking Anne McSweeny and her team in the Conference Department, Barry Lewis and his audiovisual expertise, and Tom Allum and Mary Firth in the Publications Department, without whom the 13th Advanced Medicine Conference would have been only an evanescent success.

STEPHANIE A AMIEL

December 2001

Contributors

JENNIFER ADGEY *Consultant Cardiologist, Regional Medical Cardiology Centre, Royal Victoria Hospital, Grosvenor Road, Belfast BT12 6BA*

MICHAEL ADLER *Professor of Sexually Transmitted Diseases, Department of Sexually Transmitted Diseases, Royal Free and University College Medical School, The Mortimer Market Centre, Off Capper Street, London WC1E 6AU*

STEPHANIE A AMIEL *R D Lawrence Professor of Diabetic Medicine, Department of Diabetes, Endocrinology and Internal Medicine, Guy's, King's and St Thomas' School of Medicine, King's College Denmark Hill Campus, Bessemer Road, London SE5 9PJ*

RUDY BILOUS *Professor of Clinical Medicine, Education Centre, The James Cook University Hospital, Marton Road, Middlesbrough TS4 3BW*

ANDREW K BURROUGHS *Consultant Physician and Hepatologist, Liver Transplantation and Hepatobiliary Medicine, Royal Free Hospital, Pond Street, London NW3 2QG*

A JOHN CAMM *Professor of Clinical Cardiology, Department of Cardiological Sciences, St George's Hospital Medical School, Cranmer Terrace, London SW17 ORE*

JOHN G F CLELAND *Professor, Academic Unit, Department of Cardiology, Castle Hill Hospital, University of Hull, Kingston upon Hull, East Yorkshire HU16 5JQ*

PAUL A CORRIS *Professor of Thoracic Medicine, University of Newcastle and Department of Respiratory Medicine, Regional Cardiothoracic Centre, Freeman Hospital, Newcastle upon Tyne NE7 7DN*

JOHN COSTELLO *Consultant Physician, Department of Respiratory Medicine and Allergy, Guy's, King's and St Thomas' School of Medicine, King's College Denmark Hill Campus, Bessemer Road, London SE5 9PJ*

PHILIP J COWEN *Professor of Psychopharmacology and MRC Clinical Scientist, University Department of Psychiatry, Warneford Hospital, Oxford OX3 7JX*

NICHOLAS C P CROSS *Wessex Regional Genetics Laboratory, Salisbury District Hospital, Salisbury SP2 8BJ*

ELWYN ELIAS *Professor of Hepatology, Liver and Hepatobiliary Unit, Queen Elizabeth Hospital, Nuffield House 3rd floor, Edgbaston, Birmingham B15 2TH*

MOHSEN EL KOSSI *Research Fellow, Sheffield Kidney Institute, Northern General Hospital, Herries Road, Sheffield S5 7AU*

MEGUID EL NAHAS *Professor of Nephrology, Head of the Academic Section of Medicine, Sheffield Kidney Institute, Northern General Hospital, Herries Road, Sheffield S5 7AU*

MARK FARRINGTON *Consultant Microbiologist, Public Health and Clinical Microbiology Laboratory, Box 236, Addenbrooke's Hospital, Cambridge CB2 2QW*

JOHN M GOLDMAN *Professor, Chairman, Department of Haematology, Imperial College, Hammersmith Hospital, Du Cane Road, London W12 0NN*

MARTIN GORE *Consultant Cancer Physician, Melanoma Unit, Royal Marsden Hospital, Fulham Road, London SW3 6JJ*

SIMON GRUMETT *Clinical Research Fellow, CRC Institute for Cancer Studies, University of Birmingham, Edgbaston, Birmingham B15 2TT*

PHILIP HAWKINS *Clinical Director, National Amyloidosis Centre, Royal Free and University College Medical School, Royal Free Hospital, Rowland Hill Street, London NW3 2PF*

PHILIP HOME *Professor of Diabetes Medicine, Department of Diabetes and Metabolism, University of Newcastle upon Tyne, Framlington Place, Newcastle upon Tyne NE2 4HH*

DAVID JAYNE *Consultant in Nephrology and Vasculitis, Box 157, Department of Medicine, Addenbrooke's Hospital, Cambridge CB1 2SP*

ROSE ANNE KENNY *Professor of Cardiovascular Research, Cardiovascular Investigation Unit, Royal Victoria Infirmary, Queen Victoria Road, Newcastle upon Tyne NE1 4LP*

DAVID KERR *Rhodes Professor of Therapeutic Sciences and Clinical Pharmacology; Director, National Translational Cancer Research Network, University of Oxford, Department of Clinical Pharmacology, Radcliffe Infirmary, Woodstock Road, Oxford OX2 6HE*

ROBERT LEONARD *Professor of Cancer Studies, South-West Wales Cancer Institute, University of Wales, Swansea*

SIMON LOVESTONE *Professor of Old Age Psychiatry, Departments of Old Age Psychiatry and Neuroscience, Institute of Psychiatry, De Crespigny Park, London SE5 8AF*

WILLIAM A LYNN *Consultant in Infectious Diseases, Infection and Immunity Unit, Ealing Hospital, Uxbridge Road, Southall, London UB1 3HW*

IAIN C MACDOUGALL *Consultant Nephrologist and Honorary Senior Lecturer, Department of Renal Medicine, King's College Hospital, East Dulwich Grove, London SE22 8PT*

GANESH MANOHARAN *Specialist Registrar in Cardiology, Regional Medical Cardiology Centre, Royal Victoria Hospital, Grosvenor Road, Belfast BT12 6BA*

GORDON T McINNES *Senior Lecturer in Medicine and Therapeutics, Department of Medicine and Therapeutics, Gardiner Institute, Western Infirmary, Glasgow G11 6NT*

IAN B A MENOWN *Specialist Registrar in Cardiology, Regional Medical Cardiology Centre, Royal Victoria Hospital, Grosvenor Road, Belfast BT12 6BA*

RACHEL MIDGLEY *Registrar in Medical Oncology, CRC Institute for Cancer Studies, University of Birmingham, Edgbaston, Birmingham B15 2TT*

PIOTR MILKIEWICZ *Clinical Fellow, Liver and Hepatobiliary Unit, Queen Elizabeth Hospital, Nuffield House 3rd floor, Edgbaston, Birmingham B15 2TH*

PAOLO MONTALTO *Honorary Clinical Research Fellow, Liver Transplantation and Hepatobiliary Medicine, Royal Free Hospital, Pond Street, London NW3 2QG*

MICHAEL L NICHOLSON *Professor of Surgery, Division of Transplant Surgery, Leicester General Hospital, Gwendolen Road, Leicester LE5 4PW*

PETER A O'CALLAGHAN *Department of Cardiological Sciences, St George's Hospital Medical School, Cranmer Terrace, London SW17 0RE*

CRAIG PARKINSON *Clinical Research Fellow, Department of Endocrinology, Christie Hospital, Wilmslow Road, Manchester M20 4BX*

STEPHEN J PROCTOR *Professor, Clinical Director Specialist Haematology; Head, School of Clinical and Laboratory Sciences, University Department of Haematology, Royal Victoria Infirmary, Newcastle upon Tyne NE1 4LP*

TERENCE H RABBITTS *Joint Head, Division of Protein and Nucleic Acid Chemistry, MRC Laboratory of Molecular Biology, Hills Road, Cambridge CB2 2QH*

JONATHAN RHODES *Professor of Medicine, University of Liverpool, Liverpool L69 3GA*

JOHN RIDDELL *Specialist Registrar in Cardiology, Regional Medical Cardiology Centre, Royal Victoria Hospital, Grosvenor Road, Belfast BT12 6BA*

SUSANNAH V ROWLES *Clinical Research Fellow, Department of Endocrinology, Christie Hospital, Wilmslow Road, Manchester M20 4BX*

ANDREW STEPTOE *British Heart Foundation Professor of Psychology, Department of Epidemiology and Public Health, University College London, 1-19 Torrington Place, London WC1 6BT*

ANNA STEVENSON *Clinical Research Fellow, Melanoma Unit, Royal Marsden Hospital, Fulham Road, London SW3 6JJ*

MARTYN THOMAS *Consultant Cardiologist, Department of Cardiology, King's College Hospital, London SE5 9RS*

PETER J TRAINER *Consultant Endocrinologist, Department of Endocrinology, Christie Hospital, Wilmslow Road, Manchester M20 4BX*

ALASTAIR WATSON *Professor of Medicine, Department of Medicine, University of Liverpool, Daulby Street, Liverpool L69 3BA*

A KEVIN WEBB *Professor, Clinical Director of Manchester Adult Cystic Fibrosis Unit, Wythenshawe Hospital, Manchester M23 9LT*

SIMON WESSELY *Professor, Guy's, King's and St Thomas' School of Medicine, 103 Denmark Hill, London SE5 8AF*

HAMDY ABO ZENAH *Research Fellow, Sheffield Kidney Institute, Northern General Hospital, Herries Road, Sheffield S5 7AU*

Contents

NEPHROLOGY AND TRANSPLANTATION MEDICINE

DIABETES: INCREASING LIFE EXPECTANCY

HAEMATOLOGY

PSYCHIATRY AND PSYCHOLOGY

RESPIRATORY MEDICINE AND CHEST DISEASE

THE CROONIAN LECTURE

Cardiology

Failed sudden cardiac death

Peter O'Callaghan and John Camm

☐ INTRODUCTION

Sudden and unexpected cardiac death (SCD) is estimated to cause 12% of natural deaths and accounts for approximately half of all cardiac related deaths [1]. Despite a significant reduction in total cardiac mortality in recent years, the proportion of sudden deaths has remained unchanged. In-field ECG monitoring has demonstrated that the principal cause of SCD in victims of out-of-hospital cardiac arrest is ventricular fibrillation (VF). In more than 80% of SCD there is abrupt onset of ventricular tachycardia (VT) that progresses to VF. Advances in medical technology have resulted in a contradiction of terms. Events that in the past would have resulted in death may today be successfully aborted with prompt cardiopulmonary resuscitation and defibrillation, leading to the term 'failed sudden cardiac death'. The investigation and management of SCD survivors, and in certain cases the families of SCD victims, remain a challenging and rapidly evolving clinical field.

Many disease states may result in SCD (Table 1). Structural heart disease is almost always present. Coronary artery disease (CAD) accounts for 80% of cases of SCD in Western societies. It is estimated that SCD occurs as the first clinical manifestation in up to 25% of all individuals in the community with CAD. Among patients with known CAD, about half of all cardiac deaths are sudden.

☐ SUDDEN CARDIAC DEATH INVESTIGATIONS

Following successful resuscitation from cardiac arrest, it is extremely important to establish an accurate diagnosis. It is important not only for the patient but also for relatives who may be at risk of SCD if not appropriately identified and managed. Table 2 lists the investigations that may help in establishing a diagnosis. All the investigations may be necessary in selected patients.

In practice, it is useful first to pose three questions:

1 Is there a reversible cause?

2 Is there a curable cause?

3 What is the underlying structural heart disease?

Is there a reversible cause?

Reversible causes of SCD include VF occurring in the setting of an acute myocardial infarction (MI), drug proarrhythmia, illicit drug use and others listed in Table 1. It

Table 1 Causes of sudden cardiac death.

	Cause of sudden death

Structural heart disease	Coronary artery disease:
	  atherosclerotic
	  congenital
	Dilated cardiomyopathy
	Hypertrophic cardiomyopathy
	Valvular heart disease
	Congenital heart disease
	Myocarditis
	Arrhythmogenic right ventricular cardiomyopathy
	Infiltrations (amyloid, sarcoid, tumours)
	Primary pulmonary hypertension

Structurally normal heart	Wolff-Parkinson-White syndrome Congenital long QT syndrome Brugada syndrome Bradycardia-induced *torsades de pointes* Idiopathic ventricular tachycardia
Reversible causes	Acute myocardial infarction (<48 hours) Acquired (drug-induced) long QT syndrome Toxic agents (cocaine, alcohol, etc) Severe electrolyte abnormalities Commotio cordis

Table 2 Sudden cardiac death investigations.

Index event	Reversible cause? Treatable cause? Cardiac post-mortem?
Non-invasive imaging	Echocardiogram Functional scans MRI scan
Non-invasive electrophysiological assessment	ECG x 3 24–48-hour Holter monitoring Exercise stress test Signal-averaged ECG T wave alternans? QT dispersion?
Drug challenges	Adenosine iv Ajmaline iv
Genetic screening	Hypertrophic cardiomyopathy Congenital long QT syndrome Brugada syndrome Arrhythmogenic right ventricular cardiomyopathy
Invasive tests	Cardiac catheterisation Invasive electrophysiological testing Cardiac biopsy

iv = intravenous; MRI = magnetic resonance imaging.

is important to enquire about any prodromal symptoms in the hours, days or weeks preceding a cardiac arrest. A history of increasing angina, chest pain at rest, palpitations or syncope should be sought. Other relevant aspects of the history include a detailed drug history, history of illicit drug use or heavy alcohol consumption, or a family history of sudden unexpected death. A detailed physical examination should look for evidence of chronic atherosclerosis, signs of structural heart disease and any significant co-morbid conditions. Serial ECG and cardiac enzymes are obtained to rule out an acute MI. Interpretation of these test results can be difficult in a resuscitated patient as external defibrillation may result in elevated cardiac enzymes and transient ECG changes. Blood samples should be sent for toxicology screening as soon as possible after a cardiac arrest.

Meticulous attention to detail and careful clinical, ECG and toxicological assessment should identify those patients who had a cardiac arrest as a result of a reversible and, in the future, potentially avoidable cause.

Is there a curable cause?

Curable causes of cardiac arrest are rare but accurate identification of these patients is important in order to avoid inappropriate long-term implantable defibrillator therapy. Cardiac arrest may occur secondary to Wolff-Parkinson-White syndrome (see below) or bundle branch re-entry VT, both of which can be cured by radiofrequency catheter ablation. Bundle branch re-entry VT typically occurs in a patient with dilated cardiomyopathy and His-Purkinje system disease resulting in baseline left bundle branch block. Sustained monomorphic VT is due to a macroreentry circuit, usually with slow conduction down the right bundle and retrograde activation of the left bundle. Tachycardia is easily cured by radiofrequency catheter ablation directed at the right bundle branch. These patients may require adjunctive pacemaker or antiarrhythmic therapy due to the presence of significant structural heart disease and conduction system disease.

What is the underlying structural heart disease?

After excluding a reversible or curable cause of failed SCD it is necessary to diagnose the underlying structural heart disease (Table 1). In over 90% of cases the diagnosis is obvious following echocardiography and cardiac catheterisation, usually performed as routine early investigations in the vast majority of cardiac arrest survivors. A more challenging problem is posed by the 5–10% of patients in whom these two tests are normal. However, accurate diagnosis of the cause of cardiac arrest in patients with apparently 'normal' hearts is important not only for the patient but also for relatives because of genetic causes of SCD.

☐ APPARENTLY 'NORMAL' HEART AND SUDDEN CARDIAC DEATH

In patients with 'normal' echocardiography and cardiac catheterisation it is helpful actively to consider the following diagnoses:

- ☐ Wolff-Parkinson-White syndrome

☐   Congenital long QT syndrome (LQTS)

☐   Hypertrophic cardiomyopathy (HCM)

☐   Arrhythmogenic right ventricular cardiomyopathy (ARVC)

☐   Brugada syndrome.

Wolff-Parkinson-White syndrome

Accessory atrioventricular connections (accessory pathways (APs)) may result in ventricular pre-excitation (short PR interval, delta wave and increased QRS duration) which in a symptomatic patient is known as the Wolff-Parkinson-White syndrome. Not all life-threatening APs are immediately apparent on the ECG. If the vast majority of the ventricular myocardium is activated via the AV node and His-Purkinje system, the ECG may show either subtle changes (eg loss of normal Q waves, small R wave in lead V1) or no abnormality. None the less, under the influence of increased adrenergic drive in a patient with atrial fibrillation this AP may conduct impulses so rapidly to the ventricles that there is degeneration into VF. Careful review of all available ECGs and rhythm strips may reveal evidence of intermittent ventricular pre-excitation. Intravenous adenosine, which transiently blocks AV nodal conduction, is a simple means of unmasking the presence of an AP, or a formal electrophysiological study may be undertaken.

Congenital long QT syndrome

The typical clinical presentation of congenital LQTS is syncope or cardiac arrest, precipitated by physical or emotional stress, in a young individual with a prolonged QT interval (QTc >460 ms) on the ECG. Diagnosis is difficult and complicated for two main reasons:

1   The baseline ECG may appear normal, with QT prolongation and T wave abnormalities occurring either intermittently or immediately prior to an episode of *torsades de pointes* or following a sinus pause. Analysis of multiple ECG recordings, 24–48 hour Holter recordings and exercise stress testing (QTc during tachycardia and recovery phase) may be necessary to establish the diagnosis.

2   Congenital LQTS may result from different gene mutations, not all of which are yet identified. There is incomplete penetrance and the frequent occurrence of sporadic cases. Nevertheless, screening ECGs of first-degree relatives can help establish a diagnosis.

Treatment

Beta-blockade is the mainstay of treatment in congenital LQTS. Analysis of long-term follow-up data from the international LQTS registry to determine the prognosis in patients according to their symptoms prior to treatment initiation shows that with syncope the probability of cardiac arrest or death is only 3%. By contrast, in patients with a history of cardiac arrest, the probability of a recurrent cardiac arrest or death despite beta-blocker therapy is 13% [2]. These data are limited by a lack of information on drug compliance, but nevertheless stress that patients with congenital LQTS who have survived a cardiac arrest require full-dose beta-blockade as a minimum and may have a better prognosis following defibrillator implantation.

Hypertrophic cardiomyopathy

HCM should be carefully considered in patients with cardiac arrest and apparently 'normal' hearts. Sometimes careful review of the echocardiogram or echocardiography of first-degree relatives is required to establish the diagnosis. Symptom severity correlates poorly with risk of SCD. Analysis of 78 failed SCD patients found that 71% were less than 30 years old, 54% had no functional limitations (New York Heart Association class I) and 61% were performing sedentary or minimal physical activity immediately prior to cardiac arrest [3]. Haemodynamic variables such as left ventricular outflow tract obstruction are not useful in risk stratification for SCD.

The risk factors for SCD in HCM patients are:

☐ family history of SCD

☐ syncope

☐ non-sustained VT on Holter monitoring

☐ abnormal blood pressure response to exercise.

Treatment

Survivors of cardiac arrest diagnosed with HCM are usually treated with an implantable defibrillator. In addition, family screening (echocardiography and genetic testing) and family counselling should be undertaken.

Arrhythmogenic right ventricular cardiomyopathy

ARVC is characterised by fatty or fibrofatty replacement of myocardium predominantly of the right ventricular free wall. Approximately one-third of cases are familial, with an autosomal dominant mode of inheritance. The ECG features include T wave inversion in V1–V3, right bundle branch block or right ventricular conduction delay manifest as a terminal notch on the QRS complex of right ventricular leads (epsilon wave). Patients commonly have ventricular ectopy or VT of left bundle branch block pattern suggestive of a right ventricular VT origin.

Diagnosis can be difficult due to a wide spectrum of disease severity. Careful reassessment of the echocardiogram may be useful, looking in particular at right ventricular size and function. In addition, patients tend to have a positive signal-averaged ECG unlike patients with structurally normal hearts. At our institution cardiac magnetic resonance imaging is used to assess fatty infiltration of the myocardium. The course and prognosis of ARVC are highly variable and difficult to predict. Patients who have survived a cardiac arrest are advised to undergo defibrillator implantation.

Brugada syndrome

Brugada syndrome was originally described in patients with failed SCD, no structural heart disease and a characteristic ECG consisting of right bundle branch block and ST segment elevation in V1–V3 (Fig. 1) [4]. A molecular defect in the cardiac sodium channel gene transmitted with an autosomal pattern of inheritance forms the genetic basis of this syndrome. The incidence of sudden death is estimated at 5–10% per year. Diagnosis is complicated because the baseline ECG may be entirely normal, even in patients who have suffered or are at risk of SCD. Drug challenge with a sodium channel-blocking agent such as intravenous ajmaline invariably unmasks the ECG pattern in patients who possess the genotype. Prospective evaluation of 63 patients for three years found that the Brugada syndrome is associated with a 27% incidence of syncope or sudden death, and that the probability of sudden death in asymptomatic individuals is as high as in SCD survivors. Unlike congenital LQTS, Brugada syndrome does not respond to drug therapy. At present, the mainstay of therapy is defibrillator implantation.

☐ SCREENING OF FAMILY MEMBERS

Screening is indicated for the family of a young SCD victim, and occasionally when the diagnosis is unclear despite extensive investigation in a patient with failed SCD. The exact form of family screening needs to be individualised according to both the perceived risks to the asymptomatic individual and the perceived likelihood of a given diagnosis. Echocardiography, ECG, Holter recordings and exercise stress tests are often performed. Intravenous ajmaline is frequently administered in a monitored setting to unmask Brugada syndrome. Genetic screening is starting to play a role in the identification or risk stratification of families with congenital LQTS, HCM, Brugada syndrome and ARVC.

☐ MANAGEMENT OF FAILED SUDDEN CARDIAC DEATH

Survivors of cardiac arrest, in the absence of an acute MI (first 48 hours), are at high risk of future recurrence. Data from the 1970s, which today reflect the natural history of this condition, show a 36% one-year mortality rate in patients who were successfully resuscitated, hospitalised and discharged home following an out-of-hospital VF arrest.

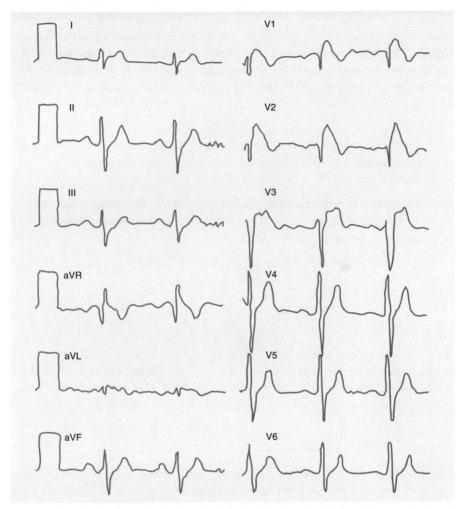

Fig. 1 ECG in Brugada syndrome. Characteristic features include right bundle branch block and convex upward ST segment elevation in V1–V3.

Although most failed SCD patients have significant CAD, the role of ischaemia in the pathogenesis of SCD is not clearly defined. Only a small proportion of patients have clinical evidence of an acute MI. None the less, transient ischaemia is suspected to be the major trigger for life-threatening ventricular tachyarrhythmias. Cardiac catheterisation identifies those survivors who have critical obstructive CAD. It is our practice to revascularise these patients whenever feasible and also to recommend implantable defibrillator therapy. In addition, patients need to be treated optimally with agents known to reduce total and sudden death mortality including, where appropriate, aspirin, beta-blockers, statins, angiotensin-converting enzyme inhibitors and spironolactone.

In patients without a reversible or curable cause the mainstay of treatment is almost always implantable defibrillator therapy.

Comparison of implantable defibrillators and antiarrhythmic agents

Three large prospective implantable cardioverter-defibrillator (ICD) trials compared implantable defibrillators with antiarrhythmic drug therapy (mainly amiodarone) in patients with life-threatening ventricular tachyarrhythmias. They consistently showed that the implantable defibrillator improves overall survival:

1   In the Antiarrhythmics versus Implantable Defibrillator (AVID) study in over 1,000 patients implantable defibrillators resulted in a 31% reduction in total mortality at three years compared with the antiarrhythmic drug therapy group (25% vs 36%, p <0.02) (Fig. 2) [5].

2   The Canadian Implantable Defibrillator Study (CIDS) [6] and the Cardiac Arrest Study Hamburg (CASH) trial [7] also found lower total mortality rates in ICD recipients.

Only the AVID trial reached clear statistical significance. A meta-analysis of these three trials was presented at the North American Society of Pacing and Electrophysiology Annual Scientific Sessions, 1999 [8]. Compared to amiodarone, the ICD reduced total mortality by 27% (p <0.05). As a result of evidence from these clinical trials, the ICD is now accepted as the therapy of first choice in failed SCD patients.

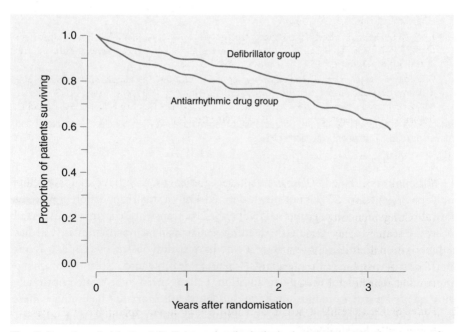

Fig. 2 Overall survival in the defibrillator and antiarrhythmic drug groups up to three years after randomisation in the Antiarrhythmics versus Implantable Defibrillator (AVID) trial. Survival was better among patients treated with the implantable defibrillator (p <0.02).

☐ CONCLUSIONS

The management and prognosis of patients following failed SCD have substantially improved since the availability of implantable defibrillators. In patients without an identifiable reversible or curable cause, any underlying structural heart disease needs to be treated aggressively by revascularisation, risk factor reduction and optimal medical therapy in addition to defibrillator implantation. Failed SCD patients with apparently normal hearts and relatives of young SCD victims need to be investigated carefully so that appropriate primary prevention strategies can be instituted in order to break the vicious cycle of SCD in a family.

REFERENCES

1   Pinto DS, Josephson ME. Sudden cardiac death. In: Hurst JW (ed). *Hurst's the heart*, 10th edn. New York: The McGraw Hill Co, 2001: 1015–48.

2   Schwartz PJ, Priori SG, Napolitano C. The long QT syndrome. In: Zipes DP, Jalife J (ed). *Cardiac electrophysiology: from cell to bedside*, 3rd edn. Philadelphia: WB Saunders Co, 2000: 597–615.

3   Maron BJ, Roberts WC, Epstein SE. Sudden death in hypertrophic cardiomyopathy: a profile of 78 patients. *Circulation* 1982; **65**: 388–94.

4   Brugada J, Brugada R, Brugada P. Right bundle-branch block and ST-segment elevation in leads V1 through V3: a marker for sudden death in patients without demonstrable structural heart disease. *Circulation* 1998; **97**: 457–60.

5   A comparison of antiarrhythmic-drug therapy with implantable defibrillators in patients resuscitated from near-fatal ventricular arrhythmias. The Antiarrhythmics Versus Implantable Defibrillators (AVID) Investigators. *N Engl J Med* 1997; **337**: 1576–83.

6   Connolly SJ, Gent M, Roberts RS, Dorian P, *et al.* Canadian implantable defibrillator study (CIDS): a randomized trial of the implantable cardioverter defibrillator against amiodarone. *Circulation* 2000; **101**: 1297–302.

7   Kuck KH, Cappato R, Siebels J, Ruppel R. Randomized comparison of antiarrhythmic drug therapy with implantable defibrillators in patients resuscitated from cardiac arrest: the Cardiac Arrest Study Hamburg (CASH). *Circulation* 2000; **102**: 748–54.

8   Connolly SJ, Hallstrom AP, Cappato R, Schron EB, *et al.* Meta-analysis of the implantable cardioverter defibrillator secondary prevention trials. AVID, CASH and CIDS studies. Antiarrhythmics vs Implantable Defibrillator study. Cardiac Arrest Study Hamburg. Canadian Implantable Defibrillator Study. *Eur Heart J* 2000; **21**: 2071–8.

☐ SELF ASSESSMENT QUESTIONS

1   The three commonest causes of sudden cardiac death (SCD) in patients over 35 years old are:
    (a) Congenital long QT syndrome (LQTS)
    (b) Coronary artery disease
    (c) Anomalous coronary arteries
    (d) Hypertrophic cardiomyopathy (HCM)
    (e) Valvular heart disease

2   Failed SCD as a result of each of the following requires implantable cardioverter-defibrillator (ICD) therapy:
    (a) Acute myocardial infarction
    (b) Wolff-Parkinson-White (WPW) syndrome

(c) Brugada syndrome
(d) HCM
(e) Congenital LQTS

3 The following are risk factors for SCD in patients with HCM:
(a) Abnormal blood pressure response to exercise
(b) Severity of left ventricular outflow tract obstruction
(c) Non-sustained ventricular tachycardia
(d) Exertional chest pain
(e) Syncope

4 Brugada syndrome:
(a) Is associated with a lower risk of sudden death than WPW syndrome
(b) Is characterised by ST segment elevation in limb leads II, III and AVF
(c) May be effectively treated with class Ic agents such as flecainide
(d) Requires ICD therapy due to the high risk of sudden death
(e) Is associated with a high risk of cardiac arrest in asymptomatic individuals

5 Congenital LQTS:
(a) Can be excluded if the corrected QT interval is above 440 ms
(b) Often results in syncope during emotional or physical stress
(c) Requires ICD therapy in patients who present with a cardiac arrest
(d) Occurs sporadically in as many as 30% of all cases
(e) Can usually be treated satisfactorily with beta-blockade, with or without cervical sympathectomy

ANSWERS

1a False	2a False	3a True	4a False	5a False
b True	b False	b False	b False	b True
c False	c True	c True	c False	c True
d True	d True	d False	d True	d True
e True	e True	e True	e True	e False

Beta-blockers for heart failure

John Cleland

☐ INTRODUCTION

It is a sad indictment of medical research that a few anecdotal reports [1] were sufficient to delay for over 30 years the acceptance of beta-blockers as a highly beneficial treatment for patients with heart failure secondary to left ventricular (LV) dysfunction. This failure highlights the need to challenge preconceptions about the management of disease wherever they are inadequately supported by data. Treatment according to some theoretical rationale or logical train of thought is necessary whenever clinicians have to manage problems that have not been addressed by randomised controlled trials (RCTs). However, it is clear that treatment according to theoretical principles has at least two major flaws:

1 If the understanding of the pathophysiology of the disease being treated is wrong, treatment is likely to be ineffective or harmful.

2 If the theoretical rationale becomes fashionable, the treatment becomes another modern medical myth, which may then impede for decades the acquisition of real knowledge.

Such myths, old and modern, abound in medicine and heart failure is no exception. Aspirin, revascularisation and nitrates are current examples of unproven, but theoretically logical, therapies for many patients with heart failure, provided that one line of theoretical reasoning is followed and not another. These are opinion-based interventions. It is also likely that many effective treatments for heart failure are overlooked or avoided because their mode of action does not fit contemporary theories about the mechanism underlying the disease in question.

Beta-blockers are a prime example of a class of drugs avoided because of untested theoretical risks. They have been rescued only recently, having been actively avoided for over 30 years by most doctors because their pharmacological profile did not fit the understanding of the pathophysiology of disease. It had been assumed that activation of the sympathetic nervous system in patients with heart failure was an important compensatory mechanism, giving inotropic support to the heart and helping maintain blood pressure, and that blocking this supporting mechanism would be deleterious. It is possible that in some extreme circumstances, for short periods of time (eg impending cardiogenic shock), sympathetic activation is helpful in supporting the failing heart, but the deleterious effects of chronic sympathetic activation on the heart appear to outweigh any short-term benefit [2].

From this pathophysiological perspective, there is a sound theoretical rationale for the use of beta-blockers in heart failure. It took randomised trials to show conclusively which theory was correct.

☐ MECHANISMS OF ACTION OF BETA-BLOCKING AGENTS

Beta-blocker therapy exerts clinical benefit by retarding or reversing the progression of heart failure and by decreasing the risk of sudden death [3]. The beneficial effects on symptoms and worsening heart failure are likely to be mediated by an improvement in ventricular function, an effect that develops gradually over a period of months. The effect on sudden death may be mediated by a reduction in arrhythmias, acute vascular occlusion or both [4].

The immediate effect of beta-blockers is to cause ventricular function to decline as sympathetic support is withdrawn from the failing heart [4] – unless the drug also has vasodilator properties, in which case there may be an immediate beneficial effect on cardiac function [5]. Long-term beta-blockade reduces cardiac volume, myocardial hypertrophy and filling pressures, and increases ejection fraction, a process termed ventricular remodelling [3,6]. These effects occur gradually over a period of months, but beta-blockers appear to have an impact on mortality even before beneficial effects on ventricular function are observed [7]. It is possible that there is protection from cardiac arrhythmias soon after initiation of a beta-blocker, although chronic therapy may exert even greater benefit. Similarly, beta-blockers may exert both immediate and long-term reduction in the risk of coronary vascular events [3,4,8]. Reduction in arrhythmias subsequent to coronary occlusion may account for an apparent increase in non-fatal myocardial infarction (MI) with beta-blockers in some studies [8,9].

The underlying cellular or subcellular mechanisms leading to the beneficial effects of beta-blockers on ventricular function are uncertain, but likely to be complex and multifactorial. Potential mechanisms include protection of adrenergic receptors, from either catecholamines or stimulatory autoantibodies [10], and neuroendocrine effects, especially suppression of renin, which may help prevent breakthrough production of angiotensin II for patients on angiotensin-converting enzyme (ACE) inhibitors [3]. Beta-blockers may improve myocardial energetics [11], either by reducing myocardial oxygen requirements or by increasing diastolic coronary blood flow, thereby reducing myocardial ischaemia which may occur even in the absence of epicardial coronary disease in patients with heart failure [11]. Reduction in heart rate is likely to play a major role in the benefits of beta-blockade [12]. An improvement in myocardial force–frequency relationships has also been reported [13]. At heart rates in the physiological range, the normal myocardium increases its force of contraction as heart rate increases. The failing heart does not respond in this manner, and the force of contraction may decline at higher heart rates. The failing heart may be more efficient at a reduced heart rate.

Possible mechanisms for an anti-arrhythmic effect of beta-blockade include:

☐   reduction in sympathetic drive, heart rate and myocardial ischaemia

☐   improvement in baroreflex function

☐   prevention of episodic hypokalaemia that results from surges in sympathetic activity during stress or exercise [14], and

☐   an overall improvement in cardiac function.

Currently, it is uncertain whether it is necessary to block only the beta-1 receptor or whether non-selective agents might prove superior. Blockade of beta-2 receptors may enhance peripheral vasoconstriction and bronchoconstriction, and therefore could be deleterious. However, it could also be advantageous either by protecting the cardiac myocyte more effectively from catecholamine excess or by preventing catecholamine-induced hypokalaemia. Agents that act non-selectively on both beta-1 and beta-2 receptors and also have peripheral vasodilator actions, such as carvedilol, may offer optimal myocardial, metabolic and haemodynamic benefit [6,15].

☐ ANCILLARY PROPERTIES OF BETA-BLOCKERS

Beta-blockers are a pharmacologically heterogeneous class of compounds and many have ancillary properties (Table 1):

☐   Some beta-blockers (eg xamoterol, pindolol, oxprenolol and possibly bucindolol) are partial agonists and may be disadvantageous to patients with heart failure.

☐   Several agents (eg carvedilol and labetolol) also block alpha receptors which may increase cardiac myocyte protection and cause peripheral vasodilatation. Alpha-blockers have not been successful in the treatment of heart failure, perhaps because they induce reflex sympathetic activation, the deleterious effects of which can be prevented by beta-blockers.

☐   Other agents (eg nebivolol) induce vasodilatation by increasing nitric oxide production.

☐   A beneficial effect of beta-blockade on the atherosclerotic process has been reported, although the effect remains controversial.

☐   Non-selective agents, in contrast to beta-1 selective agents, may decrease cardiac norepinephrine production and suppress beta receptor density [3].

☐   Carvedilol has antioxidant properties *in vitro* and inhibits vascular smooth muscle cell proliferation [3], although it was unsuccessful at reducing restenosis after coronary angioplasty in one study [16].

☐   Carvedilol has also been reported to have other potentially important effects on the vascular endothelium. These include downregulation of cellular adhesion molecules, thereby inhibiting inflammatory infiltration and reducing tissue damage in response to infarction, increasing the plasma concentrations of vascular growth factors and suppression of plasma endothelin-1, an important vasoconstrictor substance. Whether or not these properties are unique to carvedilol is controversial.

Table 1 Ancillary properties of beta-blockers.

Name	Beta-1 selective	Alpha-blockade	Lipophilic	Increased ISA	Other ancillary properties
Acebutolol	Disputed	No	No	Disputed	No
Atenolol	Yes	No	No	No	No
Betaxolol	No	No	Yes	No	No
Bisoprolol	Yes	No	Weak	No	No
Bucindolol	No	No	Yes	Disputed	Vasodilator action
Carvedilol	No	Yes	Yes	No	Anti-oxidant / Effects on endothelial function
Celiprolol	Yes	No	No	Beta-2 only	No
Labetolol	No	Yes	Yes	No	No
Metoprolol	Yes	No	Yes	No	No
Nebivolol	Yes	No	?	No	Vasodilatation through nitric oxide
Oxprenolol	No	No	Yes	Yes	No
Pindolol	No	No	Weak	Yes	No
Propranolol	No	No	Yes	No	Membrane stabilising effect (quinidine-like)
Sotalol	No	No	No	No	Class III anti-arrhythmic activity*
Timolol	No	No	Weak	No	Anti-platelet effects?
Xamoterol	Yes	No	No	Marked	No

* Early effect observed only at high dose. Class III effects may be observed with beta-blockers in general during chronic therapy.
ISA = intrinsic sympathomimetic activity.

☐ RANDOMISED CONTROLLED TRIALS

Agents studied (Table 2, overleaf)

Large, positive outcome trials have been conducted with carvedilol [7,17–20], bisoprolol [9,21] and metoprolol [22,23], while large studies of xamoterol [24] and bucindolol [25] have shown harm or lack of benefit, respectively. There are ongoing substantial trials of betaxolol, nebivolol, talinolol and probably other agents. It is likely that there are important differences in the clinical benefits between beta-blockers. Unless stated otherwise, the information presented below refers to outcomes using the beta-blockers known to be effective (carvedilol, bisoprolol and metoprolol). Caution should be used in extrapolating these data to other agents.

Populations studied (Table 3, p19)

More patients with heart failure have been included in RCTs of beta-blockers than for any other agent. Studies have been confined so far to patients with LV systolic dysfunction and an ejection fraction below 40%. Within this limitation, a broad range of patients has been included – from those with asymptomatic LV systolic dysfunction [18,19] to patients with severe heart failure requiring hospitalisation for decompensation [7]. Patients requiring intravenous (iv) inotropic therapy, and those with gross fluid retention, acute pulmonary oedema and cardiogenic shock have generally been excluded. Patients with heart rate and systolic blood pressure as low as 60 bpm and 85 mmHg, respectively, have been randomised. Most patients studied have been below 75 years and patients aged over 80 years are under-represented. Many patients with hypertension, diabetes, atrial fibrillation, ischaemic heart disease (IHD) and dilated cardiomyopathy have been included. Background therapy has generally included diuretics, digoxin and ACE inhibitors (Table 4, p19). A large placebo-controlled trial of nebivolol is focusing on patients aged over 70 years, and will include patients with preserved LV systolic function.

☐ THE MAJOR STUDIES REPORTED SO FAR (Tables 2 & 5)

USCT (see end of text for explanation of studies)

The UCST programme was the first study to show a reduction in all-cause mortality with a beta-blocker [17]. It comprised four component projects investigating the effects of carvedilol in mild, moderate or severe heart failure and a dose-ranging study [26–29]. The primary outcome was submaximal exercise tolerance, apart from one trial in which it was progression from mild to more severe heart failure using a composite end-point [27]. Projects were designed to last 6–12 months. The target dose for titration of carvedilol was 25 mg bd, increasing to 50 mg bd for patients weighing more than 85 kg. Controversy continues whether all-cause mortality was a predefined primary outcome measure of the programme.

Table 2. Design of major trials of beta-blockers in heart failure.

Trial	Ref.	Population	Design	Comparisons	Target dose	Primary outcome
USCT programme	17	Predominantly mild to moderate heart failure with LVEF ≤35%	Active run-in followed by parallel group	Carvedilol/ Placebo	25 mg bd	All-cause mortality
CIBIS-II	9,21	Predominantly moderate to severe heart failure with echocardiographic LVEF ≤35%	No run in Parallel group	Bisoprolol/ Placebo	10mg od	All-cause mortality
MERIT-HF	22,23	Predominantly mild to moderate heart failure with echocardiographic LVEF ≤40%	No run in Parallel group	Metoprolol CR/ XL/Placebo	200 mg od	All-cause mortality
BEST	25	Predominantly moderate to severe heart failure with LVEF <35%	No run in Parallel group	Bucindolol/ Placebo	<75 kg: 100 mg/day >75 kg: 200 mg/day	All-cause mortality
COPERNICUS	7	Severe heart failure with LVEF <25%	No run in Parallel group	Carvedilol/ Placebo	25 mg bd	All-cause mortality
CAPRICORN	20	Post-infarction LVEF ≤40%	No run in Parallel group	Carvedilol/ Placebo	25 mg bd	(i) All-cause mortality (ii) Death or CVS hospitalisation
COMET*	15	Mild to moderate heart failure with echocardiographic LVEF <40%	No run in Parallel group	Carvedilol/ Metoprolol	C: 25 mg bd M: 50 mg bd	(i) All-cause mortality (ii) Death or all-cause hospitalisation
SENIORS**		Mild, moderate or severe heart failure regardless of LVEF (stratified <35%>) Age >70- years	No run in Parallel group	Nebivolol/ Placebo	Unknown	All-cause mortality or hospitalisation with heart failure
CHRISTMAS*	31	Mild to moderate heart failure stratified according to myocardial hibernation volume	No run in Parallel group	Carvedilol/ Placebo	25 mg bd	Interaction of therapy with hibernation status on LVEF

* complete in 2002; ** complete in 2004.
CVS = cardiovascular; LVEF = left ventricular ejection fraction.

Table 3: Number of patients studied and their characteristics.

Patient characteristics	USCT [17]	CIBIS-II [9,21]	MERIT-HF [22,23]	BEST [25]	COPERNICUS [7]
Age (years)	58	61	64	60	63
Female (%)	23	19	22	22	20
Median LVEF	23	28	28	23	20
NYHA II	53	0	41	0	0
NYHA III	44	83	56	92	} 100*
NYHA IV	3	17	4	8	
Ischaemic heart disease	47	50	65	59	67
Hypertension	ca 50	NA	44	59	NA
Diabetes	NA	12	25	36	NA
Atrial fibrillation	12	20	17	12	19

*Combined NYHA III and IV.
LVEF = left ventricular ejection fraction; NA = not applicable; NYHA = New York Heart Association.

Table 4. Background treatment of patients in randomised controlled trials of beta-blockers (% receiving each type of drug).

Treatment	USCT [17]	CIBIS-II [9,21]	MERIT-HF [22,23]	BEST [25]	COPERNICUS [7]
Diuretics	95	99	91	94	99
Digoxin	91	52	64	93	66
ACE inhibitor	95	96	90*	91	97
Spironolactone	NA	NA	8	4	20
Amiodarone	NA	15	NA	NA	18
Statins	NA	NA	NA	23	NA
Aspirin	NA	41	NA	45	NA
Anticoagulant	NA	31	NA	46	NA

* includes angiotensin receptor blockers.
ACE = angiotensin-converting enzyme; NA = not applicable.

Results

There was a remarkable 65% reduction in all-cause mortality over a mean follow-up period of 6.7 months. The study was stopped by its data safety monitoring committee, with the recommendation that all patients should be treated with carvedilol. This implied that it was stopped because of the mortality benefits of carvedilol. However, only 53 deaths were observed, leading sceptics to doubt the result. Another criticised design feature was the active run-in period that excluded patients intolerant of beta-blockers, although adding deaths during run-in to the carvedilol arm of the study did not lead to a loss of statistical significance. This study showed similar benefits across all subgroups reported, a reduction in cardiovascular hospitalisation, particularly for worsening heart failure and good tolerance of carvedilol.

Table 5 Summary of contemporary landmark studies of beta-blockers in heart failure.

Study	Ref	Nos. randomised to:		Follow-up (months)	Deaths (1-year mortality)				Lives saved of potential lost*			Risk reduction (%)	p
		Beta-blocker	Placebo		Placebo		Beta-blocker				(NNT/year)		
					No.	%	No.	%	No.				
UCST	17	Carvedilol 696	398	6.5	31	11.1	22	3.9	72/111		14	65	0.0001
CIBIS-II	9,21	Bisoprolol 1,327	1,320	16	228	13.2	156	9.0	42/132		24	32	0.0001
MERIT-HF	22,23	Metoprolol 1,990	2,001	12	217	11.0	145	7.2	38/110		26	35	0.0062
COPERNICUS	15	Carvedilol 1,156	1,133	11	190	19.7	130	12.8	70/197		14	35	0.00014
Total of above		5,169	4,852	*ca 12*	666	16.6	453	14.9	*not calculated*			36	*0.00001*
BEST	25	Bucindolol 1,354	1,354	36	447	16.6	409	14.9	17/166		59	10	0.109
CAPRICORN	20	Carvedilol 975	984	16	151	11.5#	116	9.2#	23/115		43	23	0.031

* per 1,000 treated per year.
# recalculated.
NNT = number needed to treat.

CIBIS-I and -II

The first substantial RCT of a beta-blocker for heart failure due to ischaemic or non-ischaemic causes was CIBIS-I [30]. This study was inadequately powered to provide a conclusive answer, but suggested benefit confined to patients with dilated cardiomyopathy.

CIBIS-II [9,21], a follow-up to CIBIS-I, compared bisoprolol with placebo, and is widely regarded as the first study incontrovertibly designed as a mortality trial. It attempted to recruit patients with moderate to severe heart failure (New York Heart Association (NYHA) III/IV). The target dose of bisoprolol was 10 mg/day, twice that used in CIBIS-I.

Results

The one-year mortality in the placebo arm of the CIBIS-II study was only 13.2%, suggesting that the population was predominantly NYHA class III. There was a striking reduction in all-cause mortality and hospitalisation, and also in hospitalisation for worsening heart failure in the active treatment group.

MERIT-HF

MERIT-HF compared metoprolol and placebo in patients with predominantly mild to moderate heart failure [22,23]. The target dose was 200 mg of metoprolol CR/XL.

Results

The one-year placebo mortality (11%) was slightly less than in CIBIS-II. There was a striking reduction in all-cause mortality and hospitalisations for worsening heart failure, and a modest reduction in all-cause hospitalisation with active treatment.

BEST

In the BEST study, bucindolol, an unlicensed beta-blocker, was compared with placebo in patients with moderately severe heart failure [25].

Results

There was no reduction in overall mortality and trends to excess mortality were noted in the sickest patients. The lack of effect of bucindolol in this study led to fears that beta-blockers should not be used in patients with severe heart failure. It was also attributed to the ancillary properties of bucindolol, which may include partial agonist activity. Bucindolol showed a significant reduction in mortality among Caucasian patients, but African-American patients fared badly with this agent and it has been suggested that the large cohort of African-American patients contributed to the overall lack of effect. There is controversy about the efficacy of beta-blockers in this group of patients, although African-Americans appeared to benefit as much as Caucasians in the carvedilol trials. The CIBIS-II and MERIT-HF studies recruited patients predominantly in Europe and therefore included few patients of African descent.

COPERNICUS

Only patients with severe heart failure were recruited into the COPERNICUS study [7]. The target dose of carvedilol was 25 mg bd. Patients hospitalised with severe heart failure could be recruited into this study provided that they were not on an intensive care unit, had not received an iv inotropic or vasodilator agent within the previous four days and did not exhibit signs of gross fluid overload. Patients receiving iv diuretic infusions could also be included.

Results

One-year placebo mortality was 19.7%, indicating a large placebo effect. There were striking reductions in mortality in the carvedilol arm and in hospitalisation for both all-cause and worsening heart failure.

CAPRICORN

Patients with LV systolic dysfunction, with or without mild heart failure, up to 21 days after an MI were recruited into the CAPRICORN study [20], most being included on days 3–5. Randomisation was to carvedilol, target dose 25 mg bd, or placebo.

Results

There was a significant reduction in mortality and myocardial reinfarction, but non-significant trends towards a reduction in the development of heart failure or cardiovascular hospitalisation with active treatment.

☐ EFFECTS OF BETA-BLOCKERS

Symptoms

Compared with placebo, beta-blockers usually cause a short-term exacerbation of heart failure symptoms but a long-term benefit [22]. Symptomatic benefit is generally apparent within 2–6 months [22,27,28]. It is unclear whether this reflects a genuine long-term benefit of beta-blockers on symptoms or a slowing of the progressive deterioration in symptoms expected on placebo – albeit often masked by a placebo effect – but, whatever the means, it is clear that in the long term most patients will feel better on a beta-blocker than on a placebo.

There is some evidence to suggest that early deterioration is less likely with carvedilol than with other beta-blockers. In a substantial study of metoprolol [22,23] there were higher rates of withdrawal for worsening heart failure during the first two months before a long-term advantage on symptoms became apparent. This was not observed in the COPERNICUS study [7] – all the more remarkable as it was performed in the sickest population studied so far. It may reflect the advantages of using a beta-blocker with vasodilator properties. (Potential differences between beta-blockers are further discussed below.)

Ventricular function

One of the most consistent therapeutic outcomes in medicine is the increase in LV ejection fraction (LVEF) observed with chronic beta-blockade [6,31]. The effect appears to parallel the improvement in symptoms and becomes evident only after some months of therapy. It is accompanied by a fall in systolic and diastolic volumes, indicating that improved ejection fraction is not simply related to reductions in heart rate and ventricular mass [18]. The average increase after six months' treatment with a beta-1-selective blocker is about 5%, but some studies suggest even greater increases with longer follow-up. Carvedilol may exert a greater effect on LVEF than other agents [6].

The aetiology of the heart failure may have an important effect on the increase in ejection fraction observed in response to beta-blockade [29,31,32]. The increase is much more consistent in patients with dilated cardiomyopathy than in those with IHD [29,31,32], and the average increase may be twice as great in the former. This heterogeneity of response may reflect the fact that patients with a large volume of scar cannot respond with an increase in ejection fraction, whereas patients with extensive myocardial hibernation or ischaemia may respond similarly to those with dilated cardiomyopathy, a condition in which microvascular disease and myocardial ischaemia may be common [31,33]. However, the latter may benefit from its other effects.

In patients with dilated cardiomyopathy, higher doses of beta-blockers appear to cause a greater rise in ejection fraction over six months [29]. Whether longer-term therapy with lower doses would catch up is unknown. In patients with IHD, higher doses do not usually exert a greater effect on ejection fraction [29]; this may reflect the much greater heterogeneity in response among this group of patients.

In patients with atrial fibrillation, the addition of a beta-blocker improves ventricular rate control and ventricular function [12,34,35]. Withdrawal of digoxin results in less good heart rate control and decline in ventricular function [34].

Morbidity

The commonest major cardiovascular morbid event for patients with heart failure is hospitalisation for an exacerbation of the underlying condition. This was reduced substantially and consistently in all the large positive RCTs of beta-blockers for heart failure. Up to half such events occur in the absence of a clear precipitating factor, and benefit in these patients presumably reflects a favourable effect on ventricular remodelling. However, a substantial proportion of admissions with worsening heart failure are precipitated by rapid atrial fibrillation or coronary events and beta-blockers may also exert a favourable effect on these outcomes.

There are few data to show that beta-blockers reduce the risk of major morbid events such as MI and stroke in patients with heart failure. Indeed, the CIBIS-II study showed an increase in non-fatal stroke and no reduction in non-fatal MI on bisoprolol [9], probably reflecting a combination of two effects:

1   Beta-blockers substantially reduce mortality, so more patients were alive and at risk of non-fatal events.

2   Both MI and stroke are powerfully arrhythmogenic and common causes of sudden death. Beta-blockers may prevent early arrhythmias, allowing patients to reach hospital to receive a diagnosis and appropriate therapy.

The increase in these non-fatal events may be a sign of the efficacy of beta-blockers.

Post-infarction studies of beta-blockers including the CAPRICORN study [20] suggest that these agents can reduce recurrent infarction, reinforcing the idea that sudden death is a common manifestation of MI in patients with heart failure that may be modified by beta-blockers.

Mortality (Table 5)

Four trials, each including at least 1,000 patients (carvedilol [7,17], bisoprolol [9] and metoprolol [22,23]), have shown a reduction in mortality. This appeared to reflect both a reduction in sudden death and in death due to progressive heart failure. There was little evidence of heterogeneity across subgroups, but possibly greater consistency across subgroups with carvedilol than with the other agents. However, BEST [25] and the xamoterol severe heart failure study [24] suggest that the benefits of beta-blockers should not be considered a class effect. Questions also remain about whether some beta-blockers are effective in patients with atrial fibrillation or in some racial groups [12,25]. (These issues are further discussed below.)

The less marked improvement in ventricular function with beta-blockers in patients with IHD did not translate into a diminution of benefits on either morbidity or mortality. A trend to greater benefit in patients with IHD was observed in several trials [9,23]. This further reinforces the concept that beta-blockers have benefits on mortality mediated by mechanisms other than ventricular remodelling. A reduction in vascular and/or arrhythmic events seems likely.

It is worth emphasising that patients with diabetes, lung disease (excluding asthma) and peripheral vascular disease, common traditional contraindications to the use of beta-blockers, benefited at least as much as other patients [22].

Currently, the COMET study is comparing the effects of carvedilol and metoprolol on mortality in a study of over 3,000 patients with moderately severe heart failure and LV systolic dysfunction [15]. The study should be completed in 2002.

Tolerability

Despite theoretical concerns, beta-blockers have proved remarkably well tolerated in the clinical trials. Carvedilol was significantly less likely to be withdrawn than placebo in USCT [17] and COPERNICUS [7], and there was no significant difference in CIBIS-II [9] or MERIT-HF [22]. Tolerability of long-term beta-blocker therapy, at some dose, ranged from about 85% with bisoprolol in CIBIS-II to 91.5% with carvedilol in COPERNICUS. Greater differences were observed in the ability to tolerate target doses of drugs. Only 43% of patients randomised to bisoprolol (CIBIS-II) and 64% of those randomised to metoprolol (MERIT-HF) tolerated the target dose, whereas 78% and 74% tolerated the target dose of carvedilol in USCT and COPERNICUS, respectively. If higher doses of beta-blockers are more effective, this suggests that more patients will tolerate high doses of carvedilol.

Fewer patients may tolerate treatment in clinical practice because they are less highly selected, they have more comorbidity, and dedicated research staff are not available. However, a patient in a study with an agent not known to work for certain may be more likely to withdraw as the result of a side effect than a patient receiving a treatment known to be life saving. Also, as more evidence of benefit has appeared, some patients in the studies will have been withdrawn from trial medication in order to start open-label beta-blocker therapy.

☐ MAJOR OUTSTANDING ISSUES

Are there differences between beta-blockers?

Beta-blockers are a heterogeneous group of agents in structure, adrenergic receptor subtype, affinity and ancillary properties, so differences in their effects are likely. The failure of bucindolol [25] to reduce mortality in heart failure and the ability of xamoterol [24] to increase it suggests that these pharmacological differences may be translated into differences in efficacy. Differences in benefit might be observed in terms of tolerability and symptoms, effects on ventricular function, morbidity and mortality or effects within subgroups.

Tolerability and symptoms

As discussed above, there appear to be differences between agents in their tolerability, especially during the titration phase. Carvedilol seems to be better tolerated than other beta-blockers, perhaps because of its vasodilator actions, but vasodilatation may also account for the increase in hypotension and dizziness complicating uptitration of this agent. There is no conclusive evidence for differences between beta-blockers in their long-term symptomatic benefits, but they were more clearly observed in USCT [17] than in MERIT-HF [22] and may reflect the confounding effect of duration of follow-up.

Morbidity and mortality

CIBIS-II [9], MERIT-HF [22,23] and COPERNICUS [7] all suggested that beta-blockers confer a relative reduction in risk of death of about 35%. The reduction in death or all-cause hospitalisation with metroprolol reported in MERIT (19% reduction) is not clearly different from that reported with carvedilol in

COPERNICUS (24% reduction). It is impossible to know whether the outcomes observed in these trials reflect differences in the populations studied or the drugs used. The BEST trial [25] observed a much smaller, non-significant effect. USCT [17] suggested a larger benefit, but this may be an artefact generated by stopping a short-term trial because of an observed mortality benefit. However, patients in the placebo groups of CIBIS-II, MERIT-HF and COPERNICUS were at substantially different risks of dying. Relative risk reduction was similar in each study, but the absolute benefit in terms of number of lives saved for every 100 patients treated was much greater in COPERNICUS. One large study, COMET [15], and one medium-sized study, BETACAR [15], are currently in progress to determine whether pharmacological differences between agents translate into differences in clinical outcome.

Direct comparisons of beta-blockers

Four small studies comparing carvedilol with metoprolol have been reported:

1 A double-blind study of 67 patients followed over six months [37] suggested that carvedilol was not more effective than metoprolol in improving LVEF. However, patients randomised to carvedilol, who were sicker, older and had more IHD, did no worse than those on metoprolol.

2 In a study of 30 patients with dilated cardiomyopathy, whose LVEF remained below 40% (mean 29%) despite treatment with metoprolol for one year, those randomised to metoprolol continued to have a decline in LVEF over the subsequent year, but there was an increase to a mean value of 36% in those randomised to carvedilol [38].

3 Fifty-one patients, mainly Chinese, with dilated cardiomyopathy or hypertensive heart disease were randomised to metoprolol or carvedilol for three months [39]. Patients on carvedilol had a greater reduction in blood pressure and LV end-diastolic dimension and more benefit on LV diastolic function, although this did not translate into a greater effect on symptoms or exercise capacity.

4 The largest comparative trial so far [40] followed 150 patients for 14 months to investigate the effects of carvedilol and metoprolol on haemodynamics and exercise capacity. Reductions in heart rate and filling pressure and increases in ejection fraction were greater with carvedilol, but there was no difference between the drugs in their impact on either exercise capacity or frequency of ventricular ectopics on ambulatory ECG monitoring.

A recent meta-analysis [6] of studies that either measured change in ejection fraction in placebo-controlled trials of metoprolol or carvedilol or (four trials) compared these two agents directly included 19 trials and 2,184 patients followed for a mean of eight months. The conclusion was that the absolute increase in LVEF was 2–3% greater on carvedilol than on metoprolol ($p < 0.0001$), with similar effects in patients with or without IHD.

Placebo, metoprolol and celiprolol were compared in a small trial (50 patients) [41]. The study suggested no advantage to celiprolol over metoprolol despite its vasodilator properties.

Subgroup analyses

All the landmark clinical trials conducted subgroup analyses. Such analyses should not generally influence clinical practice because chance differences are likely in such a large number of analyses. None the less, they are a valuable test of the confidence that can be placed in a study and generate new hypotheses requiring testing.

Severe heart failure. The BEST trial showed a trend to increased mortality in the subgroup of patients with severe heart failure [25]. All the other major trials showed a reduction in mortality in this group of patients, but only COPERNICUS [7] had enough patients with sufficiently severe heart failure to be confident of benefit. Mortality and hospitalisation were reduced even in patients with recent decompensation or ejection fraction below 20% in the COPERNICUS study.

Aetiology of heart failure. Early, smaller trials had suggested that the mortality benefits of beta-blockers might be most prominent in, or confined to, patients with dilated cardiomyopathy, but relatively small numbers of patients with dilated cardiomyopathy were recruited to CIBIS-II and the MERIT studies. Also, these patients had fewer events and therefore tended to have less benefit. Consequently, neither study had sufficient events in these subgroups to be confident of benefit. In contrast, patients with or without IHD had significant and equal benefit in USCT and COPERNICUS.

Atrial fibrillation. Patients with atrial fibrillation obtained as much benefit as patients in sinus rhythm in USCT and COPERNICUS [7]. However, in CIBIS-II, in contrast to patients in sinus rhythm, those with atrial fibrillation obtained no benefit with bisoprolol, and tests for heterogeneity were statistically significant [12]. It is not clear why bisoprolol should not be effective in patients with atrial fibrillation. This group of patients may be less likely to attain good heart rate control due to a lower threshold for withdrawal of the beta-blocker or digoxin in response to bradycardia, although currently there is little evidence to support this hypothesis. Another possibility is that bradycardia combined with an irregular ventricular response increases the risk of *torsades de pointes* with bisoprolol, but that the broader spectrum of adrenergic receptor blockade with carvedilol provides additional arrhythmia protection. A pharmacokinetic interaction with bisoprolol seems unlikely as carvedilol, but not bisoprolol, is known to increase plasma digoxin levels.

Diabetes. Diabetic patients obtained similar benefits as non-diabetics in all the studies reported so far [21,22].

Ethnic differences. In the BEST study, bucindolol had benefits in Caucasians similar to those observed in the other landmark studies but an adverse effect on the prognosis of African-Americans [25]. MERIT-HF and CIBIS-II recruited most of their patients in Europe and so had insufficient non-Caucasians to provide a robust analysis of this question. USCT and COPERNICUS both suggested equal benefit in African-Americans and Caucasians [7,36].

Age and preserved left ventricular systolic function

The MERIT-HF study had an upper age limit of 80 years, while the mean age of patients in all the beta-blocker trials was about 63 years. MERIT-HF, USCT and COPERNICUS [7] suggest that older patients obtain similar benefits as younger ones. However, the risk/benefit ratio of beta-blockers in patients aged over 80 years is unknown, and it is not clear whether the drugs are effective or safe in patients with preserved LV systolic function. The SENIORS study [42] will address these issues by comparing the effects of nebivolol in patients with heart failure aged over 70 years, including patients with and without LV systolic dysfunction.

Dose

It is not clear whether large doses of beta-blockers are superior to low doses – indeed, the latter may prove superior. No trial is currently addressing this issue.

☐ TREATMENT INTERACTIONS

Beta-blockers may exert some of their benefit by reducing renin. This may enhance the ability of ACE inhibitors to suppress angiotensin II formation. Studies of ACE inhibitors and also studies comparing angiotensin receptor blockers and ACE inhibitors suggest that patients already receiving a beta-blocker [43,44] obtain greater benefit from an ACE inhibitor. However, since few patients in the beta-blocker studies were not receiving an ACE inhibitor, it is unclear whether beta-blockers are effective in the absence of an ACE inhibitor. It is also unclear whether addition of an ACE inhibitor to a beta-blocker is necessary, although this seems highly likely. Patients taking an ACE inhibitor and a beta-blocker appear to get a greater benefit from the addition of spironolactone [44] but not of an angiotensin receptor blocker [45].

Beta-blockers seem to work equally well in patients in sinus rhythm with or without digoxin. The combination of digoxin and beta-blockers appears superior to either agent alone for patients with atrial fibrillation [34]. A suggested beneficial interaction between beta-blockers and amiodarone has not been substantiated [46]. Beta-blockers may also reduce the frequency of implantable defibrillator discharge. The efficacy of levosimendan, the first in a new class of calcium-dependent calcium sensitisers, may be enhanced by beta-blockers, in contrast to the attenuation of the effects of beta-agonists or phosphodiesterase inhibitors by beta-blockers.

Beta-blockers should almost never be given to patients receiving verapamil or diltiazem, and only after consultation with a specialist.

☐ CLINICAL PRACTICE

Selection of patients with heart failure for beta-blocker therapy

Indications

Chronic heart failure. Beta-blockers are indicated for all stages of heart failure secondary to LV systolic dysfunction if the patient is free from cardiogenic shock, acute pulmonary oedema or evidence of gross fluid retention. It is vital to remember that, unlike diuretics, nitrates, digoxin or ACE inhibitors, beta-blockers are not usually effective as short-term rescue therapy for worsening *chronic* heart failure. Treatment should generally be initiated within days of achieving a moderate degree of stability in patients with severe heart failure as the COPERNICUS study suggested that the mortality benefit with carvedilol could be observed within days of initiation [7].

It is inappropriate to treat patients based on a clinical diagnosis alone. They must be investigated by an imaging technique, usually echocardiography, to establish the presence of LV systolic dysfunction and to investigate other causes of their heart failure.

Over 90% of patients in the large beta-blockers trials have also received ACE inhibitors. It is important to emphasise that the benefits of beta-blockade are *in addition* to those of ACE inhibition, and that some of those benefits may depend on the presence of the ACE inhibitor. However, it is likely that beta-blockers are also effective in patients who cannot tolerate an ACE inhibitor.

Recent onset heart failure. Studies with beta-blockers after MI indicate that patients with evidence of heart failure have a high mortality and the greatest absolute benefit from beta-blocker therapy [47] (Fig. 1). Those with tachycardia, third heart sound or marked, but asymptomatic, LV dysfunction are appropriately treated with a beta-blocker. If there is cardiogenic shock or pulmonary oedema, this should be treated before starting a beta-blocker.

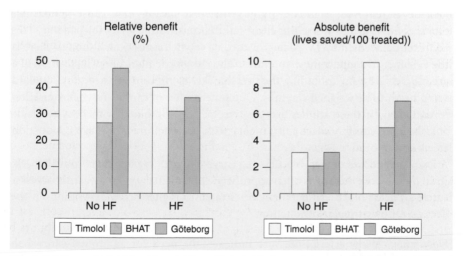

Fig. 1 Relative and absolute risk reduction with beta-blockers post-myocardial infarction with and without heart failure (HF).

Asymptomatic left ventricular dysfunction. The most common cause of asymptomatic LV dysfunction is MI. Asymptomatic LV dysfunction indicates a high risk of sudden death and progression to heart failure, both of which are targets of treatment with beta-blockers. Although patients with asymptomatic LV systolic dysfunction have not been studied specifically, the benefits observed both in long-term post-infarction trials [20] and in studies of mild heart failure [19,23] suggest that such patients should be treated. It is difficult to think of any reason why most of these patients should not be prescribed a beta-blocker.

Absolute contraindications

Asthma. Asthma is an absolute contraindication to beta-blocker treatment. Many patients with heart failure have chronic obstructive airways disease but, unless there is marked bronchodilatation with beta-agonist inhalation, such patients usually tolerate a beta-blocker.

Calcium antagonists. Some patients with dilated cardiomyopathy are treated with verapamil or diltiazem, as are some with heart failure and angina. This treatment should be withdrawn for 24 hours prior to the first dose of beta-blocker. There is no specific contraindication to the combination of dihydropyridine calcium antagonists and beta-blockers, although the indication for the former should be carefully reviewed. However, calcium antagonists should generally be withdrawn in patients with a low arterial pressure, as should other unnecessary hypotensive medications (eg nitrates).

Relative contraindications

Bradycardia and atrioventricular block. Stopping drugs that slow heart rate (eg digoxin, diltiazem and verapamil) should be considered in patients with bradycardia.

Complete heart block requires pacing, and thus the contraindication to beta-blockade is removed. Standard right ventricular pacing may cause ventricular desynchronisation and worsening heart failure, constituting a risk for patients. This may be circumvented by LV pacing or cardiac resynchronisation, although there is little evidence to support this hypothesis. The risk of pacing to allow institution of a beta-blocker versus withholding the beta-blocker to prevent the need for standard pacing needs to be weighed carefully. Outcome studies of cardiac resynchronisation are underway. If these studies are positive, pacing combined with beta-blockade could become commonplace for patients with heart failure who have conduction defects and/or bradycardia.

Even small doses of beta-blockers (eg carvedilol 6.25 mg bd) exert some benefit. A trial of low-dose therapy is often appropriate in patients with bradycardia or lesser degrees of heart block. Patients may be titrated to higher doses depending on the effect on atrioventricular conduction.

Hypotension. A low arterial pressure indicates the need for additional care when introducing a beta-blocker to avoid syncope. In addition, renal function should be monitored as it is highly dependent on perfusion pressure in patients with heart failure. Hypotension is usually a problem related to initiation of therapy. As ventricular function improves during chronic beta-blockade, an effect which may take 2–3 months to appear, arterial pressure often increases and may rise in the long term. If arterial pressure is low, hypotensive therapy should be reduced or withdrawn, starting with withdrawal of unnecessary vasodilators (eg calcium channel blockers and nitrates). Reducing the dose of diuretic can then be considered and, finally, reducing the dose of ACE inhibitors.

Renal or hepatic dysfunction. Patients with a serum creatinine above about 200 µmol/l have usually been excluded from clinical trials. Patients with renal dysfunction should be carefully monitored during initiation of a beta-blocker, especially for hypotension that may exacerbate their renal dysfunction. The beta-blockers currently being considered for the treatment of heart failure are excreted predominantly by the hepatic route and renal dysfunction usually has little impact on their plasma concentrations. Lower doses should be used in patients with severe liver dysfunction.

Generally inappropriate contraindications

Diabetes. Like heart failure, diabetes has long been considered a relative contraindication to beta-blockers because they are said to mask symptoms of hypoglycaemia and have adverse metabolic effects including increasing triglycerides. However, studies of beta-blockers post-infarction suggest that patients with diabetes benefit particularly well from beta-blockers [48]. This has been confirmed in the landmark studies of heart failure [21,22].

Peripheral vascular disease. Peripheral vascular disease is another traditional contraindication to beta-blockers, but several studies have shown that they have little impact on claudication distance [49]. Beta-blockers can be used safely, except perhaps in patients in whom the viability of the limb or digit is in doubt. These patients have a high cardiac mortality and even severe peripheral ischaemia cannot be considered an absolute contraindication to beta-blockade.

Peripheral vascular disease is a good marker of renal artery stenosis. Any treatment that reduces arterial pressure may precipitate renal failure in this setting, especially if the patient is receiving an ACE inhibitor.

When to start treatment

Treatment should be started as soon as possible after confirmation of a diagnosis of heart failure secondary to LV dysfunction, provided that there are no contra-indications. Patients with severe heart failure should now have therapy started in hospital prior to discharge, provided fluid retention has been controlled and they do not require iv therapy with a vasodilator or positive inotropic agent. The risk of adverse reactions is reduced by introducing the beta-blocker early in the course of heart failure; at that time, the patient has less severe ventricular dysfunction, a less activated sympathetic nervous system and is at lower risk of exacerbation of heart failure or hypotension during its initiation [27–29]. A logical reason to start beta-blockers early is that one of their principal effects is to slow the progression of heart failure.

Which beta-blocker?

Bisoprolol, metoprolol and carvedilol have all been shown to reduce mortality. Carvedilol may cause less worsening of heart failure during initiation and appears better tolerated in patients with severe heart failure. There is also evidence for a greater consistency of effect with carvedilol compared to beta-1-selective agents. The apparent additional benefits of carvedilol need to be weighed against increased cost. The results of the COMET study may have further impact on this balance.

Initiation and titration (Table 6)

The motto is 'start low and go slow'. Treatment should be started at low doses: for example, carvedilol 3.125 mg bd, bisoprolol 1.25 mg/day or metoprolol CR/XL about 5 mg bd (although metoprolol is not licensed for heart failure in the UK, and appropriate doses and formulations are not yet available). Treatment should be uptitrated to target doses at 2–4 week intervals (carvedilol 25 mg bd, bisoprolol 10 mg/day and metoprolol CR/XL 200 mg/day). It is not usually necessary for patients to stay in hospital for the entire initiation phase which may last several months. Beta-blockers may be started in the outpatient setting, with a 2–3 hour

Table 6 Practical tips in initiating therapy in patients with heart failure and left ventricular systolic dysfunction.

- Exclude patients with contraindications to beta-blockers
- Avoid treating patients within a few days of an exacerbation of heart failure requiring intravenous therapy
- Initiate treatment in stable patients several days prior to hospital discharge or as an outpatient
- Patients with milder degrees of heart failure generally tolerate the introduction of beta-blockers better than patients with severe heart failure. It is not a good policy to wait until a patient has progressed beyond mild symptoms before initiating a beta-blocker
- Educate patients about possible side effects, and the need to contact medical personnel *at onset* of problems. Tell them that they may feel worse, temporarily, during the titration phase
- Initiate beta-blockers at low doses
- If poorly tolerated, give after food to slow absorption
- Wait at least two weeks before uptitration, longer if side effects
- Adjust other medications (eg diuretics, vasodilators), as indicated, throughout initiation phase to maintain beta-blocker therapy
- If tolerated, titrate to target dose as used in clinical trials
- If side effects occur, dose reduction is usually preferable to stopping the beta-blocker therapy

period of observation recommended after initiation or uptitration. This is probably unnecessary for selected cases (eg younger patients with mild heart failure and without severe LV systolic dysfunction) once staff become experienced in handling these agents.

Even with such a cautious approach, 5–10% of patients may not tolerate the introduction of a beta-blocker. The greatest reported experience has been with carvedilol. In general, few adverse effects are observed with 3.125 mg bd of carvedilol, but problems are more likely with a dosage increase to 6.25 mg bd. It is not yet clear whether a protracted period of treatment (eg 4–6 weeks) with 3.125 mg bd can overcome this problem or whether use of an intermediate 3.125 mg tid or qid dose can help. These strategies should be explored in a patient who has difficulty tolerating the introduction of higher doses.

Until further evidence is available patients should be titrated to the target doses used in clinical trials, but low doses of beta-blockers appear distinctly better than none.

Management of hypotension

Asymptomatic and symptomatic hypotension are not infrequent during titration and may be more common with carvedilol due to its vasodilator properties. Blood pressure reaches its nadir 2–3 hours after dosing with a beta-blocker, and it is appropriate to monitor sicker patients for some hours after the first dose at each level of titration.

Asymptomatic hypotension

If hypotension is asymptomatic and has not led to a decline in renal function, no specific management is required other than perhaps to delay further dosage increase. With time, blood pressure will often rise, due either to tolerance to the alpha-blocking properties of carvedilol or to improvements in LV function.

Symptomatic hypotension

Minor. For patients with minor symptoms due to hypotension, reassurance and a delay in further titration will often result in spontaneous resolution of symptoms. Administration after food slows absorption and may improve symptoms. Staggering the doses of beta-blocker, diuretic and ACE inhibitor may also get round the problem by avoiding all three drugs exerting their maximum hypotensive effect at a similar time. Switching to a long-acting ACE inhibitor (eg enalapril, quinapril, ramipril bd, lisinopril, perindopril or trandolapril once daily) will smooth out the peak and trough hypotensive effects of ACE inhibition and may improve the tolerability of the beta-blocker. Patients who have just had a vigorous diuresis may be more susceptible to the hypotensive effects of a beta-blocker.

Major. Vasodilators such as calcium antagonists and nitrates should be withdrawn in patients with more severe hypotensive symptoms. If hypotension persists, the dose of diuretic should be reviewed and reduced if possible. If this fails, it is appropriate either to accept a lower dose of beta-blocker or temporarily to reduce the dose of ACE inhibitor. Bisoprolol and metoprolol, which do not cause peripheral vasodilatation, may cause less hypotension than carvedilol.

Management of bradycardia

Asymptomatic bradycardia should be managed by reassurance alone, always recognising that excessive bradycardia could manifest as increased fatigue or breathlessness. If bradycardia is symptomatic, the need for other rate-limiting medications (eg amiodarone, digoxin, diltiazem, etc) should be reviewed. Digoxin may be withdrawn in patients with mild heart failure, but in patients with more advanced heart failure digoxin withdrawal in the titration phase may increase the risk of worsening heart failure. If bradycardia develops as a problem in the maintenance phase, digoxin withdrawal should be considered. If the above are not options, the dose of beta-blocker should be reduced to relieve symptoms. As long as the patient has no symptoms attributable to the bradycardia, heart rates of 50 bpm or less are acceptable. Patients who cannot tolerate a beta-blocker because of bradycardia should be considered for pacing (see above).

Management of worsening heart failure

Increased fluid retention should be monitored by daily weighing. If the gain in weight is more than 2 kg, the patient should be instructed to increase the dose of diuretic temporarily.

For mild exacerbation of symptoms, simple reassurance, control of fluid retention with diuretics, and waiting for the benefits of beta-blockade to appear usually suffice. The beta-blocker dose should not be increased until symptoms have restabilised. More marked worsening may require a reduction in the dose, usually by 50%, and further adjustment of the doses of diuretic and ACE inhibitor or the introduction of digoxin. Beta-blockers should not be withdrawn except as a last resort as this exposes the patient to a high risk of sudden death. Any improvement due to beta-blocker withdrawal is often only temporary.

In extreme cases, hospitalisation for diuresis may be required. Levosimendan, which exerts a positive inotropic effect by sensitising troponin C to calcium, may be useful in this setting. Its actions are not diminished by beta-blockade. In two studies of heart failure it has been associated with a lower mortality than either dobutamine or placebo [50].

Other side effects

Hyperglycaemia

Both selective and non-selective beta-blockers may impair insulin sensitivity. Although carvedilol, because of its alpha-blocking qualities, has been reported not to impair insulin sensitivity [9] an increase in hyperglycaemia was observed in USCT [17]. Patients should have urine or blood glucose checked monthly for the first three months. Hyperglycaemia should be managed by intensifying the treatment for diabetes, in the same way as for patients not receiving beta-blockers. It is not appropriate to withdraw the beta-blocker.

Diarrhoea

Diarrhoea is a not uncommon side effect of carvedilol, but may improve with time. If marked, it may require a dose reduction or a switch to a beta-1-selective agent. Other causes of diarrhoea should be excluded.

Renal dysfunction

Renal dysfunction is usually a manifestation of hypotension in a patient who is already receiving a diuretic and an ACE inhibitor. Unnecessary vasodilators should be withdrawn. If there are no signs of fluid overload (eg oedema, weight gain), the diuretic dose should be cautiously reduced. If this is not effective, reduction of the dose of beta-blocker or ACE inhibitor or both may be required. Serum creatinine should be checked monthly for the first three months.

Increased serum digoxin levels

There was a small increase in serum digoxin in the carvedilol trials, possibly reflecting a small decline in glomerular filtration rate. In patients at risk of digoxin toxicity, serum digoxin levels should be checked monthly for the first three months. No adverse interaction on clinical outcomes has been observed between increasing serum digoxin concentrations and carvedilol.

☐ CONCLUSIONS

Physicians and patients need to understand the time course of the effects of beta-blocker therapy. The initial effects are often neutral or adverse, although the benefits, at least of carvedilol, may be apparent within days in patients with severe heart failure. Benefits accumulate gradually over a period of weeks to months. Patience, perseverance and education are required to allow patients to reap the full benefits of beta-blocker therapy for this malignant disease. Early treatment maximises the effectiveness and acceptance of therapy. Trials are underway to determine whether the benefits of beta-blockers extend to patients over 80 years of age and those with preserved LV systolic function. It is likely that important differences exist between beta-blockers in terms of their clinical benefit, although whether differences exist between the agents that have been reported to be effective so far awaits the outcome of a large clinical trial. It is unclear whether the target doses of beta-blockers currently recommended are optimal.

☐ TRIAL ACRONYMS

BEST   Bucindolol Evaluation of Survival Trial
BETACAR   BETAxolol versus CARvedilol in chronic heart failure
BHAT   Beta-blocker Heart Attack Trial
CAPRICORN   Carvedilol Postinfarct Survival Controlled Evaluation
CHRISTMAS   Carvedilol Hibernation Reversible Ischemia Trial: Marker of Success
CIBIS-II   Cardiac Insufficiency Bisoprolol Study-II
COMET   Carvedilol or Metoprolol European Trial
COPERNICUS   Carvedilol Prospective Randomised Cumulative Survival
MERIT-HF   Metoprolol Controlled Release Randomised Intervention Trial in Heart Failure
SENIORS   Study of Effects of Nebivolol Interventions on Outcomes and Rehospitalisation in Seniors with heart failure

REFERENCES

1   Epstein SE, Braunwald E. The effect of beta-adrenergic blockade on patterns of urinary sodium excretion. Studies in normal subjects and in patients with heart disease. *Ann Intern Med* 1966; 65: 20–7.

2   Francis GS, Rector TS, Cohn JN. Sequential neurohumoral measurements in patients with congestive heart failure. *Am Heart J* 1988; 116: 1464–8.

3   Cleland JG, Bristow MR, Erdmann E, Remme WJ, et al. Beta-blocking agents in heart failure. Should they be used and how? Review. *Eur Heart J* 1996; 17: 1629–39.

4   Cleland JG, Massie BM, Packer M. Sudden death in heart failure: vascular or electrical? *Eur J Heart Fail* 1999; 1: 41–5.

5   Basu S, Senior R, Raval U, van der Does R, et al. Beneficial effects of intravenous and oral carvedilol treatment in acute myocardial infarction. A placebo-controlled, randomized trial. *Circulation* 1997; 96: 183–91.

6   Packer M, Antonopoulos GV, Berlin JA, Chittams J, et al. Comparative effects of carvedilol and metoprolol on left ventricular ejection fraction in heart failure: results of a meta-analysis. *Am Heart J* 2001; 141: 899–907.

7   Packer M, Coats AJ, Fowler MB, Katus HA, et al. Effect of carvedilol on survival in severe chronic heart failure. *N Engl J Med* 2001; 344: 1651–8.

8   Cleland JG, Alamgir F, Nikitin NP, Clark AL, Norell M. What is the optimal medical management of ischemic heart failure? Review. *Prog Cardiovasc Dis* 2001; 43: 433–55.

9   The Cardiac Insufficiency Bisoprolol Study II (CIBIS-II): a randomised trial. *Lancet* 1999; 353: 9–13.

10 Iwata M, Yoshikawa T, Baba A, Anzai T, et al. Autoantibodies against the second extracellular loop of beta1-adrenergic receptors predict ventricular tachycardia and sudden death in patients with idiopathic dilated cardiomyopathy. *J Am Coll Cardiol* 2001; 37: 418–24.

11 Eichhorn EJ, Heesch CM, Barnett JH, Alvarez G, et al. Effect of metoprolol on myocardial function and energetics in patients with nonischemic dilated cardiomyopathy: a randomized, double-blind, placebo-controlled study. *J Am Coll Cardiol* 1994; 24: 1310–20.

12 Lechat P, Hulot JS, Escalono S, Wehrlen-Grandjean M, Dargie HJ. Relationships between nature of cardiac rhythm, heart rate and bisoprolol benefit on survival in chronic heart failure in CIBIS I and II trials. *Circulation* 2000; 102: I–779.

13 Bohm M, La Rosee K, Schmidt U, Schulz C, et al. Force-frequency relationship and inotropic stimulation in the nonfailing and failing human myocardium: implications for the medical treatment of heart failure. *Clin Invest* 1992; 70: 421–5.

14   Whyte K, Jones CR, Howie CA, Deighton N, *et al.* Haemodynamic, metabolic, and lymphocyte beta 2-adrenoceptor changes following chronic beta-adrenoceptor antagonism. *Eur J Clin Pharmacol* 1987; **32**: 237–43.

15   McGowan J, Murphy R, Cleland JGF. Carvedilol for heart failure; clinical trials in progress. *Heart Fail Rev* 1999; **4**: 89–95.

16   Serruys PW, Foley DP, Hofling B, Puel J, *et al.* Carvedilol for prevention of restenosis after directional coronary atherectomy: final results of the European carvedilol atherectomy restenosis (EUROCARE) trial. *Circulation* 2000; **101**: 1512–8.

17   Packer M, Bristow MR, Cohn JN, Colucci WS, *et al.* The effect of carvedilol on morbidity and mortality in patients with chronic heart failure. U.S. Carvedilol Heart Failure Study group. *N Engl J Med* 1996; **334**: 1349–55.

18   Left ventricular remodeling with carvedilol in patients with congestive heart failure due to ischemic heart disease. Australia-New Zealand Heart Failure Research Collaborative Group. *J Am Coll Cardiol* 1997; **29**: 1060–6.

19   MacMahon S, Sharpe N, Doughty R, Krum H, *et al.* Randomised, placebo-controlled trial of carvedilol in patients with congestive heart failure due to ischaemic heart disease. *Lancet* 1997; **349**: 375–80.

20   Effects of carvedilol on outcome after myocardial infarction in patients with left-ventricular dysfunction: the CAPRICORN randomised trial. *Lancet* 2001; **357**: 1385–90.

21   Erdmann E, Lechat P, Verkenne P, Wiemann H. Results from post-hoc analyses of the CIBIS II trial: effect of bisoprolol in high-risk patient groups with chronic heart failure. *Eur J Heart Fail* 2001; **3**: 469–79.

22   Hjalmarson A, Goldstein S, Fagerberg B, Wedel H, *et al.* Effects of controlled-release metoprolol on total mortality, hospitalizations, and well-being in patients with heart failure: the Metoprolol CR/XL Randomized Intervention Trial in congestive heart failure (MERIT-HF). MERIT-HF Study Group. *JAMA* 2000; **283**: 1295–302.

23   Effect of metoprolol CR/XL in chronic heart failure: Metoprolol CR/XL Randomised Intervention Trial in Congestive Heart Failure (MERIT-HF). *Lancet* 1999; **333**: 2001–7.

24   Xamoterol in severe heart failure. The Xamoterol in Severe Heart Failure Study Group. *Lancet* 1990; **336**: 1–6.

25   The beta-blocker evaluation of survival trial investigators. A trial of the beta-blocker bucindolol in patients with advanced chronic heart failure. *N Engl J Med* 2001; **344**: 1659–67.

26   Cohn JN, Fowler MB, Bristow MA, Colucci WS, *et al.* Effect of carvedilol in severe chronic heart failure. *J Am Coll Cardiol* 1996; **27**: 169A (abstract)

27   Colucci WS, Packer M, Bristow MR, Gilbert EM, *et al.* Carvedilol inhibits clinical progression in patients with mild symptoms of heart failure. US Carvedilol Heart Failure Study Group. *Circulation* 1996; **94**: 2800–6.

28   Packer M, Colucci WS, Sackner-Bernstein JD, Liang CS, *et al.* Double-blind, placebo-controlled study of the effects of carvedilol in patients with moderate to severe heart failure. The PRECISE Trial. Prospective Randomized Evaluation of Carvedilol on Symptoms and Exercise. *Circulation* 1996; **94**: 2793–9.

29   Bristow MR, Gilbert EM, Abraham WT, Adams K, *et al.* Carvedilol produces dose-related improvements in left ventricular function and survival in subjects with chronic heart failure. MOCHA Investigators. *Circulation* 1996; **94**: 2807–16.

30   A randomized trial of beta-blockade in heart failure. The Cardiac Insufficiency Bisoprolol Study (CIBIS). CIBIS Investigations and Committees. *Circulation* 1994; **90**: 1765–73.

31   Cleland JG, Pennel D, Ray S, Murray G, *et al.* The carvedilol hibernation reversible ischaemia trial; marker of success (CHRISTMAS). The CHRISTMAS Study Steering Committee and Investigators. *Eur J Heart Fail* 1999; **1**: 191–6.

32   O'Keefe JH Jr, Magalski A, Stevens TL, Bresnahan DR Jr, *et al.* Predictors of improvement in left ventricular ejection fraction with carvedilol for congestive heart failure. *J Nucl Cardiol* 2000; **7**: 3–7.

33   de Jong RM, Cornel JH, Crijns HJ, van Veldhuisen DJ. Abnormal contractile responses during dobutamine stress echocardiography in patients with idiopathic dilated cardiomyopathy. *Eur J Heart Fail* 2001; **3**: 429–36.

34   Khand AU, Rankin AC, Martin W, Taylor J, Cleland JGF. Digoxin or carvedilol for the treatment of atrial fibrillation in patients with heart failure? *Heart* 2000; **83**(Suppl 1): P30 (abstract).

35   Eichhorn EJ, Lukas MA, Wu B, Shusterman N. Effect of concomitant digoxin and carvedilol therapy on mortality and morbidity in patients with chronic heart failure. *Am J Cardiol* 2000; **86**: 1032–5, A10-1.

36   Yancy CW, Fowler MB, Colucci WS, Gilbert EM, *et al.* Race and the response to adrenergic blockade with carvedilol in patients with chronic heart failure. *N Engl J Med* 2001; **344**: 1358–65.

37   Kukin ML, Kalman J, Charney RH, Levy DK, *et al.* Prospective, randomized comparison of effect of long-term treatment with metoprolol or carvedilol on symptoms, exercise, ejection fraction, and oxidative stress in heart failure. *Circulation* 1999; **99**: 2645–51.

38   Di Lenarda A, Sabbadini G, Salvatore L, Sinagra G, *et al.* Long-term effects of carvedilol in idiopathic dilated cardiomyopathy with persistent left ventricular dysfunction despite chronic metoprolol. The Heart-Muscle Disease Study. *J Am Coll Cardiol* 1999; **33**: 1926–34.

39   Sanderson JE, Chan SK, Yip G, Yeung LY, *et al.* Beta-blockade in heart failure: a comparison of carvedilol with metoprolol. *J Am Coll Cardiol* 1999; **34**: 1522–8.

40   Metra M, Giubbini R, Nodari S, Boldi E, *et al.* Differential effect of beta-blockers in patients with heart failure: a prospective, randomized, double-blind comparison of the long-term effects of metoprolol versus carvedilol. *Circulation* 2000; **102**: 546–51.

41   Sanderson JE, Chan SK, Yu CM, Yeung LY, *et al.* Beta blockers in heart failure: a comparison of a vasodilating beta blocker with metoprolol. *Heart* 1998; **79**: 86–92.

42   Banerjee P, Banerjee T, Khand AL, Cleland JGF. Diastolic heart failure – neglected or misdiagnosed. *J Am Coll Cardiol* 2001 (in press).

43   Thackray SD, Witte KK, Khand A, Dunn A, *et al.* Clinical trial updates: highlights of the scientific sessions of the American Heart Association year 2000: Val HeFT, COPERNICUS, MERIT, CIBIS-II, BEST, AMIOVIRT, V-MAC, BREATHE, HEAT, MIRACL, FLORIDA, VIVA and the first human cardiac skeletal muscle myoblast transfer for heart failure. *Eur J Heart Fail* 2001; **3**: 117–24.

44   Pitt B, Zannad F, Remme WJ, Cody R, *et al.* The effect of spironolactone on morbidity and mortality in patients with severe heart failure. Randomized Aldactone Evaluation Study Investigators. *N Engl J Med* 1999; **341**: 709–17.

45   Boutite F, Boissel JP, Connolly SJ, Camm AJ, *et al.* Amiodarone interaction with beta-blockers: analysis of the merged EMIAT (European Myocardial Infarct Amiodarone Trial) and CAMIAT (Canadian Amiodarone Myocardial Infarction Trial) databases. *Circulation* 1999; **99**: 2268–75.

46   Effect of prophylactic amiodarone on mortality after acute myocardial infarction and in congestive heart failure: meta-analysis of individual data from 6500 patients in randomised trials. Amiodarone Trials Meta-Analysis Investigators. *Lancet* 1997; **350**: 1417–24.

47   Houghton T, Freemantle N, Cleland JG. Are beta-blockers effective in patients who develop heart failure soon after myocardial infarction? A meta-regression analysis of randomised trials. *Eur J Heart Fail* 2000; **2**: 333–40.

48   Jonas M, Reicher-Reiss H, Boyko V, Shotan A, *et al.* Usefulness of beta-blocker therapy in patients with non-insulin-dependent diabetes mellitus and coronary artery disease. Bezafibrate Infarction Prevention (BIP) Study. *Am J Cardiol* 1996; **77**: 1273–7.

49   Breckenridge A, Roberts DH. Antihypertensive treatment in concomitant peripheral vascular disease: current experience and the potential of carvedilol. Review. *J Cardiovasc Pharmacol* 1991; **18**(Suppl 4): S78–81.

50   Gomes UC, Cleland JG. Heart failure update. *Eur J Heart Fail* 1999; **1**: 301–2.

Intracoronary radiation therapy to treat and prevent restenosis

Martyn Thomas

☐ INTRODUCTION

The Achilles heel of percutaneous transluminal coronary angioplasty (PTCA) has traditionally been abrupt vessel closure (2–8%) [1] and the high incidence of recurrence, both clinical (13–16%) and angiographic (22–32%) even for 'simple' lesions [2]. The early use of intracoronary stents has greatly reduced the incidence of abrupt vessel closure during PTCA, and the Stress/Benestent studies showed the benefit of this type of device in reducing both angiographic and clinical restenosis following PTCA [2]. However, the population of patients studied in the Stress/Benestent studies was highly selected (focal lesions <15 mm in length, reference diameter >3mm, non-ostial, no thrombus, non-bifurcational, non-vein graft with elective deployment) and would account for only 15–20% of patients undergoing PTCA at our institution. The results of intracoronary stenting in 'non-Stress/Benestent' lesions are less impressive, with angiographic and clinical restenosis rates of 30–50% [3]. The newly produced disease process of 'in-stent restenosis' is also extremely difficult to treat. The use of simple techniques in this setting, such as redilatation by PTCA, is associated with a recurrence rate of 50–80%, especially in diffuse disease processes [4]. Restenosis, therefore, remains the greatest challenge to interventional cardiology, following either PTCA or intracoronary stent insertion.

The use of radiation therapy to treat a proliferative, non-malignant disease process has been established in the treatment of keloid scars [5]. If restenosis following coronary angioplasty is considered as a similar process, the use of radiation would seem a reasonable approach in this setting.

☐ BASIC CONCEPTS OF ANGIOPLASTY AND STENT RESTENOSIS

The pathological mechanisms of both balloon restenosis and in-stent restenosis are now well established and accepted as different [6,7]. The predominant reduction in luminal diameter at six months following PTCA is caused by adventitial constriction (70–80%), with only a small contribution by neointima, whereas the reverse is true for in-stent restenosis with which over 90% of the loss of acute gain is caused by an aggressive neointima within the stented segment. The potential mechanisms for the effect of intracoronary brachytherapy (defined as radiation therapy with the radioactive source placed in or near the target cell) may therefore be different in these two settings.

The important measures of loss of the gain following angioplasty, and therefore the way by which any potential anti-restenosis therapy may be measured, are:

- ☐ *Binary angiographic restenosis* rate: follow-up lesion diameter of less than 50% of the reference diameter. For coronary stenting, angiographic restenosis is generally in the region of 20–50% depending on the type of lesion.

- ☐ *Clinical restenosis* rate: the requirement for further revascularisation procedures because of recurrent symptoms. For stenting, this varies between 8% and 30% depending on the lesion type.

- ☐ *Angiographic late loss*: the loss of acute gain (in mm) at the lesion site at the six-month quantitative angiographic follow-up. For balloon angioplasty, this value is generally around 0.7. Clearly, the lower this number the more effective the anti-restenosis treatment.

- ☐ *Angiographic late loss index*: the late loss at the lesion site divided by the acute gain. This is accepted as the most sensitive measure of the effectiveness of any technique, and generally measures 0.4–0.6 for balloon angioplasty. Again, the lower this value the more effective the anti-restenosis treatment.

☐ BASIC CONCEPTS OF INTRAVASCULAR RADIATION THERAPY

In intracoronary brachytherapy (as defined above) the radiation may be delivered via a stent, removable solid source or fluid/gas filled balloon, each placed at the site of the coronary lesion following standard intervention. (The unit of dose of radiation therapy, the Gray (Gy), refers to the mean energy imparted by ionising radiation to matter in a given volume divided by the mass of matter in that volume.)

Broadly speaking, two types of radiation source are currently used for intracoronary brachytherapy, delivering either beta or gamma radiation:

- ☐ *Beta particles:* high-speed electrons emitted from the nucleus of an unstable atom. They are high energy but have a low penetration, so there is a rapid dose fall off distant to the source.

- ☐ *Gamma rays:* high-energy photons, again emitted from the nucleus of an unstable atom. Their penetration is much higher than that of beta particles, so the dose fall off is much less.

There are potential advantages and disadvantages of both types of source (see below). The mechanism of action of both beta and gamma radiation is identical. Radiation disrupts DNA by strand and cross-link breakage. This leads to cell death at the next cell division. The target cell for brachytherapy treatment is not entirely clear, but the most likely candidate appears to be the myofibroblast. In the adventitial layer myofibroblasts migrate into the intima and transform to smooth muscle cells [8]. Most brachytherapy systems therefore aim to administer the target dose to the adventitial layer of the coronary artery. The dose of radiation appears crucial: too low a dose is ineffective or even stimulatory to neointimal growth, while too high a dose is potentially associated with aneurysm formation due to thinning and weakening of the vessel wall. The potential for long-term fibrotic complications has not yet been seen in the human.

☐ ANIMAL DATA

The principle of using brachytherapy post-angioplasty to reduce restenosis has been proven in a number of animal models for both beta and gamma radiation [9,10]. There is, however, a major difference in the pathology of the balloon overstretch animal injury model (the mechanism used to create the lesion in the animal coronary artery) and the human atherosclerotic artery. It is likely that doses proven effective in the animal model will prove ineffective in the human because the disease process in the latter is less predictable and often markedly eccentric [11]. There has also been criticism of the animal models for the short-term follow-up and young age of the animals which may affect radiation sensitivity. Despite these concerns, human studies were started following encouraging results in the animal models.

☐ CLINICAL TRIALS

Condado *et al* [12], who performed the first intracoronary brachytherapy cases worldwide, reported an encouraging late loss index of 0.19 at six months. More recently, the five-year follow-up has shown an encouragingly low binary angiographic restenosis rate of 28% (presented at Cardiovascular Radiation Therapy V, Washington, Feb 5–7, 2001). Despite the use of relatively high doses of radiation and the occurrence of one new pseudoaneurysm at early follow-up, there has been no progression of aneurysm formation or late adverse effects in this group of patients.

The SCRIPPS trial

The SCRIPPS trial (see end of text for explanation of trials) was a landmark study which reported favourable results for the use of intracoronary gamma brachytherapy in humans [13]. It was a double-blind, randomised, placebo-controlled trial comparing gamma radiation (^{192}Ir embedded within an intracoronary guidewire) with placebo in a group of patients with coronary restenosis. Two-thirds of the patients had presented with in-stent restenosis, a particularly high risk group for repeat restenosis following further interventional therapies. The results indicated a major advantage of ^{192}Ir over placebo:

- ☐ six-month angiographic restenosis was dramatically reduced (by 37%) (Fig. 1(a))

- ☐ 63% reduction in late loss to 0.38, and

- ☐ 80% reduction in late loss index to 0.12 (Fig. 1(b)).

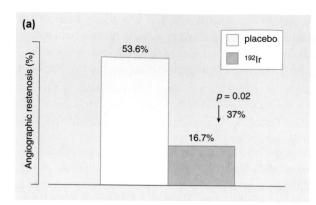

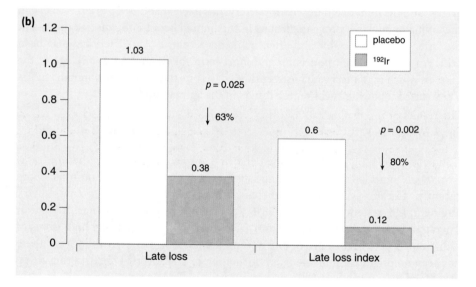

Fig. 1 The SCRIPPS trial: **(a)** six-month angiographic restenosis (stent plus border); **(b)** six-month late loss and late loss index.

These results were maintained at two years, with marked clinical benefit and a target lesion revascularisation rate of 15.4% in the ^{192}Ir group compared with 44.8% in the placebo group.

The SCRIPPS trial and the Condado data proved a major impetus to further clinical trials and to the development of multiple different brachytherapy systems by interventional cardiology companies.

The IRIS trials using the [32]phosphorus radioactive stent

The ^{32}P stent incorporates a radioactive source within the stent. Results of clinical trials so far have been disappointing [14]. The initial IRIS registry in the USA showed that the stent could be delivered with no early complications but with an angiographic restenosis rate of 39%. Subsequent dose-ranging studies in Europe have been equally disappointing. The principal difficulty with this device appears to be the so-called 'edge effect', a problem related to radiation dose which may be difficult to combat using stent-based radiation technology. When the source length does not completely cover the injured segment of coronary artery, a previously injured area receives a low dose of radiation. This leads to the so-called 'candy wrapper' lesion seen at follow-up which, as the name suggests, is a lesion with no late loss at the actual site of the lesion but with severe restenosis at the proximal and distal margins. An extension of this is 'geographic miss', which occurs when the source is not placed wholly within the injured segment at the initial procedure. The solution to both the edge effect and geographic miss is principally twofold:

1   Operators must learn the importance of positioning the source within the injured segment and ensure good overlap into non-injured segments.

2   Success will be facilitated by the industry developing a source of much greater length.

Dose-ranging studies with the ^{32}phosphorus stent

The results of the European dose-ranging studies using the ^{32}P stent are shown in Fig. 2. Within-stent restenosis of higher activity stents (3–6 μCi) was found to be low (3.5%) but restenosis at the edges of the stents was high (39.5%). No solution has currently been found to the problems of the radioactive stent.

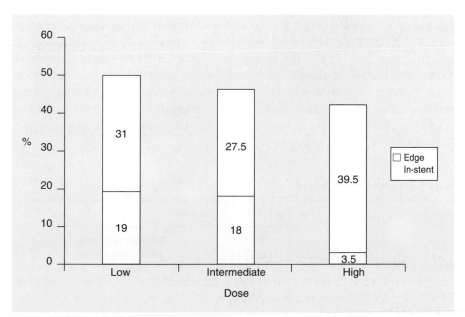

Fig. 2 Edge and in-stent angiographic restenosis in the European dose-ranging studies using the ^{32}P stent (low dose activity stents: 0.75–1.5 μCi; intermediate dose: 1.5–3.0 μCi; high dose: 3.0–6.0 μCi).

The WRIST trials

WRIST was another landmark series of trials. The first WRIST trial was a single-centre, double-blind randomised trial of gamma radiation (^{192}Ir) versus placebo for the treatment of in-stent restenosis following standard treatment [15]. The six-month outcomes were dramatically in favour of the ^{192}Ir arm, with the following reductions:

☐ angiographic restenosis: 67%

☐ target lesion revascularisation: 79%

☐ target vessel revascularisation: 61%, and

☐ major adverse cardiac events: 63%.

Subsequently, the beta-WRIST trial tested a similar strategy with a beta source and showed similar results in favour of radiation therapy [16]. These data have now been confirmed in a multicentre trial [17].

BERT

The BERT studies have investigated the use of beta radiation (^{90}Sr delivered via the Novoste Beta-Cath system) to reduce restenosis following coronary angioplasty [18]. The Novoste device is non-centred but the strontium is delivered via a blind-ending 5F catheter which tends to 'self-centre' in the artery. The original trial, which had no control group, was essentially a registry of the use of beta radiation to prevent restenosis following balloon angioplasty with no primary intention to deploy a stent. Bail out stenting was required in 13% of cases. Three different doses of radiation were used during the study (12 Gy, 14 Gy, 16 Gy). The results are shown in Table 1. For the group as a whole, the angiographic restenosis rate was 17%, with an encouraging late loss index of 0.09. In addition, the in-stent restenosis rates in the bail out stent group were low, and there was a suggestion of a dose effect with better results achieved with higher radiation doses. The results have now been confirmed in a multicentre trial of in-stent restenosis (START trial, presented at Cardiovascular Radiation Therapy V, Washington, Feb 5–7, 2001).

Table 1 Six-month angiographic data from the BERT trial.

	Patients	
Angiographic data	All (78) (%)	Patients receiving 14 Gy and 16 Gy (52) (%)
Angiographic restenosis	17	15
Late loss index	9	4
Bail out stenting	13	9
In-stent restenosis	8	0

Other beta radiation trials

The PREVENT trial delivered beta radiation via a ^{32}P source embedded in the end of a standard guidewire (Galileo system, Guidant Corporation) [19]. The ^{32}P patients again had an impressively low lesion angiographic restenosis rate and late loss index, but the edge effect was clearly demonstrated by a vessel restenosis rate of 25% (Table 2). Clinically, this led to a target lesion revascularisation rate of only 4% but a target vessel revascularisation rate of 24%.

The Schneider/Sauverwein trials used an yttrium source embedded in a guidewire delivering beta radiation via a computerised afterloader. The initial animal data with this device were encouraging but the human Phase I trial had a high restenosis rate (angiographic restenosis: 40%; target lesion revascularisation: 27%) [11], probably because it is likely that a relatively low dose of radiation was delivered. These initial results have led to a multicentre dose-ranging study, the results of which have recently been published [20]. This trial investigated the effect of four different doses of radiation (9 Gy, 12 Gy, 15 Gy, 18 Gy at 1 mm from the endoluminal surface) on angiographic restenosis rates in a group of patients undergoing balloon angioplasty in *de novo* coronary lesions without planned stent insertion. The trial reported the lowest ever restenosis rate (4%) in the 18 Gy group.

Table 2 Six-month results of the PREVENT trial in 63 patients (available data).

	No. of patients	
	^{32}P (48)	Control (15)
Treatment site angiographic restenosis rate (%)	6	33
Treatment site and adjacent site restenosis rate (%)	25	44
Late loss index (%)	5	51
Death (%)	2	0
Myocardial infarction (%)	11	6
Target lesion revascularisation (%)	4	18
Target vessel revascularisation (%)	24	29

☐ ONGOING ISSUES

Dosimetry and type of radiation (beta versus gamma)

It seems clear that there is a therapeutic window in which radiation therapy is effective. Too low a dose appears at best ineffective, and may be pro-proliferative; too high a dose may potentially lead to coronary aneurysm formation in the future due to a weakening of the vascular wall. The therapeutic dose is likely to be around 10–18 Gy at 1 mm from the endoluminal surface. Dosimetry is more difficult with the beta sources because of the low penetration of the energy but, despite this, the clinical results appear equal for beta and gamma radiation. In Europe, the majority of centres performing this type of work have decided to use beta radiation.

Beta radiation

Because of its low penetration into tissues, beta radiation has the advantage of less radiation exposure to the catheter laboratory and hospital staff and a lower total body radiation dose to the patient. The use of centring catheters to deliver a homogeneous dose to the target area is probably more important with beta radiation.

Gamma radiation

Gamma radiation has practical difficulties in the need for more extensive radiation protection measures and the increased total body dose to the patient. The dwell times of gamma sources are also much longer than beta sources (15–20 min vs 3–6 min). During the dwell time of gamma sources, interventional staff have to leave the cardiac catheter laboratory to limit their radiation exposure which is not necessary with beta radiation. However, the higher tissue penetration of gamma radiation has the advantage of easier dosing with centring of the delivery device less important.

Licensing

Currently, three factors must be in place to perform intracoronary brachytherapy in the UK. A team consisting of an interventional cardiologist, clinical oncologist and medical physics representative is required in order to fulfil these requirements:

1   *Ethics committee approval* if the patient is participating in either a clinical trial or a national/international registry.

2   *Administration of Radioactive Substances Advisory Committee licence approval.* The licence allows the therapeutic delivery of radiation and is usually held by a radiation oncologist. Given the training requirements, it is unlikely that it will be held by an interventional cardiologist in the foreseeable future.

3   *Medical Device Agency approval* of the delivery device.

Anxieties for the future

The longest follow-up of any patient who has undergone intracoronary brachytherapy is approaching six years. There are worries about potential long-term complications of this procedure, including:

☐   late fibrosis leading to delayed restenosis

☐   late thinning of the vessel wall, leading to aneurysm formation, and

☐   new tumour formation at either a local or distant site.

These potential complications have thus far not been seen, but from data in the field of radiation oncology they may be expected 10–20 years following the index procedure.

☐ CONCLUSIONS

Intracoronary brachytherapy may prove to be the greatest breakthrough for interventional cardiology since the coronary stent. It is currently unclear where this procedure will fit into the interventional armamentarium. It remains to be seen whether it will be used as a primary procedure, with or without a coronary stent, or be reserved for the treatment of in-stent restenosis. It is unlikely that intracoronary brachytherapy will be delivered twice to the same site, which may play an important part in the decision making progress. The long-term follow-up of the pioneering work of Condado and Teirstein will be pivotal in the general acceptance of this form of treatment by the interventional community.

☐ TRIAL ACRONYMS

BERT   Beta Energy Restenosis Trials
IRIS   Isostent Restenosis Intervention Studies
PREVENT   Proliferation REduction with Vascular ENergy Trial
SCRIPPS   Scripps Coronary Radiation to Inhibit Proliferation Post Stenting
START   Stents And Radiation Therapy
WRIST   Washington Radiation for In-Stent restenosis Trials

REFERENCES

1   Bergelson BA, Fishman RF, Tommaso CL. Abrupt vessel closure: changing importance, management, and consequences. Review. *Am Heart J* 1997; **134**: 362–81.

2   Serruys PW, de Jaegere P, Kiemeneij F, Macaya C, *et al.* A comparison of balloon-expandable-stent implantation with balloon angioplasty in patients with coronary artery disease. Benestent Study Group. *N Engl J Med* 1994; **331**: 489–95.

3   Moussa I, Di Mario C, Moses J, Reimers B, *et al.* Comparison of angiographic and clinical outcome of coronary stenting of chronic total occlusions versus subtotal occlusions. *Am J Cardiol* 1998; **81**: 1–6.

4   Baim DS, Levine MJ, Leon MB, Levine S, *et al.* Management of restenosis within the Palmaz-Schatz coronary stent (the U.S. multicenter experience). The U.S. Palmaz-Schatz Stent Investigators. *Am J Cardiol* 1993; **71**: 364–6.

5   Van den Brenk HAS, Minty CC. Radiation in the management of keloids and hypertrophic scar. *Br J Surg* 1959/60; **47**: 595–605.

6   Mintz GS, Popma JJ, Pichard AD, Kent KM, *et al.* Arterial remodeling after coronary angioplasty: a serial intravascular ultrasound study. *Circulation* 1996; **94**: 35–43.

7   Hoffmann R, Mintz GS, Popma JJ, Satler LF, *et al.* Chronic arterial responses to stent implantation: a serial intravascular ultrasound analysis of Palmaz-Schatz stents in native coronary arteries. *J Am Coll Cardiol* 1996; **28**: 1134–9.

8   Scott NA, Cipolla GD, Ross CE, Dunn B, *et al.* Identification of a potential role for the adventitia in vascular lesion formation after balloon overstretch injury of porcine coronary arteries. *Circulation* 1996; **93**: 2178–87.

9   Waksman R, Robinson KA, Crocker IR, Gravanis MB, *et al.* Endovascular low-dose irradiation inhibits neointima formation after coronary artery balloon injury in swine. A possible role for radiation therapy in restenosis prevention. *Circulation* 1995; **91**: 1533–9.

10 Verin V, Popowski Y, Urban P, Belenger J, *et al.* Intra-arterial beta irradiation prevents neointimal hyperplasia in a hypercholesterolemic rabbit restenosis model. *Circulation* 1995; **92**: 2284–90.

11 Verin V, Urban P, Popowski Y, Schwager M, *et al.* Feasibility of intracoronary beta-irradiation to reduce restenosis after balloon angioplasty. A clinical pilot study. *Circulation* 1997; **95**: 1138–44.

12 Condado JA, Waksman R, Gurdiel O, Espinosa R, *et al.* Long-term angiographic and clinical outcome after percutaneous transluminal coronary angioplasty and intracoronary radiation therapy in humans. *Circulation* 1997; **96**: 727–32.

13 Teirstein PS, Massullo V, Jani S, Popma JJ, *et al.* Catheter-based radiotherapy to inhibit restenosis after coronary stenting. *N Engl J Med* 1997; **336**: 1697–703.

14 Hehrlein C, Kubler W. Advantages and limitations of radioactive stents. Review. *Semin Interv Cardiol* 1997; **2**: 109–13.

15 Waksman R, White RL, Chan RC, Bass BG, *et al.* Intracoronary gamma-radiation therapy after angioplasty inhibits recurrence in patients with in-stent restenosis. *Circulation* 2000; **101**: 2165–71.

16 Waksman R, Bhargava B, White RL, Chan RC, *et al.* Intracoronary beta-radiation therapy inhibits recurrence of in-stent restenosis. *Circulation* 2000; **101**: 1895–8.

17 Leon NB, Teirstein PS, Moses JW, Tripuraneni P, *et al.* Localized intracoronary gamma-radiation therapy to inhibit the recurrence of restenosis after stenting. *N Engl J Med* 2001; **344**: 250–6.

18 King SB 3rd, Williams DO, Chougule P, Klein JL, *et al.* Endovascular beta-radiation to reduce restenosis after coronary balloon angioplasty: results of the beta energy restenosis trial (BERT). *Circulation* 1998; **97**: 2025–30.

19 Raizner AE, Oesterle SN, Waksman R, Serruys PW, *et al.* Inhibition of restenosis with beta-emitting radiotherapy. Report of the Proliferation Reduction with Vascular Energy Trial (PREVENT). *Circulation* 2000; **102**: 951–8.

20 Verin V, Popowski Y, de Bruyne B, Baumgart D, *et al.* Endoluminal beta-radiation therapy for the prevention of coronary restenosis after balloon angioplasty. The Dose-Finding Study Group. *N Engl J Med* 2001; **344**: 243–9.

☐ SELF ASSESSMENT QUESTIONS

1 Restenosis following coronary angioplasty:
   (a) Has essentially been eliminated by intracoronary stenting
   (b) Has the same pathophysiology with or without stent placement
   (c) Is dependent on pre-procedural factors such as diabetes, lesion length and vessel size
   (d) Is greater if measured angiographically rather than clinically
   (e) Is easier to treat if a stent has been placed

2 Intracoronary radiation therapy:
   (a) Has a similar mechanism whether beta or gamma radiation is used
   (b) Has a dose-dependent effect
   (c) Is most effective when delivered via radioactive stent
   (d) Reduces late loss after treatment of in-stent restenosis
   (e) Has no follow-up data longer than two years

3 In order to perform intracoronary brachytherapy:
   (a) No additional arrangements are required within a cardiac unit
   (b) Specific radiation protection issues are raised with gamma therapy
   (c) Specific licences are required

(d) Medical physics and clinical oncology personnel should be present at all cases
(e) Major structural changes to a catheter laboratory are required for the use of beta radiation

4   Potential complications of intracoronary radiation therapy include:
   (a) Hair loss
   (b) Increased late loss at six months
   (c) Intracoronary aneurysm formation
   (d) Restenosis at the margins of the original lesion at six months
   (e) Increased target vessel revascularisation at six months

5   Potential advantages of beta versus gamma radiation include:
   (a) Easier delivery of homogeneous dose to the vessel wall
   (b) Reduced radiation exposure to patient and staff
   (c) Lower 'dwell' times within the coronary artery
   (d) Improved efficacy in reducing restenosis following coronary angioplasty
   (e) Reduced licensing requirements within the UK

ANSWERS

1a	False	2a	True	3a	False	4a	False	5a	False
b	False	b	True	b	True	b	False	b	True
c	True	c	False	c	True	c	True	c	True
d	True	d	True	d	True	d	True	d	False
e	False	e	False	e	False	e	False	e	False

Modern management of unstable angina

Ganesh Manoharan, John Riddell, Ian Menown and Jennifer Adgey

☐ INTRODUCTION

Unstable angina (UA) is part of a continuum of clinical expression of acute coronary syndromes (ACS). It is defined as ischaemic chest pain of recent origin which occurs either more frequently than previously, or is more severe, more prolonged or more difficult to control with medication, or as prolonged chest pain at rest. Though previously underestimated, it is now well accepted that UA is associated with a high risk of myocardial infarction (MI) or death if treated inadequately.

Hospital admissions for UA have now exceeded those for acute MI. It is estimated that there are approximately 226 patients with UA per 100,000 population per year in the UK, or at least 130,000 patients per year. The recent PRAIS-UK registry of patients with ACS without ST elevation [1] showed that the incidence of death or MI in-hospital was 5% and by six months it was 12.2% (see end of text for explanation of trials). Assessment of death/new MI/refractory angina or readmission for UA showed that the incidence in-hospital was 7.6% and at six months 30%.

The ongoing advances in the understanding of the aetiology and pathogenesis of ACS and UA have led to the recent publication of a large number of clinical trials of new pharmacological agents and interventional techniques directed at managing patients appropriately, and ultimately reducing the incidence of acute MI and death. This chapter will review the evidence for the new management options.

☐ PATHOGENESIS

The aetiology of ACS has been shown to be associated with plaque fissure or erosion and an ensuing platelet thrombus leading to subtotal or complete occlusion of the coronary artery. Plaque disruption results in platelet adherence to the exposed extravascular tissues and initiation of platelet activation [2]. Mediators such as collagen, adenosine diphosphate, thrombin, thromboxane A2, serotonin, adrenaline and arachidonic acid are among the agents responsible for this activation [3]. It is hypothesised that, following the development of the platelet thrombus, embolisation occurs downstream. This gives rise to microvascular platelet aggregation, resulting in minimal myocardial damage and troponin release.

Platelet aggregation plays a major role in the formation of thrombus in ACS. The glycoprotein (GP) IIb/IIIa receptor represents a pathway for platelet aggregation [2]. It is the most abundant receptor found on platelet membrane surfaces

(40,000–80,000/platelet) and belongs to a family of surface receptors called integrins. Following activation of platelets, the previously dormant GP IIb/IIIa receptor undergoes structural change and becomes active [2]. It binds with the soluble ligands fibrinogen and von Willebrand factor, causing platelet-platelet adherence, promoting the generation of a platelet mass and, as a consequence, providing an ideal environment for thrombus formation [2].

The concept of inflammation as a factor in the aetiology of ACS has led to a new understanding of the pathogenesis and may result in improved pharmacological treatments. The evidence in favour of inflammation as a significant factor includes the finding of an association between raised C-reactive protein (CRP) and a worse prognosis in patients with unstable angina. Initial studies with macrolide antibiotics suggest that their use might improve prognosis [4].

☐ PRESENTATION, DIAGNOSIS AND RISK STRATIFICATION

Patients with UA represent a heterogeneous group ranging from those at low risk to those at high risk of death, MI or recurrent ischaemia both in-hospital and up to one year following the acute event. Various factors adversely affect or are associated with a worse prognosis, including:

- ☐ presence of rest pain
- ☐ age
- ☐ prior history of MI
- ☐ poor left ventricular function
- ☐ history of diabetes mellitus
- ☐ haemodynamic deterioration during pain
- ☐ pulmonary oedema
- ☐ new mitral regurgitation or third heart sound
- ☐ hypotension, and
- ☐ co-morbid conditions (which reduce life expectancy).

The initial 12-lead ECG has provided prognostic information in many studies [5,6]. Hamm *et al* [7] have shown that the initial ECG is important in the risk stratification process, which should take place in the accident and emergency (A&E) department. Of those ACS patients presenting with acute ischaemic chest pain, approximately 43% will have a normal admission ECG, 26% negative T waves, 20% ST segment depression and 11% will be non-diagnostic (either bundle branch block or pacing). About one-third will have raised cardiac troponin (cTn) T or cTnI [7]. ECG changes, in particular ST segment depression of 0.5 mm or above, reflect a worse prognosis, both short- and long-term, as shown in the GUSTO IIb and RISC studies.

The newer, more sensitive and specific serum markers of myocyte necrosis, cTnT or cTnI, provide the clinician with valuable diagnostic and prognostic information and are also helpful in identifying the higher risk subgroup of ACS patients. Hillis *et al* [8] have recently shown that patients have a favourable early prognosis if creatine kinase (CK)-Marsh-Bender (MB) (MASS), cTnI or both remain negative during the initial eight hours of hospitalisation. In a substudy of GUSTO IIa, cTnT greater than 0.1 ng/ml was associated with a 30-day mortality of 11.8% compared with 3.9% for lower levels of cTnT (p <0.001) [9]. There were similar findings in the TIMI IIIb substudy. Even in the presence of a normal CK-MB, elevation of either cTnT or cTnI is associated with a threefold increase in mortality [10]. In a substudy of TIMI IIA, an elevated CRP at presentation in patients with ACS was correlated with an increased mortality in those with a negative qualitative cTnT, but a combination of the two when positive offers a more comprehensive risk assessment [4].

A systematic approach to risk stratification allows the physician to provide more individualised care to each patient presenting with this challenging condition. Early and reliable risk stratification integrating clinical presentation, ECG findings and laboratory tests permits more effective patient care and targeting of resources. Using this integrated approach, it is possible to define low, medium and high risk groups (Fig. 1).

☐ MANAGEMENT OPTIONS

Pharmacological

There should be urgent assessment and treatment of patients with UA on first presentation, for example, by the general practitioner, paramedic crew or mobile coronary care unit team, and also at chest pain clinics or A&E departments, followed where necessary by admission to hospital. Underlying exacerbating factors such as anaemia, infection, thyrotoxicosis, tachyarrhythmia and hypoxia should be sought and treated, but control of these aggravating factors is helpful in only 10–15% of patients. Patients with UA have benefited from:

☐   anti-ischaemic therapy: for example beta-blocking drugs, nitrates, calcium antagonists and potassium channel openers (nicorandil), and

☐   antiplatelet and antithrombin treatments: for example aspirin, clopidogrel, hirudin, unfractionated heparin (UFH) and low molecular weight heparins (LMWH) (nadroparin, dalteparin, enoxaparin).

Low molecular weight heparins

LMWHs are derived from UFH by chemical or enzymatic depolymerisation to yield fragments approximately one-third the size of heparin [11]. The combination of a predictable pharmacokinetic profile, long half-life and high bioavailability results in effective anticoagulant activity after subcutaneous administration and, unlike UFH, treatment with LMWHs does not routinely require laboratory monitoring. Numerous clinical trials have found these agents to be generally safe and beneficial in the ACS

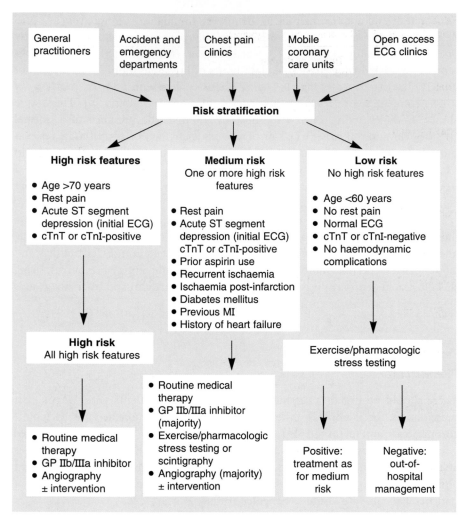

Fig. 1 Algorithm for risk stratification and management of unstable angina (cTn = cardiac troponin; GP = glycoprotein; MI = myocardial infarction).

setting (Table 1). The evidence is, however, stronger for the use of enoxaparin than for nadroparin or dalteparin [11]. Given the long half-life of LMWHs and the absence of a specific antidote, it may be best to use UFH in circumstances in which acute coronary intervention is anticipated, in order to reduce complications. Caution should also be exercised in patients with renal failure or extremes of body mass.

Glycoprotein IIb/IIIa receptor inhibitors

The drive to find a more potent antiplatelet agent has led to the discovery and development of platelet GP IIb/IIIa receptor inhibitors. The recently published National Institute for Clinical Excellence guidelines on the management of ACS

Table 1 Death/myocardial infarction (MI) rates (%) from major published trials using low molecular weight heparins (LMWH) in acute coronary syndromes.

Trial	Timing of double end-point (death/MI) (days)	Placebo	Unfractionated heparin	LMWH	
Nadroparin [11,12]	5–7	9.6	5.7	0	
FRAX.I.S 1999				6 days therapy	14 days therapy
	6	–	3.1	3.1	2.9
	14	–	4.5	5.3	4.9
	3*	–	7.9	8.6	8.9
Dalteparin [11]					
FRISC 1996	6	4.8	–	1.8	
	40	10.7	–	8.0	
	150	15.5	–	14.0	
FRIC 1997	1–6	–	3.6	3.9	
	6–45	4.7	–	4.3	
FRISC II 1999	30	5.9	–	3.1	
	3*	8.0	–	6.7	
Enoxaparin [11]					
ESSENCE 1997	14	–	6.1	4.9	
	30	–	7.7	6.2	
TIMI IIB 1999	2	–	2.1	1.7	
	8	–	5.9	4.6	
	14	–	6.9	5.7	
	43	–	8.9	7.9	
TIMI IIB-ESSENCE meta-analysis 1999	2	–	1.8	1.4	
	8	–	5.3	4.1	
	14	–	6.5	5.2	
	43	–	8.6	7.1	

* months

recommend their use in high risk patients and those undergoing percutaneous coronary intervention (PCI) (Table 2) [13]. There are similar recommendations in the British Cardiac Society and the Royal College of Physicians of London guidelines (Table 3) [14].

Commercially available GP IIb/IIIa inhibitors include abciximab (c7E3 Fab, ReoPro, Abciximab), tirofiban (Aggrastat) and eptifibatide (Integrilin). Abciximab, the first GP IIb/IIIa inhibitor was a chimeric monoclonal antibody Fab fragment compound. This has been followed by synthetic molecules of low molecular weight that differ from abciximab in that they mimic the arginine-glycine-aspartic acid sequence, and thus competitively inhibit fibrinogen binding to the GP IIb/IIIa receptor [2]. These non-antibody GP IIb/IIIa receptor inhibitors (tirofiban and eptifibatide) have a shorter duration of action and are specific to the GP IIb/IIIa receptor.

Table 2 National Institute for Clinical Excellence recommendations [13].

- For high risk patients with unstable angina or non-Q wave MI: iv GP IIb/IIIa inhibitors (consistent with current UK licensing), in addition to aspirin and low (adjusted) dose unfractionated heparin
- Raised troponin should be used to identify those at high risk
- Patients undergoing acute or elective PCI: iv GP IIb/IIIa inhibitors (consistent with current UK licensing)

GP = glycoprotein; iv = intravenous; MI = myocardial infarction; PCI = percutaneous coronary intervention.

Table 3 British Cardiac Society and the Royal College of Physicians guidelines [14].

- iv small molecule GP IIb/IIIa inhibitor for up to 96 hours should be given to patients with ACS at high risk of adverse outcome
- iv GP IIb/IIIa inhibitor should be administered to patients with ACS with elevated cardiac troponin scheduled for PCI using unfractionated heparin. This should be commenced before the intervention

ACS = acute coronary syndromes; GP = glycoprotein; iv = intravenous; PCI = percutaneous coronary intervention.

Completed clinical trials of these agents as a primary treatment for UA and as an adjunct to other interventions for UA [2] have shown improvement over existing treatments, with reductions in the incidence of death, MI, refractory ischaemia and the need for urgent revascularisation. These drugs are generally well tolerated and safe if appropriate attention is paid to dose, concomitant treatment with UFH and femoral sheath site, with no increased risk of intracranial haemorrhage compared with placebo.

Multicentre trials of glycoprotein IIb/IIIa receptor inhibitors. Four multicentre trials (PRISM, PRISM-PLUS, PARAGON A, PURSUIT) have used parenteral GP IIb/IIIa inhibitors as primary treatment in ACS (Table 4).

In the PRISM study [2], patients with ACS treated with tirofiban had a survival benefit maintained at 30 days, while in the PRISM-PLUS study (a higher risk population) death, MI or refractory ischaemia and readmission for UA at 30 days were all significantly lower for those treated with tirofiban and heparin compared with heparin alone (Table 4). Consistent benefits were seen in all patient subgroups whether treated medically or by angioplasty.

In the PRISM study, there was a 13% event rate (death or MI) at 30 days in the cTnI-positive patients treated with heparin compared with 4.3% in those treated with tirofiban [6]. In the PRISM-PLUS study, whilst there was no significant difference in the baseline cTnI levels between heparin alone (3.1 ± 6.7 ng/ml) and combination therapy with tirofiban plus heparin (1.6 ± 3 ng/ml) ($p = 0.15$), nevertheless peak levels of cTnI were statistically significantly higher in the former group than in the tirofiban and heparin group (15.5 ± 29.1 ng/ml vs 5.2 ± 8.3 ng/ml) ($p = 0.017$). Thus, treatment with tirofiban in this population prevents the increase of cTnI levels indicative of myocardial necrosis and a worse prognosis [6].

Table 4 Glycoprotein IIb/IIIa inhibitors as primary treatment in acute coronary syndromes (unstable angina (UA)) [2].

Trials	No. of patients	Outcome (30-day)	p
PRISM (tirofiban)	3,232	Mortality: heparin 3.6% tirofiban 2.3%	0.02
PRISM-PLUS (tirofiban)	1,915	Death, MI, refractory ischaemia or readmission for UA: heparin 22.3% tirofiban + heparin 18.5%	0.03
PARAGON A (lamifiban)	2,282	Death, non-fatal MI or reinfarction: low dose lamifiban 10.8% low dose lamifiban + heparin 10.3% high dose lamifiban 11.6% high dose lamifiban + heparin 12.3% placebo + heparin 11.7%	>0.05
PURSUIT (eptifibatide)	10,948	Death or MI: placebo 15.7% eptifibatide 14.2%	0.04

MI = myocardial infarction.

There was no statistically significant difference between the treatment groups in PARAGON A in composite end-point (death or non-fatal MI) at 30 days [2]. In the PURSUIT trial of 10,948 patients with UA, there was a 1.5% reduction in death or MI at 30 days ($p = 0.04$) [2].

The benefits of GP IIb/IIIa receptor inhibition with abciximab during PCI are shown in the CAPTURE trial [2]. However, the GUSTO IV ACS study (presented at the scientific meeting of the European Society of Cardiology, 2000) showed no significant difference in the primary end-point of death or MI at 30 days between 24-hour or 48-hour abciximab and placebo in the UA setting (8.2% vs 9.1% vs 8.0%). The investigators were discouraged from taking patients to the cardiac catheterisation laboratory for the first 48 hours after admission so, with both a lower risk group of patients recruited than envisaged and longer infusions of abciximab, the possibility of subtherapeutic platelet inhibition may have led to agonistic activities of the GP IIb/IIIa inhibitor rather than inhibition.

Antithrombin and antiplatelet approaches are complementary and potentially synergistic. The safety and efficacy of combination therapy with LMWHs and GP IIb/IIIa antagonists are currently being tested in UA/non-Q wave MI (NQMI) patients.

Intervention trials

In the last decade there has been an expansion in the availability of cardiac catheterisation facilities, rapid development in PCI techniques and improvement in surgical techniques (use of arterial grafts and better cardioplegia). It is not surprising, therefore, that there has been an increasing trend towards early intervention in an attempt to prevent MI, recurrent ischaemia and death in patients with UA, particularly those at high risk. However, a lack of evidence to support the benefit of a systematic invasive approach (eg OASIS Registry [15]) has resulted in much debate about the optimal management of these patients.

TIMI IIIB

The TIMI IIIB trial randomised patients to coronary angiography within 48 hours, followed by revascularisation if possible, or to a conservative approach [16]. Within six weeks, 64% of the latter group had undergone angiography. This significant crossover confounds interpretation of the results. There was a non-significant difference in death, MI or positive stress test within six weeks (16.2% vs 18.1% in the early invasive and conservative groups, respectively) ($p = 0.33$).

VANQWISH

The VANQWISH trial randomised 920 patients with NQMI to early invasive management or a conservative approach with medical therapy within 72 hours of the onset of symptoms [17]. The cross-over rate to angiography in the conservative group was 29% at 30 days. Only 44% of those randomised to early invasive management were revascularised, thus again rendering interpretation difficult. The incidence of death or non-fatal MI was higher in the invasive group at discharge, one month and one year. During follow-up, the overall mortality did not differ significantly between the conservative and invasive strategies (hazard ratio 0.72; 95% confidence intervals (CI) 0.51–1.01).

GUSTO IIb

Analysis of the GUSTO IIb trial results by Cho *et al* [18] showed that mortality at 30 days and one year was significantly lower among patients treated with an invasive strategy even after adjusting for baseline differences. However, a meta-analysis of randomised trials suggests no superiority of early invasive management [19].

FRISC II

More recently, the FRISC II study has reported the results of a comparison of an early interventional approach with a non-invasive approach in 2,457 patients with ACS following pretreatment with dalteparin [20]. Coronary angiography was performed in the invasive group in 96% of patients within seven days and revascularisation in 71% of them within 10 days. The composite end-point of death or MI at six months occurred in 9.4% of patients in the invasive group and in 12.1% of the non-invasive group (risk ratio 0.78; 95%CI 0.62–0.98; $p = 0.031$). There was a 50% reduction both in symptoms of angina and in readmission in the invasive group, with particular benefits of an invasive strategy in some groups (older patients, men, those with chest pain at rest, ST segment depression). The investigators concluded that an early invasive strategy lowers the risk of death and MI and provides better symptom relief in the subsequent six months in moderate or high risk patients with unstable coronary artery disease, particularly those with ECG changes or raised biochemical markers.

TACTICS-TIMI 18

The recently completed TACTICS-TIMI 18 study (presented at the scientific meeting of the American Heart Association, 2000) investigated an early invasive versus early conservative treatment approach in patients with UA. All received aspirin, heparin and tirofiban. There was a significant reduction in the primary end-point at six months (death, MI and rehospitalisation) for the invasively treated patients (15.9% vs 19.4%; $p = 0.025$). Further trials, including RITA-3, are underway to address this issue.

Other approaches

Intra-aortic balloon counterpulsation is a useful means of symptomatically and haemodynamically stabilising patients with refractory UA in order to optimise conditions for revascularisation, although there has never been a randomised trial. It should be noted that in a case series of patients referred to a tertiary care centre for 'refractory' UA, only 8.8% were considered to be truly refractory after their medical treatment was maximised [21].

There are currently rapid developments in percutaneous transluminal coronary angiography balloon and stent technology (eg coated stents) together with pharmacological approaches in patients with UA. At present, it seems prudent to advise an early optimal medical strategy with careful selection of high risk patients, including those with ongoing ischaemia, for angiography and potential revascularisation.

☐ CONCLUSIONS

The management of UA begins at the time of presentation with appropriate diagnosis and risk stratification. Predisposing causes should be sought and corrected. Anti-ischaemic, antithrombin and antiplatelet therapy should be commenced, and an aggressive approach with pharmacological therapies adopted without delay for those patients who fall into the high and medium risk groups, particularly with a view to follow-on angiography and revascularisation. Secondary prevention should be emphasised (eg lowering cholesterol) and modifying risk factors (smoking, hypertension, diabetes). Further developments in the understanding of UA, particularly regarding pharmacological therapies and intervention, will enable both the identification of the major factors in an individual patient (eg thrombosis or inflammation) and the optimal tailoring of therapy.

☐ TRIAL ACRONYMS

CAPTURE	c7E3 Fab AntiPlatelet Therapy in Unstable REfractory angina
ESSENCE	Efficacy and Safety of Subcutaneous Enoxaparin in Non-Q wave Coronary Events
FRAX.I.S	FRAXiparine in Ischaemic Syndrome

FRIC	FRagmin In unstable Coronary artery disease
FRISC	FRagmin and Fast Revascularisation during InStability in Coronary artery disease
FRISC II	FRagmin and Fast Revascularisation during InStability in Coronary artery disease II
GUSTO IIb	Global Use of Strategies To open Occluded coronary arteries IIb
GUSTO IV ACS	Global Use of Strategies To open Occluded coronary arteries IV Acute Coronary Syndromes
OASIS	Organisation to Assess Strategies for Ischaemic Syndromes
PARAGON A	Platelet IIb/IIIa Antagonist for the Reduction of Acute coronary syndrome events in a Global Organisation Network A
PRAIS-UK	Prospective Registry of Acute Ischaemic Syndromes in the UK
PRISM	Platelet Receptor inhibition in Ischaemic Syndrome Management
PRISM-PLUS	Platelet Receptor inhibition in Ischaemic Syndrome Management in Patients Limited by Unstable Signs and Symptoms
PURSUIT	Platelet glycoprotein IIb/IIIb in Unstable angina: Receptor Suppression Using Integrilin (eptifibatide) Therapy
RISC	Research Group on Instability in Coronary Artery Disease
RITA-3	Randomised Intervention Treatment of Angina
TACTICS-TIMI 18	Treat angina with Aggrastat (tirofiban) and determine Cost of Therapy with Invasive or Conservative Strategy – TIMI 18
TIMI IIA	Thrombolysis in Myocardial Infarction IIA
TIMI IIIB	Thrombolysis in Myocardial Infarction IIIB
VANQWISH	Veterans Affairs Non-Q-Wave Infarction Strategies in Hospital

REFERENCES

1   Collinson J, Flather MD, Fox KAA, Findlay I, *et al.* Clinical outcomes, risk stratification and practice patterns of unstable angina and myocardial infarction without ST elevation. Prospective Registry of Acute Ischaemic Syndromes in the UK (PRAIS-UK). *Eur Heart J* 2000; **21**: 1450–7.

2   Manoharan G, Maynard SJ, Adgey AAJ. The therapeutic use of glycoprotein IIb/IIIa inhibitors in acute coronary syndromes. *Exp Opin Invest Drugs* 1999; **8**: 555–66.

3   Vorchheimer D, Badimon JJ, Fuster V. Platelet glycoprotein IIb/IIIa receptor antagonists in cardiovascular disease. Review. *JAMA* 1999; **281**: 1407–14.

4   Braunwald E. Management of unstable angina based on considerations of aetiology. Review. *Heart* 1999; **82**(Suppl 1): 15–7.

5   Hyde TA, French JK, Wong CK, Straznicky IT, *et al.* Four-year survival of patients with acute coronary syndromes without ST-segment elevation and prognostic significance of 0.5-mm ST-segment depression. *Am J Cardiol* 1999; **84**: 379–85.

6   Maynard SJ, Scott GO, Riddell JW, Adgey AA. Management of acute coronary syndromes. Review. *Br Med J* 2000; **321**: 220–3.

7   Hamm CW, Goldmann BU, Heeschen C, Kreymann G, *et al.* Emergency room triage of patients with acute chest pain by means of rapid testing for cardiac troponin T or troponin I. *N Engl J Med* 1997; **337**: 1648–53.

8   Hillis GS, Zhao N, Taggart P, Dalsey WC, Mangione A. Utility of cardiac troponin I, creatine kinase-MB(mass), myosin light chain 1, and myoglobin in the early in-hospital triage of 'high risk' patients with chest pain. *Heart* 1999; **82**: 614–20.

9   Ohman EM, Armstrong PW, Christenson RH, Granger CB, *et al.* Cardiac troponin T levels for risk stratification in acute myocardial ischaemia. GUSTO-IIa investigators. *N Engl J Med* 1996; **335**: 1333–41.

10   Topol E. Patient stratification and its predictive value for cardiac events. Review. *Eur Heart J* 1998; **19**(Suppl K): K5–7.

11   Kaul S, Shah PK. Low molecular weight heparin in acute coronary syndrome: evidence for superior or equivalent efficacy compared with unfractionated heparin? Review. *J Am Coll Cardiol* 2000; **35**: 1699–712.

12   Gurfinkel EP, Manos EJ, Mejail RI, Cerda MA, *et al.* Low molecular weight heparin versus regular heparin or aspirin in the treatment of unstable angina and silent ischaemia. *J Am Coll Cardiol* 1995; **26**: 313–8.

13   Guidance on the use of glycoprotein IIb/IIIa inhibitors in the treatment of acute coronary syndromes. National Institute for Clinical Excellence 2000. www.nice.org.uk

14   Guidelines for the management of patients with acute coronary syndromes without persistent ECG ST segment elevation. British Cardiac Society Guidelines and Medical Practice Committee, and Royal College of Physicians Clinical Effectiveness and Evaluation Unit. *Heart* 2001; **85**: 133–42.

15   Yusuf S, Flather M, Pogue J, Hunt D, *et al.* Variations between countries in invasive cardiac procedures and outcomes in patients with suspected unstable angina or myocardial infarction without initial ST elevation. OASIS (Organisation to Assess Strategies for Ischaemic Syndromes) Registry. *Lancet* 1998; **352**: 507–14.

16   Effects of tissue plasminogen activator and a comparison of early invasive and conservative strategies in unstable angina and non-Q-wave myocardial infarction. Results of the TIMI IIIB Trial. Thrombolysis in Myocardial Ischaemia. *Circulation* 1994; **89**: 1545–56.

17   Boden WE, O'Rourke RA, Crawford MH, Blaustein AS, *et al.* Outcomes in patients with acute non-Q-wave myocardial infarction randomly assigned to an invasive as compared with a conservative management strategy. Veterans Affairs Non-Q-Wave Infarction Strategies in Hospital (VANQWISH) Trial Investigators. *N Engl J Med* 1998; **338**: 1785–92.

18   Cho L, Marso SP, Bhatt DL, Hsu C-H, Topol EJ. An early invasive strategy is associated with decreased mortality: GUSTO IIb trial. *Circulation* 1999; **100**: I-359.

19   Mehta S, Yusuf S, Hunt D, Natarajan M. Invasive versus conservative management of unstable angina and non-Q-wave infarction: a meta-analysis. *Circulation* 1999; **100**: I-755.

20   Invasive compared with non-invasive treatment in unstable coronary-artery disease: FRISC II prospective randomised multicentre study. FRagmin and Fast Revascularisation during InStability in Coronary artery disease investigators. *Lancet* 1999; **354**: 708–15.

21   Grambow DW, Topol EJ. Effect of maximal medical therapy on refractoriness of unstable angina pectoris. *Am J Cardiol* 1992; **70**: 577–81.

☐ SELF ASSESSMENT QUESTIONS

1   The following are responsible for platelet activation following plaque disruption:
    (a) Adenosine triphosphate
    (b) Thrombin
    (c) Collagen
    (d) Fibrinogen
    (e) Serotonin

2   The glycoprotein (GP) IIb/IIIa inhibitor receptor:
    (a) Undergoes structural change following activation, and promotes adherence of platelets to the endothelium
    (b) Is the most abundant receptor found on the platelet membrane surfaces (5,000–10,000/platelet)
    (c) Binds with the soluble ligands von Willebrand factor and fibrinogen
    (d) Belongs to a family of surface receptors called integrins
    (e) Following activation, promotes generation of platelet mass and consequently thrombus formation

3   During risk stratification for patients presenting with suspected unstable angina, the following are 'high risk' features for unstable angina:
(a) Chest pain at rest
(b) Age >70 years
(c) Female gender
(d) Acute persistent ST segment elevation
(e) Cardiac troponin (cTn) T or I-positive

4   When comparing low molecular weight heparins (LMWHs) with unfractionated heparin (UFH):
(a) LMWHs have a longer plasma half-life (8 hours) than UFH (1 hour)
(b) LMWHs have a superior bioavailability on subcutaneous administration than UFH (>90% vs 30%)
(c) LMWHs, but not UFH, exert their anticoagulant activity by activating antithrombin III
(d) LMWH is mostly composed of 'above critical length molecules' (>18 monosaccharide units >5.4 kDa), whereas less than half the UFH chains contain them
(e) LMWHs have lower rates of platelet activation, heparin-induced thrombocytopenia and osteoporosis than UFH

5   The recently published National Institute for Clinical Excellence guidelines on the management of acute coronary syndromes recommend:
(a) Use of intravenous (iv) GP IIb/IIIa receptor inhibitors in high risk patients with unstable angina or non-Q wave myocardial infarction (MI), in addition to aspirin and low (adjusted) dose UFH
(b) Use of GP IIb/IIIa receptor inhibitors in combination with thrombolytic therapy during acute ST segment elevation MI
(c) Use of LMWH in conjunction with GP IIb/IIIa receptor inhibitors
(d) Raised cTn should be used to identify those at high risk
(e) In patients undergoing acute or elective percutaneous coronary intervention, iv GP IIb/IIIa inhibitors should be used (consistent with current UK licensing)

ANSWERS

1a False	2a False	3a True	4a False	5a True
b True	b False	b True	b True	b False
c True	c True	c False	c False	c False
d False	d True	d False	d False	d True
e True	e True	e True	e True	e True

Psychological factors in cardiovascular disease

Andrew Steptoe

☐ INTRODUCTION

The notion that psychological factors contribute to the development of coronary heart disease (CHD) and other cardiovascular disorders has a long history. Many physicians can cite cases from their experience in which stress or other psychological factors have appeared to influence a patient's condition. Over recent years the evidence for connections of this kind has been put on a sounder footing, and there have been notable advances in the systematic investigation of psychological and social (or psychosocial) factors. This has resulted from improved methodology and an integration of knowledge from epidemiological, experimental laboratory and clinical investigations [1,2]. Conclusions about the role of psychosocial factors can therefore be drawn with increasing confidence. These data are now being applied to patient care in a limited fashion, although there is a need for broader dissemination leading to more effective research and practice. This chapter outlines some of the main developments in this field and the avenues of research that appear particularly relevant to clinical care.

☐ STAGES OF THE CARDIOVASCULAR DISEASE PROCESS

CHD is a progressive condition and psychosocial factors may be involved at a number of stages in the development of disease:

1   *Promotion of long-term aetiology.* Psychosocial factors may contribute to the risk of CHD through influences on the progression of atherosclerosis and the promotion of risk factors such as hypertension and abdominal obesity. In the search for factors influencing aetiology, emphasis has been placed on psychosocial adversities that are sustained for many years, such as chronic work stress and social isolation.

2   *Provocation of acute cardiac events.* Psychosocial factors are also implicated in triggering cardiac events in vulnerable individuals with CHD. The biological processes involved may be different from those operating in long-term aetiology; they may relate to the influence of acute emotions on the vascular and conduction phenomena underlying thrombus formation and rhythm disturbances.

3   *Influence on prognosis and quality of life.* It is now recognised that the impact of psychological factors does not cease when a person experiences an acute myocardial infarction (MI) or other serious event, but that emotional reactions to events are themselves significant, affecting long-term adjustment, quality of life and future prognosis.

☐ EPIDEMIOLOGICAL EVIDENCE

The newly developed field of behavioural or social epidemiology has been central in establishing the role of psychosocial factors in cardiovascular disease. Modern studies use all the panoply of analytic epidemiology to rule out the influence of other risk factors, including:

☐   large cohorts with hard disease end-points

☐   prospective designs

☐   standardised measurement, and

☐   multivariate statistics.

Acute stresses such as major life events are probably less important to disease aetiology than long-term psychosocial adversities. The latter may promote damaging lifestyles and sustained changes in neuroendocrine and autonomic nervous system activity over months or years that may in turn promote atherogenesis. The evidence for an aetiological role of psychosocial factors is strongest for experiences such as stressful work involving low job control, social isolation and lack of social support, and hostile personality profiles [3]. For example, data from the Whitehall II study of British civil servants [4] indicate that having a job over which an individual has little control increases the likelihood of future CHD by more than 50%, independently of standard risk factors. Associations between future disease and limited social networks, and with proneness to anger and hostility, have also been described. Figure 1 summarises data from a sample of 2,886 men and 5,007 women who completed a standard measure of depression and were tracked for up to 10 years [5]. After adjustment for poverty, smoking, hypertension, diabetes and body mass index, the risks for CHD were elevated in depressed respondents.

These psychosocial variables appear to be risk factors in the same way as blood pressure or cholesterol levels: the higher the level, the greater the risk. However, it is also true that many patients may have high risk profiles without succumbing to CHD, and vice versa, just as with physical risk factors.

☐ UNDERLYING MECHANISMS

Epidemiological observations have been coupled with investigations of mechanisms through which associations are mediated. One possibility is that habitual behaviours are responsible. People who are socially isolated or who are depressive or hostile in their dispositions may be at greater risk because of lifestyle factors such as smoking,

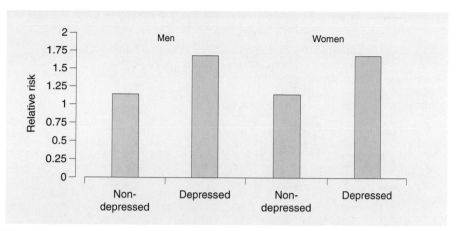

Fig. 1 Relative risk of coronary heart disease over 10 years in men and women who were depressed compared with those who were not depressed at baseline. Risk is adjusted for poverty, smoking, hypertension, diabetes and body mass index (data from [5]).

physical inactivity and dietary preferences. However, many studies have shown that associations between psychosocial factors and cardiac risk persist even after lifestyle has been taken into account, indicating that other pathways are also involved. There is new evidence that psychosocial factors may have more direct influences on vascular processes relevant to atherogenesis [6]. Psychological factors can stimulate disturbances of vascular endothelial function, eliciting increased production of inflammatory cytokines and activation of platelets, together with alterations in lipid metabolism and impairment of the parasympathetic control of cardiac function.

These discoveries have come from animal studies and experimental work with healthy groups and clinical populations. An example is a recent study of the influence of acute stress on vascular endothelial function indexed with flow mediated dilatation [7]. Healthy volunteers were stressed with a short simulated public speech task and endothelial function was assessed over the next four hours. The results summarised in Fig. 2 show that the speech induced the expected increase in the stress hormone cortisol. In addition, flow mediated vascular dilatation was impaired up to 90 minutes after the speech, returning to reference values only several hours later. This pattern of results is important in showing that a relatively mild emotional stimulus can induce sustained changes in the vascular endothelium that could presage an increased risk of vascular damage. If this pattern were repeated or sustained over years in adult life, it can be envisaged that enduring changes in risk might emerge.

☐ ACUTE CARDIAC EVENTS

Studies of the influence of psychological factors on the provocation of acute cardiac events have blossomed with the application of cardiac imaging techniques [1]. Assessments with angiography or radionuclide techniques can be carried out in alert

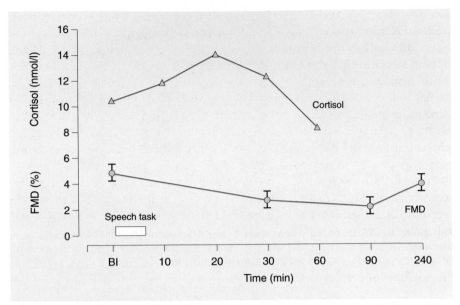

Fig. 2 Mean changes in vascular endothelial function as assessed with salivary cortisol (▲) and flow-mediated dilatation (FMD) (●) in response to a three-minute speech task. The speech task induced increases in the stress hormone cortisol and reductions in FMD after 30 min and 90 min (data derived from [7]) (Bl = baseline).

patients, allowing responses to emotional stimuli to be monitored. A number of studies have found that a proportion of individuals with coronary artery disease show signs of acute ischaemia in response to stressful tasks, including:

- ☐ ventricular wall motion abnormalities

- ☐ coronary artery spasm

- ☐ myocardial perfusion deficits, and

- ☐ QT dispersion.

Interestingly, these responses are seldom accompanied by angina-like chest pain, and they occur at a lower double-product threshold (calculated by multiplying blood pressure by heart rate) than with exercise-induced ischaemia. Psychological stress-induced responses are reversible and are particularly prominent when patients are confronted by social, conversational stressors rather than with abstract problem-solving tasks. They may be related to heightened sympathetic nervous system activity, or to momentary changes in coronary artery vascular tone.

Relevance of psychologically induced acute cardiac events

The question arises whether these responses are of academic interest only, or whether they are relevant to the vulnerability of cardiac patients to ischaemia in their ordinary lives. Although comparatively few studies have been carried out, it appears that patients who manifest stress-induced ischaemia during clinical investigations are also likely to experience episodes of ischaemia (ST segment depression) during Holter monitoring. In addition, measurements of mood and social activity during Holter monitoring have led to the identification of associations between episodes of 'silent' ischaemia and emotional distress during everyday life. Small-scale follow-up studies indicate that patients who show mental stress-induced ischaemia during standardised testing may be at higher risk for disease progression and future cardiac events. For example, Krantz and co-workers [8] found that 45 (57%) of 79 patients with coronary artery disease showed stress-induced myocardial dysfunction during echocardiography or radionuclide ventriculography. Over a 3½-year period, 20 (44%) of the stress-positive group suffered cardiac death, MI or revascularisation, compared with eight (23%) of the stress-negative group ($p = 0.05$). It is possible therefore that these laboratory studies identify patients who are particularly vulnerable to cardiac dysfunction in the presence of emotional upset.

Prognosis following acute events

Levels of psychological distress are high in the period immediately following hospitalisation for acute MI or unstable angina but tend to diminish as people come to terms with their condition. However, it is unwise to consider emotional upset merely to be a transient phenomenon with no lasting effects because some patients experience enduring increases in anxiety and depression. There is also considerable evidence that depressive symptoms in the days following acute cardiac events are indicative of poor prognosis and diminished survival [9]. For example, in one study [10] a standard depression questionnaire (the Beck Depression Inventory) was administered to 896 patients who survived acute MI at least until discharge from hospital. Over the following 12 months, 7% of men with elevated depression scores died of cardiac-related causes, compared with 2.4% of non-depressed men (women: 8.3% vs 2.7%). The odds of not surviving were more than three times higher in the depressed group, after adjusting for age, smoking, disease severity and cardiac function. Patients who were socially isolated seemed to be particularly at risk.

The mechanisms underlying these effects have not yet been established, although it is thought that psychological distress may influence autonomic pathways that stimulate cardiac arrhythmia. Intervention studies are currently underway which will help to establish the optimal management of emotional distress in cardiac patients. The largest of these is probably the ENhancing Recovery In Coronary Heart Disease (ENRICHD) trial [11], a randomised study comparing psychosocial intervention with standard medical care in 3,000 survivors of acute MI who were either depressed or had low social support.

□ WHY ARE PSYCHOSOCIAL FACTORS NOT RECOGNISED CLINICALLY?

If the evidence for a relationship between psychosocial factors and CHD is so compelling, why are these influences not recognised clinically to a greater extent? One obvious possibility is that disturbances of emotional and social function are not noticed because clinicians are not looking for them – after all, medicine is full of instances in which factors are ignored because the physician is concentrating on a different area of investigation and enquiry. A number of other factors may also be important:

☐ Psychosocial factors are risks rather than inevitable causes. They are associated with heart disease in general but may vary widely in importance. One patient may have a severe psychosocial risk profile with no signs of cardiovascular disease, while another may have severe disease with no psychosocial risk.

☐ Some psychosocial factors may be difficult to identify during clinical interviews. Patients often put on a positive face during consultations and not admit to isolation or depression without specific enquiries.

☐ There is a tendency to search for psychosocial explanations only when patients do not have other clear risk factors such as hypertension, diabetes or smoking.

Many clinicians work from implicit models in which biological and psychosocial influences are thought of as alternatives, not cofactors. However, the evidence is that psychosocial adversity clusters with other risk factors. Problems such as low control at work, hostility and social isolation are more common in people of lower socio-economic status in whom smoking, insulin resistance and other factors are also clustered [2]. The better recognised biological risk factors may disguise the role of psychosocial factors. At the same time, there is a need for brief validated measures to be more readily available to clinicians, so that psychosocial factors can be better assessed.

☐ CONCLUSIONS

The study of psychosocial factors involves the integration of evidence from epidemiological, laboratory and animal studies. Psychological factors can contribute both to the development of CHD and to prognosis in patients with established disease. The evidence is strongest for the impact of work stress, social isolation, anger, hostility and depressive symptoms. The biological mechanisms underlying these effects are beginning to be understood, and may involve the promotion of vascular inflammatory processes, alterations in autonomic regulation and the promotion of the metabolic syndrome. Psychological factors are poorly recognised in clinical practice partly because of the lack of widely available simple measures. Monitoring the psychological aftermath of acute cardiac events is particularly important since it can have an impact on survival and quality of life.

REFERENCES

1   Rozanski A, Blumenthal JA, Kaplan J. Impact of psychological factors on the pathogenesis of cardiovascular disease and implications for therapy. Review. *Circulation* 1999; **99**: 2192–217.

2   Stansfeld S, Marmot MG (eds). *Stress and heart disease.* London: *British Medical Journal* Books (in press).

3   Hemingway H, Marmot M. Evidence based cardiology: psychosocial factors in the aetiology and prognosis of coronary heart disease. Systematic review of prospective cohort studies. Review. *Br Med J* 1999; **318**: 1460–7.

4   Bosma H, Marmot MG, Hemingway H, Nicholson AC, *et al.* Low job control and risk of coronary heart disease in Whitehall II (prospective cohort) study. *Br Med J* 1997; **314**: 558–65.

5   Ferketich AK, Schwartzbaum JA, Frid DJ, Moeschberger ML. Depression as an antecedent to heart disease among women and men in the NHANES I study. National Health and Nutrition Examination Survey. *Arch Intern Med* 2000; **160**: 1261–8.

6   Steptoe A, Marmot M. The role of psychobiological pathways in socio-economic inequalities in cardiovascular disease risk. *Euro Heart J* (in press).

7   Ghiadoni L, Donald A, Cropley M, Mullen MJ, *et al.* Mental stress induces transient endothelial dysfunction in humans. *Circulation* 2000; **102**: 2473–8.

8   Krantz DS, Santiago HT, Kop WJ, Bairey Merz CN, *et al.* Prognostic value of mental stress testing in coronary artery disease. *Am J Cardiol* 1999; **84**: 1292–7.

9   Musselman DL, Evans DL, Nemeroff CB. The relationship of depression to cardiovascular disease: epidemiology, biology, and treatment. *Arch Gen Psychiatry* 1998; **55**: 580–92.

10 Frasure-Smith N, Lésperance F, Juneau M, Talajic M, Bourassa MG. Gender, depression, and one-year prognosis after myocardial infarction. *Psychosom Med* 1999; **61**: 23–37.

11 Enhancing recovery in coronary heart disease patients (ENRICHD): study design and methods. The ENRICHD investigators. *Am Heart J* 2000; **139**: 1–9.

Gastroenterology

Advances in inflammatory bowel disease

Jonathan Rhodes

☐ ADVANCES IN UNDERSTANDING OF PATHOGENESIS

Interaction between genetic and environmental factors

An individual whose identical twin has Crohn's disease has approximately one chance in two of developing Crohn's disease, whereas someone with an identical twin with ulcerative colitis has about one chance in 10 of developing that disease [1]. This implies that environmental and genetic factors are approximately equally important in the pathogenesis of Crohn's disease, while environmental factors are substantially more important for ulcerative colitis. The first Crohn's disease associated gene, *Nod2*, has recently been described. It encodes a protein that is involved in the macrophage response to bacterial lipopolysaccharide and it is abnormal in about 29% of Crohn's disease patients [2]. The environmental factors have been frustratingly elusive with the single exception of smoking. Genetic studies in affected sibling pairs suggest that probably one or more genes simultaneously confer an increased risk for both forms of inflammatory bowel disease (IBD) [3]. In mixed disease families, in which some individuals have ulcerative colitis and others have Crohn's disease, smoking seems a strong determinant of phenotype, with smokers more likely to get Crohn's disease and non-smokers more likely to develop ulcerative colitis.

It is clear that other environmental factors remain to be determined, particularly in view of the marked increase in incidence of Crohn's disease over the past 50 years. Nevertheless, a model can now be accepted in which genetic and environmental factors interact to yield a spectrum of phenotypes which range from typical Crohn's disease to typical ulcerative colitis. The important practical conclusion from this model is that it is inappropriate always to attempt to make a dogmatic distinction between the two forms of IBD. Up to 30% of cases of colitis may be difficult to categorise and are better labelled as 'indeterminate colitis', explaining to the patient that there is a spectrum of disease – rather than risk the inevitable confusion and mistrust when the diagnosis is changed (usually from ulcerative colitis to Crohn's disease when a granuloma is found) after many years of what is then presumed to have been inappropriate management.

The impact of smoking on phenotype has important practical implications. Cessation of smoking in a patient with Crohn's disease is likely to reduce the relapse rate by about 40% (Fig. 1) [4]. This is probably at least as great an improvement as can be gained by immunosuppressive therapy, and certainly better than the rather modest (ca 6%) reduction in relapse rate for Crohn's disease

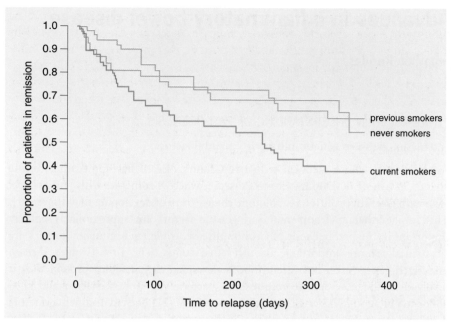

Fig. 1 Relapse rates, expressed as the proportion of Crohn's disease patients remaining in remission over time, illustrating the deleterious effects of smoking (from [4], with permission).

demonstrated for maintenance 5-aminosalicylate preparations [5]. Moreover, smoking is associated with a higher risk for perforating Crohn's disease, with abscess and fistula development.

Anti-*Saccharomyces cerevesiae* antibody in Crohn's disease, oligomannan, phagocyte dysfunction and granuloma formation

Crohn's disease is typified histologically by the presence of granulomas which are found in about 50% of cases. A granuloma is a coalescence of macrophages which occurs when macrophages either phagocytose an indigestible particle or microbe or when the macrophages themselves are dysfunctional. It is interesting that two conditions, chronic granulomatous disease and glycogen storage disease type 1b, in which well-defined congenital abnormalities in phagocytic cell function are associated with changes in the intestine, closely mimic Crohn's disease. Chronic granulomatous disease, which is most commonly X-linked, has been characterised at the molecular level and shown to be a mutation in a cytochrome gene. As a result of the mutation, the phagocytic cells cannot mount an adequate respiratory burst and are unable to generate the hypochlorite needed to kill phagocytosed bacteria. The IBD in these disorders has been shown to improve, not with immuno-suppression but by stimulation of phagocyte function with granulocyte colony-stimulating factor, an approach also reported to be successful in pilot studies in Crohn's disease [6].

Between half and two-thirds of patients with Crohn's disease have circulating antibodies (ASCA) against baker's yeast, *Saccharomyces cerevisiae*. This was initially thought to indicate a form of food allergy, but it was subsequently shown that the epitope for the antibody is mannose-α1,3 mannose, present in the oligomannan of the yeast cell wall [7]. This structure is known also to be present in the cell wall of bacteria such as mycobacteria. Intriguingly, oligomannan was already known to inhibit phagocytic function *in vitro* by blocking myeloperoxidase, thus mimicking closely the defect found in chronic granulomatous disease. It therefore seems highly plausible that shedding of cell wall oligomannan by intramucosal bacteria can lead to a local defect in phagocytic cell function within the intestinal mucosa, and that this in turn leads to the typical Crohn's phenotype with granuloma, abscess and fistula formation [8].

Adherent and invasive *Escherichia coli* in Crohn's disease

Escherichia coli were isolated from the ileal biopsies of patients with Crohn's disease by a French group [9]. Despite lacking conventional markers of pathogenicity, these *E. coli* are capable of adhering to and invading cultured epithelial cell lines (Fig. 2). It is not yet known whether they are able to express the mannose-α1,3 mannose ASCA epitope, nor is there any direct evidence that these bacteria are intramucosal or intra-epithelial in Crohn's disease tissue. If they are intra-epithelial, therapy should logically be targeted towards the use of antibiotics which achieve good penetration into cells. It is therefore interesting that good preliminary, but as yet uncontrolled, results are being reported for the treatment of Crohn's disease with clarithromycin (Fig. 3) [10], an antibiotic which achieves particularly good tissue penetration.

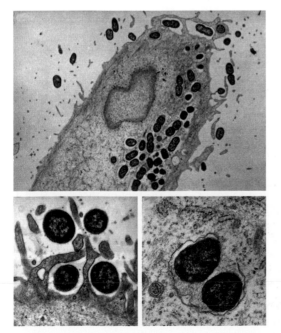

Fig. 2 Mucosa-associated *Escherichia coli* obtained from Crohn's disease tissue, demonstrating their ability to invade intestinal cells (from [9], with permission).

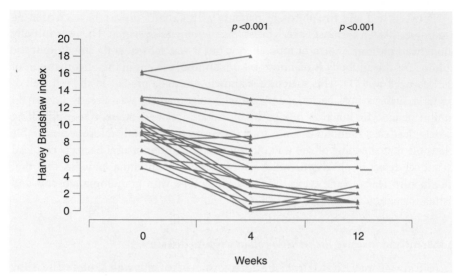

Fig. 3 Efficacy of oral clarithromycin in active Crohn's disease. A score of 5 or above on the Harvey Bradshaw index indicates active disease (from [10], with permission).

The role of non-pathogenic bacteria in IBD is further supported by the genetically engineered models of IBD, all of which have so far proved dependent on the presence of non-pathogenic bacteria for the development of intestinal inflammation.

□ ADVANCES IN TREATMENT: CROHN'S DISEASE

Cytokines, T helper 1 and T helper 2 responses and response to cytokine-targeted therapy

It has been known for many years that circulating autoantibodies tend to be more commonly associated with ulcerative colitis than with Crohn's disease. The most specific of these is the perinuclear antineutrophil cytoplasmic antibody (pANCA), present in about three-quarters of patients with ulcerative colitis. The epitope of this antibody has not been clearly resolved, but seems to be a nuclear protein that becomes perinuclear on fixation of neutrophils [11]. It is distinct from the anti-myeloperoxidase form of pANCA associated with vasculitis. Antibodies against goblet cells, other epithelial antigens such as tropomyosin, red cell membranes and other epitopes are also found in ulcerative colitis. The assumption therefore is that ulcerative colitis is mediated mainly by the humoral immune system, suggesting a T helper (Th) 2 dominated inflammatory response. The tissue cytokine profile is in keeping with this (Fig. 4).

Anti-tumour necrosis factor α antibody therapy

In Crohn's disease there is a predominantly cellular response, indicating a Th1-dominated response, with tumour necrosis factor (TNF) α as a central

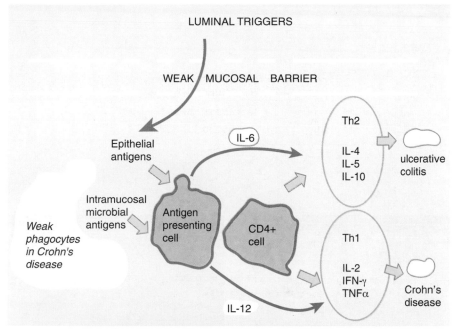

Fig. 4 The differences in cytokine profile between Crohn's disease (T helper (Th) 1 predominant inflammatory process) and ulcerative colitis (Th2 predominant process). Crohn's disease is thus seen as predominantly cell-mediated inflammation with tumour necrosis factor (TNF) α as a dominant cytokine and ulcerative colitis as predominantly humoral (IFN = interferon; IL = interleukin).

cytokine. Proof of concept of this hypothesis has been demonstrated by the dramatically effective therapeutic response to infusion of humanised monoclonal antibodies to TNFα [12].

The effect of anti-TNFα antibody therapy in Crohn's disease is remarkable on at least two counts:

1   It has been shown endoscopically to heal Crohn's disease ulcers (Fig. 5), a property shared by azathioprine and by enteral feeding but not by corticosteroids.

2   Its effect is much longer lasting than would be assumed from the half-life of the antibody. It has been suggested that this may be the result of stimulation of apoptosis via the mitochondrial pathway in a subset of T lymphocytes that express transmembrane (uncleaved) TNFα.

The dose response to anti-TNFα antibody is bell-shaped, with 5 mg/kg consistently more effective than 10 mg/kg [13] (of importance to budget holders since a single infusion at 5 mg/kg in the average adult costs nearly £2,000).

Repeated therapy has also been shown to be effective for short-term maintenance [14], but it has yet to be shown whether the dose or duration of therapy can be reduced by the addition of some other form of conventional immunosuppression such as azathioprine or, as in rheumatological patients, methotrexate. The antibody

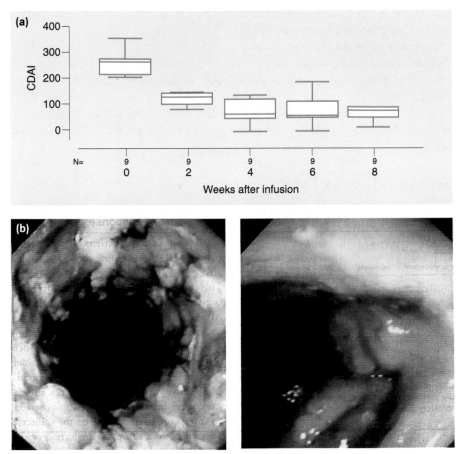

Fig. 5 (a) The beneficial effects of a single intravenous infusion of anti-tumour necrosis factor (TNF) α antibody (infliximab) on active Crohn's disease showing **(b)** healing of colonic ulcers (from [12], with permission).

has already been used in over 100,000 patients (including those with rheumatoid arthritis). Its safety profile seems remarkably good:

☐ Serious allergic reactions are uncommon (the first antibody to be licensed is a chimeric antibody with approximately one-third mouse immunoglobulin).

☐ Earlier fears about a possible increased risk for lymphoma have not so far been substantiated.

TNFα antibody therapy with infliximab (Remicade®) has also been shown to heal fistulas [15], albeit only temporarily as the fistulas open again after stopping therapy.

The main indication for anti-TNFα therapy in the UK is severe disease unresponsive to conventional therapy. A summary of the properties of anti-TNFα therapy is listed in Table 1. Guidelines are in the process of being drawn up by the National Institute for Clinical Excellence.

It should be noted that the abilities to heal ulcers, close fistulas, and work as effective maintenance therapy are not shared by corticosteroids. An increasingly widely held opinion is that corticosteroids often cause more harm than good in Crohn's disease [16], and it can be argued that in no other condition are high-dose corticosteroids prescribed in the knowledge that they will provide only short-term (eg 3 months) symptomatic benefit with no effect on the long-term course of the disease.

Table 1 Summary of the properties of anti-tumour necrosis factor α antibody treatment in Crohn's disease.

* ≤81% response
* ≤50% remission
* Plateau dose response
* Effect of single dose lasts ≥8 weeks (half-life 2 weeks)
* No clear difference in response at different sites
* Repeated courses maintain remission
* Fistula closure in ca two-thirds of patients for ca 3 months
* Good safety profile

Remaining questions:
* Cost
* Advantage over azathioprine/6-mercaptopurine

Dietary therapy and the particle hypothesis

The classical trial by O'Morain *et al* showed that enteral feeding with an amino acid-based feed is as effective as high-dose steroids at inducing remission in Crohn's disease [17]. Subsequent studies have shown that the feeding regimen also allows healing of ileal ulceration. although the mechanism remains unclear. The rising incidence of Crohn's disease in the 20th century has led to speculation that intolerance to a food additive might be the explanation. Some intriguing work has recently come from a group in London who have shown that titanium dioxide (TiO_2), an insoluble pigment used in the food industry as a whitener (E171), forms particles of a size (nanoparticles) which act as haptens. *In vitro* studies have shown that TiO_2 particles enhance by approximately one hundred-fold the response of lymphocytes to bacterial lipopolysaccharide (Fig. 6) [18]. A small preliminary controlled trial has shown remarkable results in Crohn's disease patients as a consequence of avoidance of TiO_2.

Summary of therapeutic options in Crohn's disease

All patients with Crohn's disease should be strongly encouraged to avoid smoking. The range of therapeutic options for patients with Crohn's disease is gradually

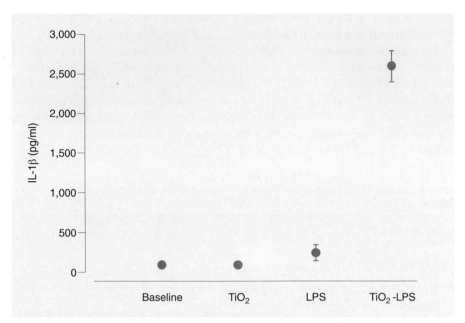

Fig. 6 The effect of titanium dioxide (TiO$_2$) particles on the stimulation of lymphocytes by bacterial lipopolysaccharide (LPS). TiO$_2$, which is insoluble, is commonly used in the food industry as a whitener (E171) (IL = interleukin) (from [18], with permission).

increasing (Table 2). No longer is there a simple choice between corticosteroids and surgery, and corticosteroids can increasingly be avoided. Different options will suit different patients:

☐ Surgery will be a good option in a patient with limited stricturing disease who has not had previous surgery, but it is a less satisfactory option in a patient with extensive disease or previous surgery.

☐ Antibiotics are increasingly used as first-line therapy, even though the evidence base is not yet strong.

☐ Azathioprine seems effective in its own right and not just as a steroid-sparing agent.

Table 2 Treatment options in Crohn's disease: the steadily increasing list.

- Corticosteroids
- Azathioprine
- Antibiotics
- Diet
- Surgery
- Anti-tumour necrosis factor α antibodies
- 5-aminosalicylates

☐   TNFα antibody therapy is dramatically effective – but dramatically expensive and generally reserved at present for patients with severe persistent disease.

☐   5-aminosalicylates are of doubtful therapeutic efficacy in Crohn's disease, but they seem to reduce the cancer risk [19] and probably should be prescribed on that account at least.

☐ ADVANCES IN TREATMENT: ULCERATIVE COLITIS

Cyclosporin therapy for severe ulcerative colitis

Approximately 20% of patients with ulcerative colitis eventually need colectomy. In a severe acute attack (defined by systemic parameters such as fever >37.5°C, tachycardia >100 beats/min and serum albumin <35 g/dl), about one in three fail to respond to intravenous corticosteroids and have in the past always needed colectomy. A small, but highly influential, trial showed that the colectomy rate may be reduced by the addition of cyclosporin therapy [20]. Subsequent studies have shown that some of these patients still need colectomy because of active disease within the next six months [21] so that the colectomy rate is probably reduced by about one-third overall. Most clinicians now start azathioprine shortly after the cyclosporin in the hope of reducing the risk of later relapse.

There remains some controversy about the use of cyclosporin. Deaths have been reported due to pneumocystis infection, while some degree of nephrotoxicity, paraesthesiae or tremor affects about 20% of patients so treated. It has been argued that the mortality related to cyclosporin therapy (probably ca 2%) may be greater than that associated with severe colitis (generally reported as <1% from large centres). This has been enough to dissuade this author so far from using cyclosporin for severe colitis. Further trials are in progress to look at lower dose cyclosporin and cyclosporin monotherapy (without corticosteroids) in the hope that these approaches may be safer.

Azathioprine and prediction of serious side effects

Corticosteroids have been shown to be of no benefit as maintenance therapy in either Crohn's disease or ulcerative colitis. Azathioprine is increasingly used for maintenance therapy in both conditions, and it is clear that it has more than just a steroid-sparing effect. Careful audit of IBD patients treated with azathioprine has shown no obvious increase in risk of malignant disease. However, azathioprine is well established as a risk factor for lymphoma in transplant recipients and it seems unlikely that it will prove completely free from risk in IBD in the very long term.

There has recently been a much greater awareness of the importance of genetic polymorphisms in determining the rate of metabolism of azathioprine. The enzyme thiopurine S-methyltransferase is particularly critical. About 3% of the population are homozygous for mutations in the gene for this enzyme and these individuals are extremely sensitive to azathioprine-induced bone marrow toxicity [22]. The enzyme can now be readily assayed and it is likely that most units will move quite rapidly towards routine assay. In the absence of the assay, treatment should always be initiated at a low dose (50 mg/day for an adult) and full blood count checked after one week before increasing the dose. It should also be noted that allopurinol therapy greatly reduces the rate at which the drug is cleared and can result in dangerous toxicity.

☐ INFLAMMATORY BOWEL DISEASE AND COLON CANCER

It has long been known that there is an increased risk of colon cancer in colitis, but many questions remain unanswered – some of which are beginning to be resolved.

Is there an increased risk of colon cancer in Crohn's disease?

All the recent evidence suggests that the risk of colon cancer in Crohn's disease is similar to that in ulcerative colitis. Cancers tend to occur at sites of inflammation, the risk is greater for patients with colonic Crohn's disease than in those with isolated ileal disease, and the age of onset (as in colitis-associated cancer) is young (median age ca 45 years). There also seems to be a similar association with dysplasia.

What is the mechanism for cancer development?

The molecular biology of colitis-associated cancer has been shown to be different from that of sporadic colon cancer. There are p53 changes relatively early in the course of the colitis-dysplasia-cancer sequence, whereas *ras* mutations occur relatively late (Fig. 7) [23]. Given the importance of intact p53 in facilitating apoptosis, it seems likely that failure of apoptosis is particularly important in colitis-associated cancer. This is also borne out by the marked frequency of major chromosomal abnormalities in colon epithelial cells in the colitic colon [24], and also by the observation that dysplastic changes seen low in crypts are not associated with increased cancer risk whereas dysplastic changes affecting the surface mucosa are highly predictive.

Similar glycosylation changes occur in colon epithelial glycoconjugates in both IBD and colon cancer. Our group has speculated that the increased expression of exposed galactose on the luminal aspect of colon epithelial cells allows interaction with intraluminal lectins of dietary or microbial origin, which in turn increases proliferation and hence cancer risk [25].

Can anything be done to reduce the risk?

There is now evidence from three independent studies that regular maintenance therapy with 5-aminosalicylates (mesalazine) reduces the risk for cancer substantially, probably by about 75% [19]. This is in accord with data from Copenhagen demonstrating no increased risk of colon cancer within their IBD population when mesalazine therapy was used widely over a long period. The

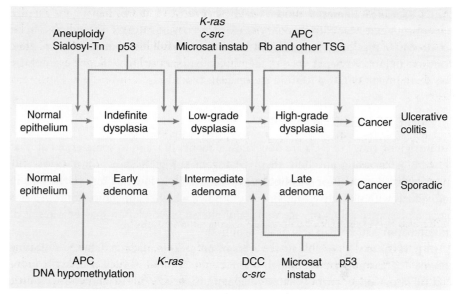

Fig. 7 Comparison between the molecular biology of colitis-associated cancer, in which p53 changes occur relatively early and APC changes late, and sporadic colon cancer (APC = adenomatous polyposis coli; DCC = deleted in colon cancer; Microsat instab = microsatellite instability; Rb = retinoblastoma gene; Tn = a blood group; TSG = tumour suppressor gene) (from [23], with permission).

mechanism for this effect is not known, but seems quite likely to be via inhibition of inducible cyclo-oxygenase (COX2), which is known to have inhibitory effects on colon cancer development that are mediated by enhanced apoptosis and inhibition of angiogenesis.

Is surveillance worthwhile?

It remains highly controversial whether surveillance is worth doing. Studies have suggested that only about 50% of cancers occurring in a colitic population are picked up on regular colonoscopic surveillance – at considerable cost. Conversely, I would argue that the potential benefit per patient is so great that surveillance remains justified so long as there continues to be an increased risk in the colitic population. It is increasingly considered that screening the normal risk, healthy population is worthwhile to prevent sporadic cancers. It is easy to calculate that prevention of all deaths from sporadic colorectal cancer (which is responsible for about 3% of all deaths at an average age of about 65, thus shortening life in an affected individual by an average of approximately 10 years) would prolong life for the average screened individual by only 3% of 10 years (ie 4 months). Occult blood screening, which reduces mortality by 15–33%, would therefore prolong life by only 4–6 weeks in the average screened individual. In patients with extensive colitis, the lifetime risk of dying of colorectal cancer is about 20% at an average age of 50. If all deaths from colitis-associated colorectal cancer could be prevented, the benefit to the average patient with extensive colitis would therefore be 20% of 25 years (ie 5 years). This is so substantial that it seems imperative to continue surveillance but, at the same time, continue to look for better ways of identifying patients at high risk, for example by the development of faecal tests for cancer gene mutations.

□ WHERE DO WE GO FROM HERE?

An intriguing range of facts are now known about IBD, and to some extent all that remains is to work out how these fit together. Fig. 8 shows one, necessarily oversimplified, model for this (including the strikingly low risk for appendicitis in individuals with ulcerative colitis). It is unknown whether appendicectomy protects against ulcerative colitis or vice versa, and altered glycosylation may be a result of inflammation rather than genetically acquired.

A guess as to the possible future areas of progress is made in Table 3, indicating the major areas of current research interest, not all of which will necessarily prove fruitful in the longer term. Whatever happens, there is good reason to be optimistic about the chances of major advances in the understanding and treatment of IBD within the next 5–10 years.

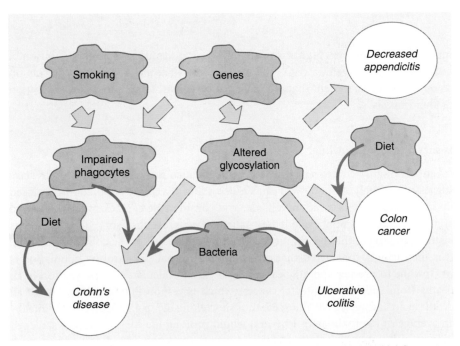

Fig. 8 A possible model linking the genetic and environmental factors associated with inflammatory bowel disease. There is evidence in the literature that smoking impairs phagocytic cell function and that ulcerative colitis is uncommonly associated with a history of appendicectomy (from [8], with permission).

Table 3 Possible areas of progress in inflammatory bowel disease.

Direction	Objective of research	Estimate of time to achieve (years)
Genetics	Identification of susceptibility genes	present–10
Microbiology	Characterisation of mucosa-associated flora	2–4
Therapy	Cytokine inhibitors	present–5
	Antibiotics with high tissue penetration	present–5
	Particle-free diet	??2–4
	Colony stimulating factors	??2–4
	Probiotics and prebiotics	?2–10
	Neuropeptide inhibitors	??5–10
	Reduced use of steroids in Crohn's disease	**now**

REFERENCES

1 Tysk C, Lindberg E, Jarnerot G, Floderus-Myrhed B. Ulcerative colitis and Crohn's disease in an unselected population of monozygotic and dizygotic twins. A study of heritability and the influence of smoking. *Gut* 1988; 29: 990–6.

2 Hugot JP, Chamaillard M, Zouali H, Lesage S, et al. Association of NOD2 leucine-rich repeat variants with susceptibility to Crohn's disease. *Nature* 2001; 411: 599–603.

3 Satsangi J, Parkes M, Louis E, Hashimoto L, et al. Two stage genome-wide search in inflammatory bowel disease provides evidence for susceptibility loci on chromosomes 3, 7 and 12. *Nat Genet* 1996; 14: 199–202.

4 Timmer A, Sutherland LR, Martin F. Oral contraceptive use and smoking are risk factors for relapse in Crohn's disease. The Canadian Mesalamine for Remission of Crohn's Disease Study Group. *Gastroenterology* 1998; 114: 1143–50.

5 Camma C, Giunta M, Rosselli M, Cottone M. Mesalamine in the maintenance treatment of Crohn's disease: a meta-analysis adjusted for confounding variables. *Gastroenterology* 1997; 113: 1465–73.

6 Vaughan D, Drumm B. Treatment of fistulas with granulocyte colony-stimulating factor in a patient with Crohn's disease. *N Engl J Med* 1999; 340: 239–40.

7 Young M, Davies MJ, Bailey D, Gradwell MJ, et al. Characterization of oligosaccharides from an antigenic mannan of *Saccharomyces cerevisiae*. *Glycoconj J* 1998; 15: 815–22.

8 Rhodes JM. Lectins, colitis and colon cancer. Review. *J R Coll Physicians Lond* 2000; 34: 191–6.

9 Boudeau J, Glasser AL, Masseret E, Joly B, Darfeuille-Michaud A. Invasive ability of an *Escherichia coli* strain isolated from the ileal mucosa of a patient with Crohn's disease. *Infect Immun* 1999; 67: 4499–509.

10 Leiper K, Morris AI, Rhodes JM. Open label trial of oral clarithromycin in active Crohn's disease. *Aliment Pharmacol Ther* 2000; 14: 801–6.

11 Eggena M, Cohavy O, Parseghian MH, Hamkalo BA, et al. Identification of histone H1 as a cognate antigen of the ulcerative colitis-associated marker antibody pANCA. *J Autoimmun* 2000; 14: 83–97.

12 van Dullemen HM, van Deventer SJ, Hommes DW, Bijl HA, et al. Treatment of Crohn's disease with anti-tumor necrosis factor chimeric monoclonal antibody (cA2). *Gastroenterology* 1995; 109: 129–35.

13 Targan SR, Hanauer SB, van Deventer SJ, Mayer L, et al. A short-term study of chimeric monoclonal antibody cA2 to tumor necrosis factor alpha for Crohn's disease. Crohn's Disease cA2 Study Group. *N Engl J Med* 1997; 337: 1029–35.

14   Rutgeerts P, D'Haens G, Targan S, Vasiliauskas E, *et al.* Efficacy and safety of retreatment with anti-tumor necrosis factor antibody (infliximab) to maintain remission in Crohn's disease. *Gastroenterology* 1999; 117: 761–9.

15   Present DH, Rutgeerts P, Targan S, Hanauer SB, *et al.* Infliximab for the treatment of fistulas in patients with Crohn's disease. *N Engl J Med* 1999; 340: 1398–405.

16   Present DH. How to do without steroids in inflammatory bowel disease. *Inflamm Bowel Dis* 2000; 6: 48–57.

17   O'Morain C, Segal AW, Levi AJ. Elemental diet as primary treatment of acute Crohn's disease: a controlled trial. *Br Med J* 1984; 288: 1859–62.

18   Powell JJ, Harvey RS, Ashwood P, Wolstencroft R, *et al.* Immune potentiation of ultrafine dietary particles in normal subjects and patients with inflammatory bowel disease. *J Autoimmun* 2000; 14: 99–105.

19   Eaden J, Abrams K, Ekbom A, Jackson E, Mayberry J. Colorectal cancer prevention in ulcerative colitis: a case-control study. *Aliment Pharmacol Ther* 2000; 14: 145–53.

20   Lichtiger S, Present DN, Kornbluth A, Gelernt I, *et al.* Cyclosporine in severe ulcerative colitis refractory to steroid therapy. *N Engl J Med* 1994; 330: 1841–5.

21   Hyde GM, Thillainayagam AV, Jewell DP. Intravenous cyclosporin as rescue therapy in severe ulcerative colitis: time for a reappraisal? *Eur J Gastroenterol Hepatol* 1998; 10: 411–3.

22   Colombel JF, Ferrari N, Debuysere H, Marteau P, *et al.* Genotypic analysis of thiopurine S-methyltransferase in patients with Crohn's disease and severe myelosuppression during azathioprine therapy. *Gastroenterology* 2000; 118: 1025–30.

23   Itzkowitz SH. Inflammatory bowel disease and cancer. Review. *Gastroenterol Clin North Am* 1997; 26: 129–39.

24   Rabinovitch PS, Dziadon S, Brentnall TA, Emond MJ, *et al.* Pancolonic chromosomal instability precedes dysplasia and cancer in ulcerative colitis. *Cancer Res* 1999; 59: 5148–53.

25   Rhodes JM. Unifying hypothesis for inflammatory bowel disease and related colon cancer: sticking the pieces together with sugar. Review. *Lancet* 1996; 347: 40–4.

☐ SELF ASSESSMENT QUESTIONS

1   In the pathogenesis of inflammatory bowel disease (IBD):
   (a) Smoking is associated with an increased risk for Crohn's disease
   (b) Genetic factors have a stronger influence on the risk for Crohn's disease than for ulcerative colitis
   (c) Most patients with ulcerative colitis have antibodies against baker's yeast (*Saccharomyces cerevesiae*)
   (d) Pathogenic *Escherichia coli* can commonly be isolated from mucosal biopsies in Crohn's disease
   (e) Genetic defects in phagocyte function can be associated with intestinal disease which mimics Crohn's disease

2   With regard to immunomodulatory therapy:
   (a) Anti-tumour necrosis factor (TNF) α antibody therapy has been shown to reduce the colectomy rate in ulcerative colitis
   (b) The effect of a single infusion of anti-TNFα antibody therapy is limited by the half-life of the antibody
   (c) Corticosteroids have no effect on the long-term course of Crohn's disease

(d) Allopurinol may dangerously enhance the effect of concomitant azathioprine therapy

(e) Cyclosporin therapy in patients with severe ulcerative colitis reduces the colectomy rate by about one-third within six months of the attack

3   Mucosal ulcers associated with Crohn's disease have been shown to heal with the following treatments:
   (a) Corticosteroids
   (b) Enteral feeding
   (c) Azathioprine
   (d) Anti-TNFα antibody
   (e) Cyclosporin

4   With regard to the risk of IBD-associated cancer:
   (a) The risk of colon cancer in a patient with colonic Crohn's disease is similarly increased to that in a patient with a similar extent of ulcerative colitis
   (b) A similar dysplasia-cancer sequence occurs in both ulcerative colitis and Crohn's disease
   (c) Surveillance is likely to prolong life more per individual than screening for colon cancer in normal risk individuals
   (d) Mutations in p53 are a common early event
   (e) Regular mesalazine treatment may lower the risk of cancer by over 70%

5   The following interventions are likely to cause a substantial reduction in the relapse rate when initiated in patients with Crohn's disease in remission:
   (a) Corticosteroids
   (b) Smoking cessation
   (c) Mesalazine
   (d) Cyclosporin
   (e) Azathioprine

ANSWERS

1a True	2a False	3a False	4a True	5a False
b True	b False	b True	b True	b True
c False	c True	c True	c True	c False
d False	d True	d True	d True	d False
e True	e True	e False	e True	e True

Portal hypertension

Andrew Burroughs and Paolo Montalto

☐ INTRODUCTION

Portal hypertension is the most important clinical consequence of liver cirrhosis. It is the cause of major complications in cirrhotic patients, particularly haemorrhage from gastro-oesophageal varices or portal hypertensive gastropathy and the development of ascites with renal failure, both of which are leading causes of death in cirrhotic patients.

Haemodynamic factors

Portal pressure (P) is determined by the magnitude of flow (Q) and the resistance to this flow (R). (Ohm's law: $P = Q \times R$.) Resistance is expressed by Poiseuille's formula as $R = 8nL/\pi r^4$ (n = blood viscosity; L = length of the system; r = vessel radius). Since n and L are constant values, resistance changes in proportion to the fourth power of the radius. Thus, even very small changes in vessel size produce large changes in pressure.

Mechanical and structural changes, consequences of the development of fibrosis, are the basis of this phenomenon. Currently, fibrosis cannot be reversed, but there is increasing evidence of a 'reversible' intrahepatic tissue component responsible for portal hypertension. Several classes of vasodilators administered in the portal vein of cirrhotic rats have decreased portal pressure and favourably influenced microvascular exchange and function [1]. Hepatic stellate cells may constitute a key element in this context. Other contractile cell types likely to be involved include activated portal myofibroblasts and activated smooth muscle cells in the proximity of arterial structures.

The rationale for drug therapy is to act on these haemodynamic factors. Drugs could act by:

☐ reducing the portal collateral blood flow (eg by splanchnic vasoconstriction)

☐ decreasing the vascular resistance of the intrahepatic and portal circulation (eg by vasodilatation)

☐ a combination of the two.

Natural history of varices and causes of bleeding

When cirrhosis is diagnosed, varices are present in about 60% of decompensated and 30% of compensated patients [2]. The threshold portal pressure gradient or its equivalent hepatic venous pressure gradient (HVPG) for the development of varices is 10–12 mmHg, but not every patient above this limit has oesophageal varices. The incidence of development of new oesophageal varices is estimated at about 8% per year, but 70% of patients are still free of varices after six years [3]. Less data are available on the rate of enlargement of oesophageal varices. Pagliaro *et al* [3] reported that after six years 4% of 225 patients without varices and 25% of 118 patients with small varices developed large varices. Discrepancies in the literature may be caused by different definitions of 'large' varices. Sustained abstinence from alcohol may result in decreasing size or even disappearance of varices in alcoholic liver disease, with improvement in survival rate [4].

The mortality for an acute episode of variceal haemorrhage is 5–50%, depending on the severity of liver disease. Death is mainly due to the high rate of failure to control bleeding during the first days after the initial episode [2]. Most deaths occur within 7–10 days of bleeding, so prompt and effective treatment for the control of acute variceal bleeding and prevention of early rebleeding is essential. Since the risk of rebleeding after an acute episode is about 70%, all patients need to have therapy to prevent this. Prevention of the development of varices is an important issue, currently being assessed in clinical trials.

At present, prevention of first bleeding is the best therapeutic option. All cirrhotics need to be screened for the presence of varices and assessed for prophylactic treatment. An upper endoscopy is recommended every two years in cirrhotic patients without varices, and annually in patients with small varices or non-abstinent alcoholics.

The risk factors for the first episode of variceal bleeding in cirrhotics are:

☐ severity of liver dysfunction

☐ large size of varices

☐ presence of endoscopic red colour signs (North Italian Endoscopic Club (NIEC) index) [5].

However, only one-third of patients with variceal bleeding have these risk factors. Efforts have been made to improve the efficiency of the NIEC index, and there is a need to define new predictive factors that could be combined in this index to improve its validity. Two recent issues have added to the current knowledge:

1   Haemodynamic evaluation of portal pressure and the risk of bleeding.

2   Bacterial infections in the pathogenesis of variceal bleeding.

Haemodynamic factors and variceal bleeding

Although no bleeding occurs if HVPG falls below 12 mmHg, the degree of HVPG elevation is not so well correlated with bleeding [6]. Moreover, the level of variceal pressure (at the site of bleeding) has been shown to be a major predictive factor for variceal haemorrhage [7].

Echo-Doppler techniques allow non-invasive and repeated measurements of various relevant parameters (eg portal blood velocity, portal blood volume). The problem is that these measures have significant intra- and interobserver error unless extensive training is carried out.

Bacterial infections and variceal bleeding

Goulis *et al* [8] postulated that bacterial infections in patients with liver cirrhosis may be the critical factor that triggers bleeding through the release of endotoxins. Bacterial infections occur commonly in variceal bleeding (35–66% of patients) [9] and are an independent prognostic factor for early rebleeding within five days of admission for variceal bleeding [10,11]. Our group has recently demonstrated that bacterial infections impair coagulation [12] by a heparin effect [13]. The hypothesis that antibiotic treatment in combination with oral non-selective beta-blockers may prevent variceal bleeding requires formal testing.

☐ TREATMENT OF ACUTE VARICEAL BLEEDING

The data from randomised trials of treatment for acute variceal bleeding show significant heterogeneity, mainly due to the failure to achieve consensus in definitions despite an international collaborative effort [14].

General measures

Patients with acute gastrointestinal bleeding must be strictly monitored for cardiovascular and respiratory function. Circulating volume must be restored as soon as possible via a central venous line. When resuscitation is adequate, the patient should undergo diagnostic endoscopy.

The goals of therapy are to:

☐   stop bleeding as soon as possible

☐   prevent early rebleeding

☐   prevent and treat complications

☐   prevent deterioration of liver function.

A recent meta-analysis [15] demonstrated that antibiotic prophylaxis significantly increased both the mean survival rate and the mean percentage of patients free of infection. All cirrhotics with upper gastrointestinal bleeding should receive prophylactic antibiotics whether or not sepsis is suspected. The optimal regimen has yet to be decided, but oral or intravenous quinolones have been used. All new studies on acute variceal bleeding will need to include data on therapeutic use of antibiotics and diagnosis of infection.

Somatostatin, octreotide and analogues

Somatostatin, a 14 amino acid peptide, has been used in the pharmacological treatment of variceal bleeding because of its ability to reduce splanchnic blood flow,

HVPG and azygous blood flow in cirrhotic patients. The haemodynamic effects may be mediated by the inhibition by somatostatin of the release of vasodilatory peptides such as glucagon, vasoactive intestinal polypeptide and substance P. Bolus injection of somatostatin (standard dose 250 µg) appears to have a greater haemodynamic effect than continuous infusion.

Octreotide, a synthetic analogue of somatostatin, shares four amino acids with the native compound which are responsible for its biological activity. The longer half-life is achieved by the addition of a phenylalanine residue at the N-terminal end and the elongation of the C-terminal end with threonine. The recommended dose is 25–50 µg/h continuous infusion.

A recent meta-analysis [16] (820 patients) found that somatostatin and octreotide did not improve survival or reduce the number of blood transfusions in patients with active bleeding from oesophageal varices. Fewer units were transfused in the patients on active drug, but the difference between experimental and control therapy was only 1.2 units of blood products saved per patient. There were no significant differences in the use of balloon tamponade or in the number of patients failing initial haemostasis or rebleeding. It was calculated that the therapeutic effect corresponded to one unit of blood saved per patient – a small effect, so treatment with these drugs in acute bleeding oesophageal varices is of doubtful value.

Vasopressin

Vasopressin has been in use for over 30 years. At pharmacological doses, it induces smooth muscle contraction, particularly in splanchnic arterioles, which reduces total portal blood flow. Four randomised placebo-controlled trials of vasopressin [17] (157 patients) showed a clear trend in favour of vasopressin, but the result was not significant and there was no difference in mortality.

In addition to doubts regarding efficacy, vasopressin causes systemic vasoconstriction, leading to serious side effects such as severe abdominal colic, cardiac arrhythmia, myocardial ischaemia and cerebrovascular episodes, and the drug has to be stopped in up to 25% of cases. Concomitant nitroglycerin has been used to minimise the systemic side effects.

Terlipressin

Terlipressin (triglycyl lysine vasopressin), a synthetic analogue of vasopressin, is converted *in vivo* into vasopressin by enzymatic cleavage of the triglycyl residues. This prolongs its biological half-life and makes continuous intravenous infusion unnecessary. The standard dose is 2 mg every four hours for the initial 24 hours, followed by 1 mg every four hours for the next 24 hours.

The clinical efficacy of terlipressin has been evaluated in four placebo-controlled trials [17] (225 patients), in one of which terlipressin was given while the patient was transferred to hospital. There was a statistically significant reduction in failure to control bleeding compared with placebo. More importantly, terlipressin significantly reduced mortality – the only vasoconstrictor to do so. There are some caveats. The sample sizes were small in the first three studies, and in the early administration trial the three doses of 2 mg, at 0, 4 and 8 hours, did not reduce the transfusion rate at 12 hours. The reduction in mortality in Child-Pugh grade C patients may therefore not be causally related to control of bleeding and needs to be reproduced in other studies. Whether terlipressin may be acting via other mechanisms (eg maintenance of renal perfusion) needs to be assessed.

Comparison of vasopressin and terlipressin

Vasopressin and terlipressin were compared in five unblinded studies [17]. Failure to control bleeding was less frequent with terlipressin, but the difference was not statistically significant, there was no difference in mortality in the two arms and there was a significantly lower complication rate with terlipressin even when nitroglycerin was given with vasopressin.

Currently, terlipressin is one of the first-choice agents for the treatment of acute variceal bleeding. Comparative studies of terlipressin against other drugs in combination with endoscopic interventions (see below) need to be done in the future.

Emergency sclerotherapy

In the best study exhibiting the benefit of emergency sclerotherapy [18] the procedure not only stopped bleeding in active bleeders but also caused less early rebleeding than sham endoscopy. A recent evaluation [17] of 33 randomised clinical trials (RCTs) found that sclerotherapy with concomitant drugs was more effective than drugs alone, although there was no difference in mortality. Sclerotherapy was significantly better than drugs alone in preventing failure to control bleeding and death with no significant difference in complications, and sclerotherapy plus drugs (including a recent study of vapreotide [19]) was more effective than sclerotherapy alone, but with no difference in mortality.

There was no difference in efficacy in studies comparing sclerotherapy with variceal ligation. New studies are needed to evaluate the role of the drugs adjunctive to sclerotherapy. If such a regimen is significantly effective, mortality should be reduced compared to sclerotherapy alone; this has not been shown to date.

Gastric variceal bleeding

The optimal treatment of gastric varices is not known. Limited information is available on vasoactive drugs, and balloon tamponade has been used with little success. Standard sclerosants are associated with unacceptable rebleeding, particularly from necrotic ulcerations. Alternative sclerosants have been evaluated. The tissue glue isobutyl-2-cyanoacrylate (bucrylate), mixed with lipiodol to delay premature hardening, has been efficacious in non-randomised studies. Alternatively, thrombin could be considered.

Uncontrolled variceal bleeding

One of the biggest problems with uncontrolled variceal bleeding is the lack of an accepted definition. The diminishing efficacy of repeated sclerotherapy is well established, with bleeding control achieved cumulatively in 70% and 85% of cases after the first and second session, respectively, with little benefit from subsequent injections [20]. We recommend using the definition of continued bleeding as bleeding which does not stop despite two sessions of therapeutic endoscopy within a five-day period of the index bleed. Patients who continue to bleed despite a correctly positioned Sengstaken tube can also be considered to have uncontrolled variceal bleeding.

No randomised studies have evaluated different salvage therapies in uncontrolled variceal bleeding. The advent of transjugular intrahepatic portosystemic shunt (TIPS) offers a valuable option in patients who have uncontrolled oesophageal or gastric variceal bleeding [21]. This is the best option for patients with poor liver function, particularly those awaiting liver transplantation.

☐ RECOMMENDED GUIDELINES IN ACUTE VARICEAL BLEEDING

The only treatment that does not require sophisticated equipment or the skill of a specialist and is immediately available is vasoactive drug therapy. Pharmacological treatment should be started as soon as variceal bleeding is suspected, even before endoscopic confirmation of diagnosis. It can be administered while the patient is transferred to hospital. Drug therapy can no longer be considered only a 'stop gap' therapy until definitive endoscopic therapy is performed, but appears to have its own therapeutic benefit.

Terlipressin should be first-choice treatment because it reduces mortality. Somatostatin and octreotide can also be considered first-line agents, but the evidence for these is far less. Endoscopic sclerotherapy or ligation should be used at diagnostic endoscopy.

☐ PREVENTION OF RECURRENT VARICEAL BLEEDING

Patients surviving the first episode of variceal bleeding are at very high risk of recurrent bleeding ($\geq$70%) and death (30–50%). The general consensus is that all patients who have previously bled from varices should have secondary therapy to prevent further variceal bleeding [17].

Beta-blockers

Meta-analysis of 12 trials (769 patients) [17] showed that beta-blockers significantly decreased the risk of rebleeding, and survival was significantly improved. Five patients and 14 patients need to be treated to prevent one rebleeding episode and one death, respectively.

The use of recently proposed haemodynamic targets to identify patients who are non-responders to drug therapy [22] could be a useful tool in the planning of treatment for secondary prevention of variceal bleeding. These patients could be offered alternative therapy such as variceal ligation or combination drug therapies if target pressure reductions are not achieved. This strategy has not been tested in a randomised study.

Beta-blockers in association with oral nitrates have been shown to induce a greater drop in portal pressure than beta-blockers alone. Other drugs that may work in combination with beta-blockers include molsidomine (a nitric oxide (NO) donor), serotonin antagonists and spironolactone. None has as yet been evaluated in an RCT.

Sclerotherapy versus beta-blockers

In 11 trials (971 patients) comparing sclerotherapy and beta-blockers for the prevention of recurrent bleeding [17] there was a striking heterogeneity in the evaluation of rebleeding, with no significant difference between the two treatment modalities. More patients on sclerotherapy survived, but the result was not statistically significant. The number of patients free of adverse events was higher in the drug group. These results demonstrate that beta-blockers are a first-choice treatment for prevention of rebleeding, provided that there are no contraindications.

Twelve trials of sclerotherapy and beta-blockers versus sclerotherapy alone (853 patients) [17] showed statistically significantly less rebleeding in the combined treatment arm – although there was significant heterogeneity both in the direction and size of effect – and fewer deaths.

Sclerotherapy versus banding

Variceal banding ligation was developed with the aim of providing an endoscopic therapy at least as effective as sclerotherapy but with fewer complications – the most common with sclerotherapy being oesophageal strictures and bleeding from treatment-induced ulcers.

Meta-analysis [17] of 18 studies (1,509 patients) comparing sclerotherapy and variceal ligation for secondary prevention found that rebleeding was significantly less common with variceal ligation, without significant heterogeneity. Variceal ligation was associated with lower mortality, but the difference was not statistically significant. Complications were less common in patients treated with variceal ligation in all but one of the studies. Overall, meta-analysis showed a statistically significant difference in favour of variceal ligation. There was no difference between the endoscopic modalities in the number of patients with varices obliterated, while recurrence was statistically significantly more frequent in patients treated with variceal ligation. However, rebleeding after initial eradication seems unusual, especially if patients have regular endoscopic follow-up and recurrent varices are re-obliterated. Variceal recurrence after sclerotherapy eradication may be predicted by endoscopic ultrasound detection of extensive peri-oesophageal collateral veins and large perforating veins of the oesophagus.

Transjugular intrahepatic portosystemic shunt versus endoscopic therapies

Analysis of 11 trials (811 patients) [23] showed that variceal bleeding was significantly more frequent in the patients receiving endoscopic treatment (47%) than TIPS (19%), but there was no difference in mortality. Post-treatment encephalopathy was less frequent after endoscopic treatment (19% vs 34%). Since TIPS has the same results as surgical shunting it cannot be recommended as the first-choice treatment for secondary prevention; it should be reserved for patients in whom secondary prevention treatment fails.

Surgical shunts

An increasing indication for a surgical shunt is in patients who have had TIPS without major encephalopathy but have had recurrent symptomatic TIPS stenosis. Ongoing trials are comparing TIPS to distal splenorenal shunts.

☐ PREVENTION OF FIRST UPPER GASTROINTESTINAL BLEEDING

Use of non-selective beta-blockers is the current, but not universal, therapeutic approach to prevent the first upper gastrointestinal bleeding in cirrhotic patients. Data from RCTs are nearly all based on patients with large varices. New therapeutic regimens of combination drug therapy and endoscopic banding ligation have recently been evaluated.

Beta-blockers

The optimal prophylactic regimen should be easy to administer, have relatively few side effects and be reasonably effective. These criteria are potentially best fulfilled by drug therapy which also protects against bleeding from portal hypertensive gastropathy [24]. Non-selective beta-blockers (propranolol, nadolol) are first-line therapy. They decrease splanchnic blood flow by reduction of cardiac output and reflex splanchnic arterial constriction. They also have a direct effect on porto-collateral resistance, decreasing azygous and gastro-oesophageal collateral blood flow, although wide individual variation in the reduction of portal pressure is achieved.

Nine prophylactic trials used beta-receptor blockade (propranolol 7, nadolol 2) in cirrhotic patients (996) with large varices [17]. The bleeding risk reduction with beta-blockers was statistically significant [17]. On average, 11 patients need to be treated to prevent one bleeding episode. There was no heterogeneity in the evaluation of mortality which was non-statistically significantly reduced with beta-blockers.

Beta-blockers have been shown to be effective independent of cause and severity of cirrhosis, presence of ascites and variceal size in an analysis of individual patient data from four of the above trials [25]. Current recommendations are that patients with large varices who have not bled should be offered prophylactic beta-blocker therapy. Bleeding may occur after stopping beta-blocker therapy, suggesting that therapy should be maintained lifelong.

There are insufficient data to make recommendations for patients with small varices but, since deteriorating liver function increases the risk of small varices bleeding, a reasonable therapeutic strategy is to treat all patients with a degree of liver dysfunction independent of the size of the varices [3].

Contraindications to beta-blocker therapy

As many as 25% of patients may have contraindications or intolerance to beta-blockers. Relative contraindications to their use are:

☐   severe and moderate heart failure

☐   severe obstructive lung disease

☐   peripheral vascular disease.

Side effects are experienced by 3–27% of patients, half of whom require withdrawal of therapy. Care should be taken in diabetic patients with severe hypoglycaemic problems.

Hepatic venous pressure gradient

About one-third of patients do not exhibit any decrease in HVPG on beta-blockers, but possibly fewer among those who have never bled. Optimal protection from the risk of bleeding is reported when the HVPG is decreased below 12 mmHg or at least by 20% from baseline [22]. HVPG is the best predictor of efficacy of prophylaxis of variceal bleeding, although this monitoring technique is not feasible when considering universal use of beta-blockade for all or most patients with varices. Empirical titration of propranolol dose (as in the original trials) is still current practice in many centres (ie administering as much as the patient can tolerate).

Combination with nitrates

Nitrates given alone in elderly patients have been associated with higher mortality than propranolol alone [26] and a recent trial has shown no difference versus placebo. The combination of isosorbide-5-mononitrate (ISMN) and beta-blocker (nadolol) was more effective in reducing bleeding, with only a small increase of side effects. The long-term results after a seven-year follow-up from this study [27] found cumulative bleeding risks of 29% and 12% in the nadolol and combination therapy groups, respectively. Addition of ISMN did not increase the incidence of liver failure, ascites or renal insufficiency. Five patients requested discontinuation because of side effects.

Combination with endoscopic sclerotherapy

The addition of endoscopic sclerotherapy was recently shown not to increase the effectiveness of beta-blockers in primary prophylaxis, and reinforced its possible harmful effect in patients with varices which have never bled.

Beta-blockers versus variceal ligation

Meta-analysis of four randomised trials [17] (290 patients) comparing endoscopic band ligation of high-risk oesophageal varices with beta-blockers (propranolol) showed a significant reduction in bleeding in the variceal ligation groups, but this was a small effect and mortality was unchanged. The theoretical advantages of variceal ligation over beta-blockers are the following:

☐   there are no contraindications except for the endoscopic procedure

☐   compliance is better (provided that the patient attends for endoscopic sessions)

☐   the therapy is effective in all patients (provided that varices are eradicated).

However, a widespread programme of prophylactic ligation would be costly and require repeated endoscopies to treat and monitor reappearance of varices.

This consideration, added to the conflicting results of the randomised trials and the small number of patients and events, does not warrant any change in the current practice of propranolol as the treatment of first choice for the primary prevention of variceal bleeding.

☐ RECOMMENDED GUIDELINES IN PRIMARY PROPHYLAXIS

Data from prophylactic trials indicate that screening for varices in cirrhotics should be part of routine clinical practice. In this author's opinion, all patients with varices should be offered prophylactic treatment to prevent first variceal bleeding. The current treatment of choice is non-selective beta-blockers.

Variceal ligation might be a reasonable alternative in patients with contra-indications to beta-blockers and those who cannot tolerate, or have no haemodynamic response to, drug therapy. However, this needs to be shown in controlled trials.

Banding is unlikely to become a routine prophylactic treatment as it is much more expensive and less applicable than beta-blockers and will not prevent gastric mucosal bleeding.

In the future there is a need to improve current medical therapy and to validate easily measured surrogate markers of portal pressure response.

☐ DRUGS NOT EVALUATED IN RANDOMISED THERAPEUTIC STUDIES

Endothelin receptor antagonists

Recent evidence indicates that stellate cells, resident perisinusoidal mesenchymal cells with an microanatomical position in the sinusoids analogous to vasoregulatory pericytes, may regulate sinusoidal blood flow. This is most evident in the context of liver injury when these cells transform into myofibroblasts (activated stellate cells). The role in normal liver is less defined. Endothelins (ET) and NO play important roles in modulating this cell contractility, and their interplay is a determinant factor of local sinusoidal blood flow, especially in injured liver [28].

ET levels are increased in injury, and activated stellate cells have the ability to respond to ET. Their exposure to ET-1 results in dramatic cellular spreading, proliferation and the acquisition of myofibroblast-like appearance typical of the activated phenotype. Induction of smooth muscle alpha-actin, a marker of activation, is prominent and dose-dependent after exposure to ETs. Enhanced stellate cell contractility in the setting of liver injury may lead to perisinusoidal constriction and increased intrahepatic resistance. Administration of a mixed ET_A/ET_B receptor antagonist (bosentan) in high concentration to isolated perfused cirrhotic livers reduced portal pressure by 15–20% [29]. ET receptor antagonists are currently undergoing phase I clinical trials, opening new perspectives for the treatment of portal hypertension.

Nitric oxide

NO exerts its vasodilator action locally and balances the effects of humoral and local vasoconstrictors such as ET. Vascular beds with defective NO synthesis demonstrate an abnormally increased vascular resistance. A recent experimental study in rats demonstrated a deficit in NO production in the cirrhotic liver associated with impairment in the intrahepatic vasodilatory response to an endothelial agonist such as acetylcholine [30]. Elevation of hepatic NO is another approach that holds promise as a way to reduce activated stellate cell contractility. Orally administered nitrates may serve this purpose but have so far been shown to be beneficial only in combination with beta-blockers.

Angiotensin-converting enzyme inhibitors and angiotensin II-receptor antagonists

The haemodynamic effects of angiotensin-converting enzyme (ACE) inhibitors and angiotensin II-receptor antagonists are controversial in patients with cirrhosis [31,32]. Acute administration of captopril induced a significant decrease in arterial pressure but no change in portal pressure, adversely affecting renal function. In contrast, infusion of the ACE inhibitor enalapril significantly decreased the HVPG.

Angiotensin II is considered a potential mediator of intrahepatic portal hypertension because its plasma level is elevated in cirrhosis and its administration induces a rise in portal pressure. Mechanisms that contribute to this effect are:

☐ enhancement of the adrenergic vasoconstrictor influence on the portal systems

☐ direct contractile influence on stellate cells (which serve as regulators of the sinusoidal blood flow)

☐ sodium and fluid retention induced by stimulation of aldosterone secretion.

Losartan

The effect of losartan (an angiotensin II-receptor antagonist) on portal pressure in patients with cirrhosis was evaluated in a prospective study [32]. The initial study group of 30 patients (24 alcoholics) with severe portal hypertension (HVPG >20 mmHg) was later augmented by 15 patients (13 alcoholics) with moderate portal hypertension (HVPG 12–20 mmHg). Untreated patients with either severe (15 patients) or moderate (10) portal hypertension were used as controls. Losartan induced a significant decrease of HVPG in all patients with severe and moderate portal hypertension, with no non- responders. One patient treated with losartan had a short symptomatic reaction after the first dose which did not recur despite continued treatment.

Irbesartan

Similar results were described in abstract for irbesartan, another angiotensin II-receptor antagonist [33]. There was a fall in HVPG in all 11 patients and no change in renal function when assessed at two months. One patient discontinued the treatment for symptomatic arterial hypotension.

Before considering the use of losartan or irbesartan in therapeutic trials, confirmatory randomised, double-blind haemodynamic studies are needed in patients with non-alcoholic cirrhosis (in whom spontaneous improvement of portal pressure is not expected) and also studies investigating the mechanism of losartan-induced portal pressure reduction [34]. The long-term effect on renal function also needs to be evaluated.

Alpha-adrenoceptor antagonists

Prazosin

Prazosin, an alpha-1-adrenergic blocker, is another vasodilator that reduces portal pressure in patients with cirrhosis and may have synergism with propranolol. Prazosin enhances peripheral vasodilatation, increasing plasma renin activity and favouring sodium and water retention [35]. In an RCT comparing propranolol plus prazosin with propranolol plus ISMN, the former combination caused a greater reduction in HVPG than propranolol plus ISMN, but there were more side effects in that group (46% vs 25%). These side effects may preclude its use.

Carvedilol

Carvedilol, a novel vasodilating non-selective beta-blocker, is a weak alpha-1-adrenoceptor antagonist and exhibits some calcium channel antagonism [36]. Carvedilol has been shown in three non-randomised studies in patients with cirrhosis to decrease HVPG to more than 20% of the baseline value before therapy and to less than 12 mmHg in over 50% of patients [36]. However, it has a greater arterial hypotensive effect than propranolol in patients with cirrhosis (without compromising hepatic blood flow or renal function) so patient intolerance may be frequent. It is a good candidate drug as a portal hypotensive agent.

Clonidine

Clonidine, a central alpha-2-adrenoceptor agonist, may also act directly on arterial tone in cirrhotic patients. It induces a sustained decrease in sympathetic nervous activity and portal pressure without adverse effects on hepatic blood flow and liver function. Short- and long-term administration did not modify renal haemodynamics or induce natriuretic responses in patients with ascites. Side effects were common, with significant hypotension precluding routine clinical use.

Diuretics

Anti-aldosterone drugs

Most patients with portal hypertension have an expanded plasma volume associated with peripheral vasodilatation. The use of anti-aldosterone drugs aims at decreasing portal pressure through a decrease in blood volume. Loop diuretics cause acute depletion of plasma volume, with a reduction of the porto-hepatic gradient, promptly followed by an increase in sodium retention. Chronic administration of spironolactone in patients with cirrhosis without ascites leads to a significant reduction in the HPVG and variceal pressure [37], both as a single agent and in combination with propranolol in non-responders to beta-blockers. Anti-aldosterone agents, already widely used in cirrhotic patients for the treatment of ascites, could be useful adjunctive therapy in the treatment of portal hypertension.

5-Hydroxytryptamine receptor antagonists

A serotonin mechanism has been reported to contribute to the hyperdynamic circulation of portal hypertension. Serotonin antagonists also decrease portal pressure in experimental animal models and in portal hypertensive patients. However, these agents are not available for clinical use.

□ CONCLUSIONS

Future trials can be significantly improved if the standardised definitions of critical end-points (eg bleeding or rebleeding episodes, treatment failure, etc) agreed in recent consensus conferences [14] are applied. This will aid both the reduction of the heterogeneity in RCTs of drugs and other treatment modalities in portal hypertension and the clarification of the best and widely accepted treatment options. New drugs should be evaluated within this framework.

REFERENCES

1 Marteau P, Ballet F, Chazouilleres O, Chretien Y, et al. Effect of vasodilators on hepatic microcirculation in cirrhosis: a study in the isolated perfused rat liver. Hepatology 1989; 9: 820–3.
2 D'Amico G, Pagliaro L, Bosch J. The treatment of portal hypertension: a meta-analytic review. Hepatology 1995; 22: 332–54.
3 Pagliaro L, D'Amico G, Pasta L, Politi F, et al. Portal hypertension in cirrhosis: natural history. In: Bosch J, Groszmann R (eds). Portal hypertension. Pathophysiology and treatment. Cambridge, MA: Blackwell Scientific, 1994: 72–92.
4 Vorobioff J, Groszmann RJ, Picabea E, Gamen M, et al. Prognostic value of hepatic venous pressure gradient measurements in alcoholic cirrhosis: a 10-year prospective study. Gastroenterology 1996; 111: 701–9.

5   Prediction of the first variceal haemorrhage in patients with cirrhosis of the liver and esophageal varices. A prospective multicenter study. The North Italian Endoscopic Club for the Study and Treatment of Esophageal Varices. *N Engl J Med* 1988; 319: 983–9.

6   Armonis A, Patch D, Burroughs A. Hepatic venous pressure measurement: an old test as a new prognostic marker in cirrhosis? Review. *Hepatology* 1997; 25: 245–8.

7   Nevens F, Bustami R, Scheys I, Lesaffre E, Fevery J. Variceal pressure is a factor predicting the risk of a first variceal bleeding: a prospective cohort study in cirrhotic patients. *Hepatology* 1998; 27: 15–19.

8   Goulis J, Patch D, Burroughs AK. Bacterial infection in the pathogenesis of variceal bleeding. *Lancet* 1999; 353: 139–42.

9   Bleichner G, Boulanger R, Squara P, Sollet JP, Parent A. Frequency of infections in cirrhotic patients presenting with acute gastrointestinal haemorrhage. *Br J Surg* 1986; 73: 724–6.

10 Goulis J, Armonis A, Patch D, Sabin C, *et al.* Bacterial infection is independently associated with failure to control bleeding in cirrhotic patients with gastrointestinal haemorrhage. *Hepatology* 1998; 27: 1207–12.

11 Bernard B, Cadranel JF, Valla D, Escolano S, *et al.* Prognostic significance of bacterial infection in bleeding cirrhotic patients: a prospective study. *Gastroenterology* 1995; 108: 1828–34.

12 Papatheodoridis GV, Patch D, Webster GJ, Brooker J, *et al.* Infection and hemostasis in decompensated cirrhosis: a prospective study using thromboelastography. *Hepatology* 1999; 29: 1085–90.

13 Montalto P, Vlachogiannakos J, Pastacaldi S, Cox D, *et al.* Bacterial infection in cirrhosis impairs coagulation by a heparin like effect. *J Hepatol* 2000; 32(Suppl 2): 68A.

14 de Franchis R. Updating consensus in portal hypertension: report of the Baveno III Consensus Workshop on definitions, methodology and therapeutic strategies in portal hypertension. *J Hepatol* 2000; 33: 846–52.

15 Bernard B, Grange JD, Khac EN, Amiot X, *et al.* Antibiotic prophylaxis for the prevention of bacterial infections in cirrhotic patients with gastrointestinal bleeding: a meta-analysis. *Hepatology* 1999; 29: 1655–61.

16 Gotzsche PC. Somatostatin or octreotide for acute bleeding oesophageal varices (Cochrane review). *The Cochrane Library*, Issue 1. Oxford: Update Software, 1999.

17 Goulis J, Burroughs AK. Portal hypertensive bleeding: prevention and treatment. In: McDonald J, Burroughs AK, Feagan B (ed). Evidence based gastroenterology and hepatology. London: *British Medical Journal* Books, 1999: 389–426.

18 Hartigan PM, Gebhard RL, Gregory PB. Sclerotherapy for actively bleeding esophageal varices in male alcoholics with cirrhosis. Veterans Cooperative Variceal Sclerotherapy Group. *Gastrointest Endosc* 1997; 46: 1–7.

19 Cales P, Masliah C, Bernard B, Garnier PP, *et al.* Early administration of vapreotide for variceal bleeding in patients with cirrhosis. French Club for the Study of Portal Hypertension. *N Engl J Med* 2001; 344: 23–8.

20 Bornman P, Terblanche J, Kahn D, Jonker MA, Kirsch RE. Limitations of multiple injection sclerotherapy sessions for acute variceal bleeding. *S Afr Med J* 1986; 70: 34–6.

21 Chau TN, Patch D, Chan YW, Nagral A, *et al.* 'Salvage' transjugular intrahepatic portosystemic shunts: gastric fundal compared with esophageal variceal bleeding. *Gastroenterology* 1998; 114: 981–7.

22 Feu F, Garcia-Pagan JC, Bosch J, Luca A, *et al.* Relationship between portal pressure response to pharmacotherapy and risk of recurrent variceal haemorrhage in patients with cirrhosis. *Lancet* 1995; 346: 1056–9.

23 Papatheodoridis GV, Goulis J, Leandro G, Patch D, Burroughs AK. Transjugular intrahepatic portosystemic shunt compared with endoscopic treatment for prevention of variceal rebleeding: a meta analysis. *Hepatology* 1999; 30: 612–22.

24 Perez-Ayuso RM, Pique JM, Bosch J, Panes J, *et al.* Propranolol in prevention of recurrent bleeding from severe portal hypertensive gastropathy in cirrhosis. *Lancet* 1991; 337: 1431–4.

25   Poynard T, Cales P, Pasta L, Ideo G, *et al.* Beta-adrenergic-antagonist drugs in the prevention of gastrointestinal bleeding in patients with cirrhosis and esophageal varices. An analysis of data and prognostic factors in 589 patients from four randomized clinical trials. Franco-Italian Multicenter Study Group. *N Engl J Med* 1991; **324**: 1532–8.

26   Angelico M, Carli L, Piat S, Gentile S, Capocaccia L. Effects of isosorbide-5-mononitrate compared with propranolol on first bleeding and long-term survival in cirrhosis. *Gastroenterology* 1997; **113**: 1632–9.

27   Merkel C, Marin R, Sacerdoti D, Donada C, *et al.* Long-term results of a clinical trial of nadolol with or without isosorbide mononitrate for primary prophylaxis of variceal bleeding in cirrhosis. *Hepatology* 2000; **31**: 324–9.

28   Rockey D. The cellular pathogenesis of portal hypertension: stellate cell contractility, endothelin, and nitric oxide. Review. *Hepatology* 1997; **25**: 2–5.

29   Sogni P, Moreau R, Gomola A, Gadano A, *et al.* Beneficial haemodynamic effects of bosentan, a mixed ET(A) and ET(B) receptor antagonist, in portal hypertensive rats. *Hepatology* 1998; **28**: 655–9.

30   Gupta TK, Toruner M, Chung MK, Groszmann RJ. Endothelial dysfunction and decreased production of nitric oxide in the intrahepatic microcirculation of cirrhotic rats. *Hepatology* 1998; **28**: 926–31.

31   Gentilini P, Romanelli RG, La Villa G, Maggiore Q, *et al.* Effects of low-dose captopril on renal haemodynamics and function in patients with cirrhosis of the liver. *Gastroenterology* 1993; **104**: 588–94.

32   Schneider AW, Kalk JF, Klein CP. Effect of losartan, an angiotensin II receptor antagonist, on portal pressure in cirrhosis. *Hepatology* 1999; **29**: 334–9.

33   Debernadi-Venon D, Barletti C, Marzano A, Alessandria C, *et al.* Efficacy of irbesartan, an angiotensin II receptor selective antagonist, in the treatment of portal hypertension. *Hepatology* 1999; **30**: 219A.

34   Garcia-Tsao G. Angiotensin II receptor antagonist in the pharmacological therapy of portal hypertension: a caution. *Gastroenterology* 1999; **117**: 740–2.

35   Albillos A, Lledo JL, Rossi I, Perez-Paramo M, *et al.* Continuous prazosin administration in cirrhotic patients: effects on portal hemodynamics and on liver and renal function. *Gastroenterology* 1995; **109**: 1257–65.

36   Banares R, Moitinho E, Piqueras B, Casado M, *et al.* Carvedilol, a new nonselective beta-blocker with intrinsic anti-Alpha1-adrenergic activity has a greater portal hypotensive effect than propranolol in patients with cirrhosis. *Hepatology* 1999; **30**: 79–83.

37   Nevens F, Lijnen P, VanBilloen H, Fevery J. The effect of long-term treatment with spironolactone on variceal pressure in patients with portal hypertension without ascites. *Hepatology* 1996; **23**: 1047–52.

☐ SELF ASSESSMENT QUESTIONS

1   The threshold portal pressure gradient (hepatic venous pressure gradient) for the development of oesophageal varices is:
(a) 5–6 mmHg
(b) 10–12 mmHg
(c) 19–20 mmHg
(d) 15–17 mmHg
(e) 17–18 mmHg

2   Prophylactic antibiotics need to be administered in cirrhotic patients with upper gastrointestinal bleeding:
(a) Always
(b) Only if active bleeding at endoscopy

(c) Only in decompensated cirrhotics
(d) Never
(e) According to individual clinical practice

3   The following drugs have some evidence for reducing mortality from randomised controlled trials in acute variceal bleeding:
(a) Vasopressin
(b) Somatostatin
(c) Terlipressin
(d) Octreotide
(e) Vapreotide

4   The following groups of cirrhotic patients who have not bled and have varices should be evaluated for primary prevention of bleeding with non-selective beta-blockers:
(a) All patients
(b) Only if large varices are present
(c) Only if there is decompensated liver disease
(d) Only non-alcoholics
(e) Only if portal vein is patent

5   The following have portal hypotensive effects and can be easily used clinically:
(a) Spironolactone
(b) Carvedilol
(c) Clonidine
(d) Prazosin
(e) Losartan

ANSWERS

1a False	2a True	3a False	4a False	5a True
b True	b False	b False	b True	b True
c False	c False	c True	c False	c False
d False	d False	d False	d False	d False
e False	e False	e False	e False	e False

Regulation of apoptosis in the normal and diseased gastrointestinal tract

Alastair Watson

☐ TYPES OF CELL DEATH: APOPTOSIS VERSUS NECROSIS

It is essential that cell number is tightly controlled in multicellular organisms. This is particularly true in gastrointestinal epithelium as this tissue has one of the most rapid turnover rates in the body. To balance cell division, a number of programmed cell death mechanisms have evolved collectively called 'apoptosis'. This term was coined in 1972 to denote a form of cell death fulfilling particular morphological features best seen under electron microscopy [1], including:

☐ condensation in nuclear chromatin

☐ cell shrinkage

☐ compaction of intracellular organelles

☐ cell surface blebbing

☐ fragmentation into apoptotic bodies that are cleared rapidly by phagocytosis.

These morphological features served as criteria for the definition of apoptosis for a number of years, but more recently it has become accepted that apoptosis can be defined as a cell death regulated by members of the Bcl-2 gene family and/or mediated by a family of cysteine proteases, the caspases.

Apoptosis is not the only form of programmed cell death. Sperandio and colleagues recently defined another form, 'paraptosis', which does not fulfil the criteria for apoptosis [2]. This occurs in the brain in a number of degenerative conditions and is neither mediated by caspases nor regulated by Bcl-2 family members.

The pattern of apoptosis in tissues contrasts strongly with that of necrosis:

☐ *Necrosis* is not genetically regulated, but is a direct consequence of physical damage to the cell. It typically occurs synchronously in large populations of cells and is associated with inflammation. It is the main form of cell death found in any inflammatory reaction or abscess.

☐ By contrast, *apoptosis* occurs in single cells asynchronously. Thus, even in tissues where apoptosis rates are high, the numbers of apoptotic cells seen on histological sections are very low. Histological sections are snapshots in time, so short-lived events such as apoptosis are rarely seen. Furthermore, as apoptotic cell death does not provoke inflammation, apoptosis is inconspicuous.

Apoptosis is not an inevitable consequence of cellular damage – a crucial contrast to necrosis. The cell makes a decision whether or not to execute itself following cellular damage. This can be illustrated by the effect of the anti-apoptotic gene Bcl-2 (Fig. 1). If CEM-C7 cells are transfected with Bcl-2 or vector control and the cells challenged with the DNA damaging agent VP-16, apoptosis ensues in a time-dependent manner in the control cells, but those transfected with Bcl-2 do not undergo apoptosis in response to the DNA damage. It is important to emphasise that the degree of DNA damage is identical in the two cell lines. The difference is that Bcl-2 has prevented the engagement of an apoptosis death programme.

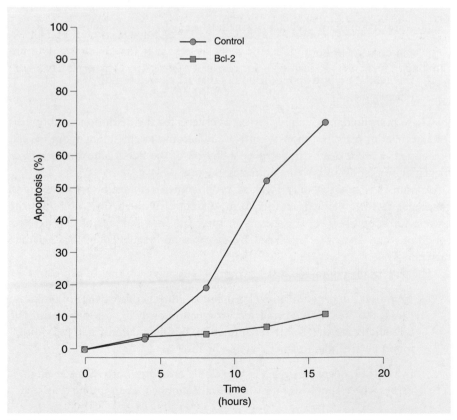

Fig. 1 Inhibition by Bcl-2 of the induction of apoptosis in CEM-C7 cells by the DNA damaging agent VP-16 (10 μmol).

☐ MOLECULAR MECHANISMS OF APOPTOSIS (Fig. 2)

The role of mitochondria

The molecular mechanisms underlying apoptosis have been the subject of intense investigation over the last 15 years. A number of apoptotic pathways have now been defined in mammalian cells. In one pathway, mitochondria play a central role in sensing any of a diverse range of cellular stresses and orchestrating them into a single signal-transduction pathway. For example, removal of growth factors from receptors at the plasma membrane causes the translocation of pro-apoptotic Bcl-2 family members such as Bax to the mitochondria. This causes the release of cytochrome c from the intermembrane space of mitochondria into the cytosol.

The mechanism by which this release is achieved is currently the subject of much debate. In one model, pro-apoptotic Bcl-2 family members such as Bax and Bak come together to form large multimolecular complexes in the outer plasma membrane, resulting in the formation of a pore sufficiently large to allow the efflux of cytochrome c. In this model, anti-apoptotic Bcl-2 family members can also participate in the formation of the multimolecular complex, thus preventing pore formation. Other models suggest cytochrome c is released through a large pore in mitochondrial membranes, the permeability transition pore. Released cytochrome c forms another multimolecular complex, the apoptosome, that includes the cytochrome c-binding protein APAF1, procaspase 9 and d-adenosine triphosphate. This causes the processing of the inactive procaspase 9 into its active subunit, initiating activation of a cascade of other caspases culminating in proteolysis and cell death.

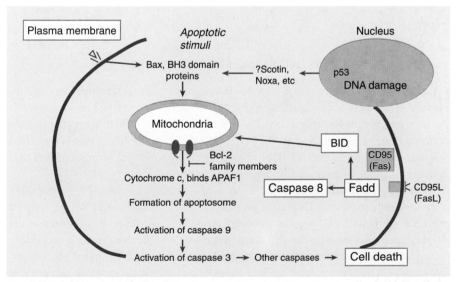

Fig. 2 Schematic representation of the mitochondrial and CD95-mediated pathways of apoptosis.

DNA damage

Another potent inducer of apoptosis is DNA damage which modifies the activities of enzymes such as ATM kinase and DNA-dependent kinase that modify p53 and its negative regulator MDM-2. This results in increased levels of activated p53 protein, a transcription factor which activates several target genes able to induce apoptosis, including Scotin, Noxa and Bax. These pathways are of great complexity and are not fully understood. Nevertheless, regardless of the precise molecular mechanisms, they culminate in the release of cytochrome c from mitochondria with formation of the apoptosome leading to processing and activation of the caspase family.

Cell surface receptor CD95

Another distinct apoptotic pathway of great importance in the functioning of the immune system, both in the elimination of immature T cells and in the T cell-mediated killing of target cells, involves the cell surface receptor CD95 (Fas) and its cognate ligand CD95L (Fas ligand). The CD95 receptor is a member of the tumour necrosis factor (TNF) superfamily of proteins. A cytoplasmic 'death domain', a protein-protein interaction motif critical for engaging downstream components of the CD95 signal-transduction pathway, is shared by a subset of these receptors. On receptor activation, the death domain interacts with a death domain in the adapter proteins FADD or TRADD. Caspase 8 is processed and activated by this interaction, with subsequent cleavage of downstream caspases and cell death. In its pure form, this pathway is poorly inhibited by Bcl-2. However, in many cell types there is insufficient caspase 8 to activate downstream caspases fully, and caspase 8 instead activates the BH3-only domain protein BID. This translocates to mitochondria and binds to Bcl-2 and Bax, causing the release of cytochrome c and the formation of the apoptosome. This mitochondrial branch of the CD95 pathway can be seen as an amplification loop resulting in the more efficient induction of cell death.

☐ APOPTOSIS IN NORMAL INTESTINAL EPITHELIUM

A number of types of apoptosis can be discerned in normal intestinal epithelium (Fig. 3). At the base of the unstressed crypt there is a constant low rate of apoptosis (perhaps one apoptosis per ten crypts in the small intestine) which serves to regulate the number of cells migrating up the crypt/villus axis. In the colon, this is regulated by Bcl-2, but not by Bax or Bcl-w. No Bcl-2 family member has been identified that regulates this type of apoptosis in the small intestine.

Cells are shed from the tip of the villus in the small intestine and from the table of the colonic epithelium (Fig. 4). Once detached from their extracellular matrix, intestinal epithelial cells rapidly undergo apoptosis. However, it is controversial whether apoptosis initiates the shedding process or whether apoptosis is secondary to unrelated processes causing the extrusion of cells from the epithelial monolayer. This issue will not be resolved until an apoptotic regulating protein or caspase can be shown to regulate the shedding process.

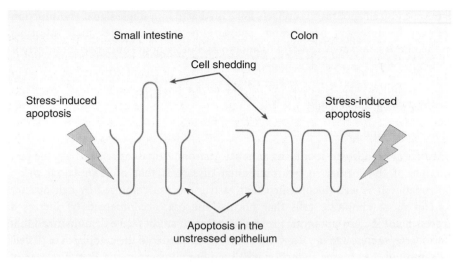

Fig. 3 Types of apoptosis in the small and large intestines.

Apoptosis can be readily induced in intestinal epithelium by DNA-damaging agents including gamma radiation and 5-fluorouracil (5-FU). However, a remarkable feature of this form of apoptosis not currently understood is that it is restricted to the lower half of the crypts and is completely absent from the villi. Studies with knockout mice have demonstrated that DNA damage-induced apoptosis is mediated by p53 but not by Bax [3]. Bcl-2 and Bcl-w inhibit this form of apoptosis. Other studies with p53 knockout mice show that DNA

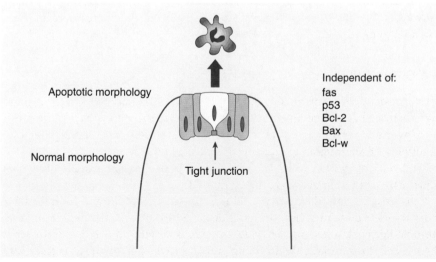

Fig. 4 Cell shedding process at the tip of the small intestinal villi (human, mouse and rat). Apoptotic bodies are seen only in the lumen. It is currently unknown whether apoptosis triggers the shedding process.

damage-induced apoptosis is unlikely to be mediated by a single signal-transduction pathway because 4½ hours after exposure to radiation the small intestinal epithelium is completely resistant to apoptosis, but 24 hours after radiation there is a low rate of p53-independent apoptosis.

☐ EXCESSIVE APOPTOSIS

Helicobacter and gastric cancer

Excessive or inadequate apoptosis can cause gastrointestinal cancer. Perhaps the best example of the former in gastrointestinal disease is that of *Helicobacter pylori* gastropathy. It is well documented that gastric mucosa colonised by helicobacter contain more apoptotic cells that normal mucosa, accompanied by increased expression of the pro-apoptotic protein Bak. Recent studies have demonstrated that helicobacter secrete a toxin, VacA, which is translocated into the cytoplasm of gastric cells and localises to the mitochondrial membrane where it causes the release of cytochrome c and the induction of apoptosis (Fig. 5) [4]. These and other studies indicate that apoptosis may well underlie the gastric atrophy seen following long-standing helicobacter infection. Chronic inflammation will also contribute to apoptosis through the production of interferon-γ, the release of CD95L and the induction of apoptosis. Atrophy is the major precursor lesion of gastric cancer, so apoptosis may well play a role in gastric carcinogenesis. More studies are required, in particular to determine:

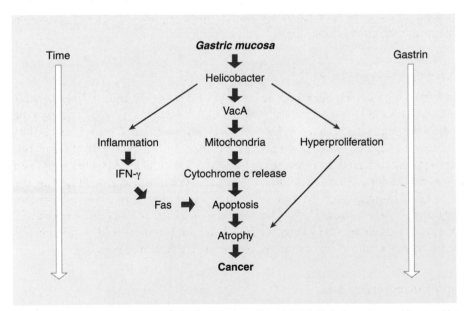

Fig. 5 Helicobacter induces apoptosis through a number of mechanisms causing gastric atrophy, the major precursor lesion of gastric cancer. Gastrin accelerates the progression of the epithelium from normality to hyperproliferation to atrophy to cancer (IFN = interferon).

☐   which cells in the gastric epithelium undergo apoptosis

☐   whether the apoptotic process promotes the production of genetically unstable stem cells prone to producing malignant mutations.

☐ INADEQUATE APOPTOSIS

Colorectal cancer

Colorectal cancer and Crohn's disease exemplify the role of deficient apoptosis in gastrointestinal disease. Failure of apoptosis of stem cells with potentially malignant mutations may well play an important role in colonic carcinogenesis. A number of the genes that are characteristically mutated during colonic carcinogenesis, including APC, MYC, DCC and p53, normally function to induce apoptosis. Furthermore, cyclooxygenase (COX)-2 is overexpressed early during colonic carcinogenesis. COX-2 expression tends to put the cells into an anti-apoptotic state by upregulating Bcl-2 and downregulating Bax, which may partly explain the potent chemopreventive effects of COX-2 inhibitors against colorectal cancer [5]. Furthermore, differential rates of apoptosis in the small and large intestines may explain why colonic cancer is over one hundred times more common than small intestinal cancer. In a study of the effects of a panel of carcinogens on apoptosis rates in the small and large intestines, Potten and colleagues [6,7] found that in the small intestine apoptosis was induced with maximal rates at the cell positions where stem cells are believed to reside. In contrast, in the large intestine, maximal apoptosis rates were found at cell positions significantly displaced from the stem cells. This relative lack of apoptosis at the stem cell position may indicate that colonic stem cells occasionally fail to undergo apoptosis following mutation, thereby founding potentially malignant clones.

Apoptosis and chemotherapeutic drugs

Apoptosis is also important in the action of chemotherapeutic drugs against colorectal cancer. It is well established that 5-FU, the mainstay of chemotherapy for colonic cancer, causes apoptosis in both small and large intestinal epithelium [8], but the relationship between apoptosis and destruction of intestinal epithelium is not straightforward. Standard therapeutic doses of 5-FU induce substantial apoptosis. However, this loss of cells is insufficient to damage epithelial integrity [9] because the loss of cells through apoptosis is immediately balanced by an increase in cell division. Interestingly, if the dose of 5-FU is increased tenfold, the rate of apoptosis in intestinal epithelium increases by only 30%. However, high-dose 5-FU causes mitotic arrest, as well as apoptosis, and subsequent tissue destruction is severe.

Apoptosis and mitotic arrest

Both apoptosis and mitotic arrest are p53-dependent. Thus, even extremely high doses of 5-FU fail to cause significant tissue destruction in p53 knockout mice. This combination of apoptosis and mitotic arrest may explain the enteropathy experienced by a small proportion of patients with colorectal cancer treated with 5-FU. More significantly, it may also explain the role of apoptosis in colonic cancers themselves. Although apoptosis can be induced, it occurs in insufficient cells to cause tumour shrinkage unless mitotic arrest is also achieved. Ways of increasing apoptotic rates in colonic tumours is now a major goal of experimental therapeutics.

Crohn's disease

Crohn's disease is a chronic inflammatory disease of the gut wall. The identity of the triggers of this inflammation is currently unknown, although it may simply be an abnormal response to normal gut flora. Whatever the trigger, a chronic inflammatory state is set up, with high levels of the cytokines TNF, interleukin (IL)-1, IL-2, IL-6 and IL-8. Recent investigations have shown that a key element in the pathogenesis of Crohn's disease is defective resolution of this inflammatory response. Apoptosis of T cells is an important mechanism in terminating normal inflammatory responses. Animal models with defective triggering of apoptosis in lymphocytes show a number of chronic autoimmune inflammatory and lymphoproliferative disorders. Recent evidence suggests that Crohn's disease may be one of these. Indeed, one of the effects of corticosteroids, the principal therapeutic agent used in Crohn's disease, is to induce apoptosis in T cells thereby terminating inflammatory reactions.

The role of tumour necrosis factor

Over the last decade a remarkable series of discoveries has shown that TNF plays a central role in the pathogenesis of Crohn's disease [10]. First, 60% of patients treated with blocking antibodies to TNF (infliximab) showed a remarkable improvement. This is probably the single most important therapeutic advance in Crohn's disease since the introduction of azathioprine in the 1970s.

Secondly, overexpression of the TNF gene in mice leads to arthritis and enteritis with skip lesions, transmural inflammation and granuloma formation highly reminiscent of human Crohn's disease. The TNF receptor is a member of the same family as the CD95 receptor discussed above. Its activation by binding of soluble TNF activates a complex signal-transduction pathway which promotes the inflammatory response through activation of the transcription factor NF-κB (Fig. 6). The effect of TNF on apoptosis is ambiguous. Its receptor binds to FADD which directly induces apoptosis in cells expressing the receptor, but in many cases the induction of NF-κB will tend to inhibit apoptosis. Thus, the effect of TNF on apoptosis will depend on the ratio of these competing mechanisms.

Interleukin-6 and Crohn's disease

Recent investigation on the effects of IL-6 in Crohn's disease provides much more direct evidence for the importance of apoptosis in terminating the inflammatory reaction of Crohn's disease (Fig. 7) [11]. T cells and macrophages of Crohn's disease

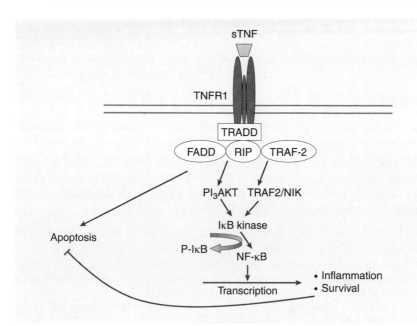

Fig. 6 Signal-transduction pathways triggered by tumour necrosis factor (TNF) binding to the TNF receptor (TNFR). The effect of TNF on apoptosis in tissue is ambiguous depending on the balance between signals directly inducing apoptosis and signals from NF-κB inhibiting apoptosis.

patients secrete IL-6 and a soluble IL-6 receptor, respectively. Recent studies have shown that IL-6 and its receptor form complexes in the intracellular matrix through a process called trans-signalling. The complexes bind to glycoprotein (GP) 130 receptors in T cells, activating the STAT-3 pathway which upregulates the expression of Bcl-2 and Bcl-x_l in T cells. Another remarkable series of experiments has shown that specific neutralisation of the soluble IL-6 receptor will cause apoptosis in lymphocytes from Crohn's disease patients and resolve inflammation within a

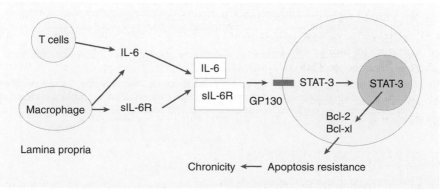

Fig. 7 Proposed mechanism to explain how interleukin (IL-)6 blocking antibodies heal animal models of Crohn's disease (from [11], with permission) (GP = glycoprotein).

number of animal models of Crohn's disease [11]. These experiments demonstrate for the first time the importance of apoptosis in terminating the inflammatory response in Crohn's disease and point the way to a major new therapeutic modality.

☐ CONCLUSION

Although remarkable advances have been made in understanding the molecular mechanisms of apoptosis, much remains to be discovered about the regulation of apoptosis in gastrointestinal epithelial cells. Nevertheless, important advances have been made in the role of apoptosis and in the treatment of malignancies, including colorectal cancer. Specific apoptosis therapies are likely to be developed for the treatment of inflammatory bowel disease.

REFERENCES

1   Kerr JFR, Wyllie AH, Currie AR. Apoptosis: a basic biological phenomenon with wide-ranging implications in tissue kinetics. Review. *Br J Cancer* 1972; **26**: 239–57.

2   Sperandio S, de Belle I, Bredesen DE. An alternative, nonapoptotic form of programmed cell death. *Proc Natl Acad Sci USA* 2000; **97**: 14376–81.

3   Watson AJM, Pritchard DM. Lessons from genetically engineered animal models. VII. Apoptosis in intestinal epithelium: lessons from transgenic and knockout mice. Review. *Am J Physiol Gastrointest Liver Physiol* 2000; **278**: G1–5.

4   Galmiche A, Rassow J, Doye A, Cagnol S, *et al.* The N-terminal 34 kDa fragment of *Helicobacter pylori* vacuolating cytotoxin targets mitochondria and induces cytochrome c release. *EMBO J* 2000; **19**: 6361–70.

5   Watson AJM, DuBois RN. Lipid metabolism and APC: implications for colorectal cancer prevention. *Lancet* 1997; **349**: 444–5.

6   Li YQ, Fan CY, O'Connor PJ, Winton DJ, Potten CS. Target cells for the cytotoxic effects of carcinogens in the murine small bowel. *Carcinogenesis* 1992; **13**: 361–8.

7   Potten CS, Li YQ, O'Connor PJ, Winton DJ. A possible explanation for the differential cancer incidence in the intestine, based on distribution of the cytotoxic effects of carcinogens in the murine large bowel. *Carcinogenesis* 1992; **13**: 2305–12.

8   Pritchard DM, Watson AJ, Potten CS, Jackman AL, Hickman JA. Inhibition by uridine but not thymidine of p53-dependent intestinal apoptosis initiated by 5-fluorouracil: evidence for the involvement of RNA perturbation. *Proc Natl Acad Sci USA* 1997; **94**: 1795–9.

9   Pritchard DM, Potten CS, Hickman JA. The relationships between p53-dependent apoptosis, inhibition of proliferation, and 5-fluorouracil-induced histopathology in murine intestinal epithelia. *Cancer Res* 1998; **58**: 5453–65.

10 Papadakis KA, Targan SR. Tumor necrosis factor: biology and therapeutic inhibitors. *Gastroenterology* 2000; **119**: 1148–57.

11 Atreya R, Mudter J, Finotto S, Mullberg J, *et al.* Blockade of interleukin 6 trans signaling suppresses T-cell resistance against apoptosis in chronic intestinal inflammation: evidence in Crohn disease and experimental colitis *in vivo*. *Nat Med* 2000; **6**: 583–8.

☐ SELF ASSESSMENT QUESTIONS

1   Characteristic features of apoptosis are:
    (a) Cell swelling
    (b) Clearance of apoptotic cells

(c) Oligonucleosomal cleavage

(d) Condensation of nuclear chromatin rarely

(e) Phosphatidylserine redistributes to the outer surface of the cell membrane

2   Features of genetic regulation of apoptosis include:

(a) Bcl-2 family members can either prevent or induce apoptosis

(b) p53 prevents apoptosis

(c) Bcl-2 family members are found only in mammals

(d) CD95L participates in the killing of target cells by killer T cells

(e) Bcl-2 family members do not regulate the release of cytochrome c from mitochondria

3   In the intestine:

(a) Apoptotic bodies are found at the top of the villus following radiation-induced DNA damage

(b) Apoptotic bodies can be seen only by immunohistochemistry

(c) Cells in the stem cell zone are very sensitive to apoptotic stimuli

(d) Apoptosis without cell cycle arrest causes architectural destruction of the mucosa

(e) p53 is a major determinant of apoptosis in the normal intestine

4   *Helicobacter pylori:*

(a) Promotes apoptosis in gastric epithelium

(b) VacA toxin can cause cytochrome c release

(c) Gastric atrophy protects against gastric cancer

(d) Helicobacter and gastrin act synergistically to promote gastric cancer

(e) Helicobacter may promote apoptosis through CD95/CD95L

5   In Crohn's disease: .

(a) Apoptotic bodies are easily seen in inflammatory lesions

(b) One of the actions of prednisolone may be to induce apoptosis in T cells

(c) Tumour necrosis factor (TNF) can directly induce apoptosis

(d) Interleukin-6 may promote resistance to apoptosis in lamina propria T cells

(e) Blocking antibodies to TNF can be used for the treatment of Crohn's disease

ANSWERS

1a False	2a True	3a False	4a True	5a False
b True	b False	b False	b True	b True
c True	c False	c True	c False	c True
d False	d True	d False	d True	d True
e True	e False	e True	e True	e True

New challenges and opportunities in human health

Molecular biology, target identification and new therapeutics

Terence Rabbitts

☐ INTRODUCTION

Molecular biology is a branch of biological sciences which reduces biological phenomena to molecular explanation, determining what molecules look like, how they function and how they interact with other molecules. The molecular understanding of biological pathways will explain not only how cells carry out their autonomous functions but also the many interactions needed for the correct development and tissue homeostasis. Organisms develop by processes dictated by their genetic information, and diseases result from alterations in this information. Thus, molecular biologists hope to explain how diseases not originating from infections occur by interpreting the mistakes in the pathogenesis of disease at the molecular level.

The search for altered genes in human disease is a major objective. The initial aim is to identify a mutated gene and determine its nucleotide sequence, facilitating a comparison of the functions of normal and mutant proteins and thereby indicating the basis of the disease process. This in turn will allow an evaluation of whether a mutant protein is a suitable drug target. For the purposes of this review, a drug is any agent which can intervene in a biological process through its specific binding to a target molecule. This chapter will discuss:

☐ the current status of gene discovery

☐ target identification, and

☐ molecular technology developments which may in some cases be required to develop drugs.

☐ GENE DISCOVERY AND DRUG TARGET IDENTIFICATION

Molecular cloning, in particular cDNA cloning techniques, has led to the identification of many genes involved in diseases. In cancer, the study of chromosomal translocations in tumours has been a productive area as the break points of these somatically arising chromosomal aberrations pinpoint areas of the genome where genes must be located which are important for cancer (reviewed in [1]). Thus, the first cancer-specific chromosomal translocation break points in the Philadelphia chromosome and the t(8;14) chromosomal translocation of Burkitt's lymphoma resulted in the cloning of the *BCR-ABL* fusion gene and the translocated *CMYC* gene, respectively. This demonstrated that cellular proto-oncogenes are activated by chromosomal translocations in cancer and illustrated the two most common outcomes of chromosomal translocations (Fig. 1). These findings paved the way for the identification of many novel genes whose protein products are targets for drug therapy.

The Human Genome Project

Gene discovery on a much greater scale is provided by the Human Genome Project (HGP) and the mouse genome equivalent, in which the aim is to identify all human and mouse genes. Achieving this goal in man has been slow but sure. It has come closer with the publication of drafts of the human gene sequences [2,3]. The cDNA cloning technologies [4–6] which first allowed direct cDNA sequencing were established from work done in 1975–76, and this in turn led to indirect protein sequencing. There have now been 21,076 mouse cDNAs published from the work of one consortium [7]. Meanwhile, the HGP has progressed to the complete sequence in 2001, a landmark which will provide molecular biologists with the complete set of human genes and facilitate the discovery of many more disease genes [2,3].

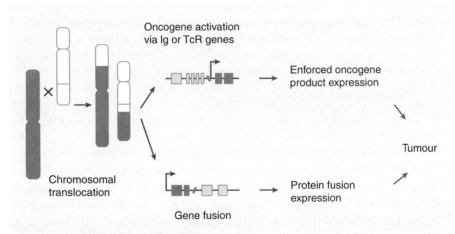

Fig. 1 Two major consequences of chromosomal translocations in cancer leading to tumour formation. When a chromosomal translocation occurs in lymphoid cells or precursors the aberrant chromosome can involve immunoglobulin (Ig) genes or T cell receptor (TcR) genes which are normally undergoing rearrangement in lymphopoiesis. In this type of chromosomal translocation (upper section), a proto-oncogene near the chromosomal translocation break point becomes associated with the rearranging gene locus and an enforced oncogene expression results because of this new transcriptional environment (eg the *CMYC* gene in Burkitt's lymphoma). In the second type of chromosomal translocation (lower section), which occurs widely in haematopoietic tumours and sarcomas, the break points occur within a gene on each chromosome. When the translocated chromosome is formed, exons of each gene are now linked resulting in a fusion protein being made from the mRNA (eg the *BCR-ABL* fusion gene in chronic myelogenous leukaemia).

The human genome sequence

The ultimate target identification information package is the human genome sequence itself:

☐ *Bioinformatics* is the analysis of complex sequence data to reveal genes and hints about genome evolution and organisation. There are about 50,000 human genes and many more proteins (>200,000). This discrepancy is largely attributable to differences in RNA splicing which contributes variable amounts of genetic information to mRNA, and thus in turn to proteins.

☐ *Functional genomics* will be used to determine what all the genes do.

☐ *Comparative proteomics*, the direct study of expressed protein profiles (or DNA micro-arrays) will determine tissue-specific expression profiles.

These combined efforts will identify disease-associated drug targets. The next tasks will be:

☐ drug design

☐ development of technologies for therapy, and

☐ development of technologies for drug delivery.

☐ TROJAN HORSE THERAPEUTICS: RECRUITING CELLULAR PATHWAYS FOR THERAPY

Abnormal proteins found in disease cells such as cancer cells are specific because of their origin in somatic mutations. A strategy for treating disease is to use these mutant antigens to recruit and activate destructive endogenous pathways. Many complex interactive mechanisms in the cell could be recruited for the benefit of therapeutics (Fig. 2). Cells can respond to the binding of ligands to cell surface receptors, causing signal transduction. This transfers the external stimulus through cytoplasmic pathways to the cell nucleus to affect DNA transcription. In addition, transcription itself is a controllable process involving multiple protein interactions as well as specific and non-specific DNA binding. After transcription, RNA splicing and transport mechanisms come into play and mRNA (and other RNAs like tRNA) are transferred to the cytoplasm for protein synthesis. Underlying this cell physiology is a dynamic system of protein turnover [8] through the proteosomes, providing for cell metabolism stability and ultimately the homeostasis of tissues. Another control system is the apoptosis (or programmed cell death) pathway [9] which responds to cell senescence or cellular damage (eg DNA damage) by cell death through activation of zymogens.

All these pathways – and indeed any other used by the cell – can be recruited by linking chimeric antigen-specific exogenous effector molecules ('drugs') to selected components of the pathway to be activated (the 'Trojan horse' strategy). These chimeric molecules are the exogenous molecules which trick the cell into activating

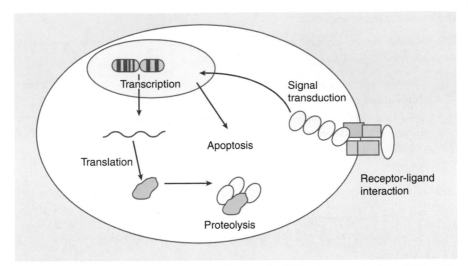

Fig. 2 Endogenous cellular pathways accessible for the Trojan horse technology. Multiprotein complexes are involved in many cellular activities such as signal transduction, transcription, proteolysis and apoptosis. These pathways can be recruited and activated by exogenous introduction of one or more components linked to antigen-specific moieties, such as intracellular antibodies. The pathways can thereby be controlled by the exogenous factor for therapeutic needs.

an endogenous mechanism to cause a change in the cell. Proof of principle of this concept has been achieved using an antibody-antigen interaction dependent apoptosis (Aida) technique (Fig. 3) [10].

Functional intracellular antibodies

Recruiting endogenous proteins to perform their normal function in response to an exogenous reagent requires specificity and affinity. Antibodies have evolved both these qualities but are designed for extracellular functions, so in their normal form are not ideal for intracellular use. We have recently described a selection procedure, intracellular antibody capture [11,12], which facilitates direct isolation of functional intracellular antibodies (ICAbs) in the form of single-chain (sc) Fv (ie immuno-globulin VH and VL segments held together by a flexible linker, allowing the formation of an antibody-combining site). This method allows selection of any antigen-specific ICAb which can be linked to an intracellular component in an appropriate expression system for the Trojan horse therapeutic strategy.

Demonstration of the Trojan horse strategy

Recruitment of the apoptosis pathway has been used to demonstrate the Trojan horse strategy. Apoptosis occurs by activation of zymogens, of which activation of procaspase 3 (Fig. 3) (the so-called executioner of the cell death pathway) is an irreversible step to cell death. The experimental therapeutic strategy combines expression of ICAbs fused to procaspase 3 inside cells (Fig. 4(a)), which bind to two

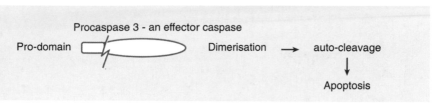

Fig. 3 Procaspase is the executioner of the cell death pathway. Caspase is involved in apoptosis after it is cleaved from its inactive state called procaspase 3. This can occur by dimerisation of procaspase 3 and cleavage of the pro-domain to yield the active form.

close sites on the target antigen (Fig. 4(b)). The binding of antibody to antigen effectively dimerises the caspase 3 and leads to auto-activation and apoptosis. β-galactosidase was used as test antigen because it forms a natural tetramer and thus provides naturally occurring proximal antigenic sites for the ICAb-caspase 3 fusion to bind [10].

Data illustrating the effectiveness of this approach, in which β-galactosidase activity was a measure of cell viability, are shown in Fig. 5. When β-galactosidase antigen alone was expressed the score was the equivalent of 100% cell viability, but this dropped to about 10% when anti-β-galactosidase ICAb-caspase 3 fusion was expressed because of the activation of the apoptosis pathway. This effect is antibody-specific. A non-relevant ICAb (F8) had no effect on viability and required active exogenous caspase 3 fused to the ICAb because an inactivating mutant version was ineffective.

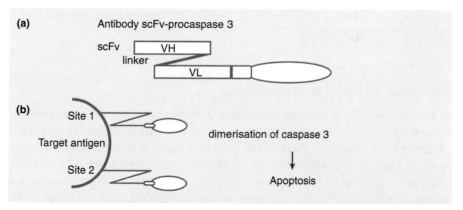

Fig. 4 Antibody-antigen interaction dependent apoptosis (Aida) technology, an example of recruitment of endogenous pathways for therapy: **(a)** The exogenous intracellular antibody (ICAb)-caspase fusion molecule comprises an antigen-specific single-chain (sc) Fv fused to procaspase 3 which can be introduced into a cell after expression from a vector (eg a virus), protein transduction or other physical methods. **(b)** The target antigen in the cell can have one or more sites for the scFv-caspase 3. If binding to one or more sites causes procaspase 3 activation, cell death will occur by apoptosis. In other forms of the approach, natural dimerisation of the target protein will be sufficient for auto-activation of procaspase 3. An alternative version of the strategy is the use of other pathways to produce an effect in the target cell, such as recruiting proteosomes through exogenous scFv fusion molecules. In much the same way as with procaspase, one or more binding sites on the target antigen will suffice to activate the pathway.

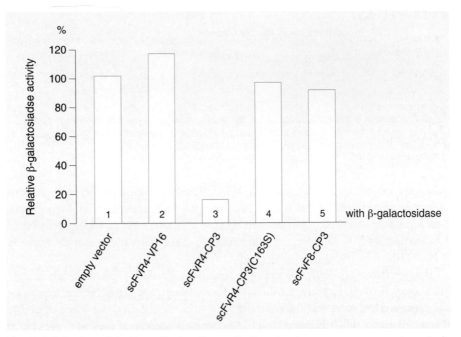

Fig. 5 Cell death mediated by antibody-antigen activation of endogenous caspases and apoptosis (Aida technology). Viability of cells expressing β-galactosidase and various single-chain (sc) Fv-fusion proteins was determined by measuring β-galactosidase activity. Cell death was observed in cells expressing β-galactosidase (antigen) and specific antibody fused to procaspase 3 (scFvR4-CP3). No other form of scFv fusion caused cell death, including the same scFv fused to an inactive mutant form of caspase 3 (scFvR4-CP3(C163S)) or a non-relevant intracellular antibody (ICAb) fused to procaspase 3 (scFvF8-CP3). The authenticity of apoptosis was confirmed by assessment of DNA laddering and by detection of the specific procaspase 3 cleavage product.

Future developments of the Trojan horse strategy

Antibodies have been used in our model experiments to bind to intracellular antigen, demonstrating the effectiveness of the Trojan horse strategy for recruitment of cellular pathways. Any molecule capable of mediating a specific molecular interaction will suffice, for instance peptides or even small molecules which can be adapted to the needs. Further development of the strategy for clinical use will require effective delivery systems tailored to specific cell types. The inherent specificity of the Aida method or variants using non-antibody recognition, however, provides the ultimate specificity for this recruitment strategy. A possible application of this technology might be in cancer treatment where a fusion molecule from a chromosomal translocation is the target antigen. For instance, a site on either side of the fusion junction of a molecule like BCR-ABL in Philadelphia chromosome-positive chronic myelogenous leukaemia would provide suitable antigenic sites for binding and activating the apoptosis pathway. This could be carried out *ex vivo* as part of bone marrow transplantation treatment.

☐ CONCLUSION

Molecular biology has provided the means to identify the complete set of human genes [2,3] and, in turn, the immense potential for identifying new disease-associated proteins as potential drug targets. The invention of novel approaches to using these targets therapeutically is a major challenge and should see the advent of a new era in therapeutics with significant benefit for treatment of disease. The Trojan horse technological approach is just one of the new strategies opening up as a result of molecular biological discoveries. We hope to see these ideas translated into clinical practice in a short time.

REFERENCES

1   Rabbitts TH. Chromosomal translocations in human cancer. *Nature* 1994; **372**: 143–9.

2   Human genome issue. *Nature* 2001; **409**: 813–958.

3   Human genome issue. *Science* 2001; **291**: 1279–304.

4   Maniatis T, Kee SG, Efstratiadis A, Kafatos FC. Amplification and characterisation of a beta-globin gene synthesized in vitro. *Cell* 1976; **8**: 163–82.

5   Rabbitts TH. Bacterial cloning of plasmids carrying copies of rabbit globin messenger RNA. *Nature* 1976; **260**: 221–5.

6   Rougeon F, Kourilsky P, Mach B. Insertion of a rabbit beta-globin gene sequence into an *E. coli* plasmid. *Nucleic Acids Res* 1975; **2**: 2365–78.

7   Kawai J, Shinagawa A, Shibata K, Yoshino M, *et al.* Functional annotation of a full-length mouse cDNA collection. *Nature* 2001; **409**: 685–90.

8   Hunt RT, Nasmyth KA, Diffley J (ed). *Programmed proteolysis and the control of cell division.* Philosophical Transactions, vol 354. London: Royal Society, 1999.

9   Apoptosis special issue. *Science* 1998; **281**: 1305–26.

10 Tse E, Rabbitts TH. Intracellular antibody-caspase-mediated cell killing: an approach for application in cancer therapy. *Proc Natl Acad Sci USA* 2000; **97**: 12266–71.

11 Visintin M, Tse E, Axelson H, Rabbitts TH, Cattaneo A. Selection of antibodies for intracellular function using a two-hybrid *in vivo* system. *Proc Natl Acad Sci USA* 1999; **96**: 11723–8.

12 Tse E, Chung G, Rabbitts TH. Protocols for isolating antigen-specific intracellular antibody fragments as single chain Fv for use in mammalian cells. In: Turksen K (series ed). *Methods and Protocols.* Humana Press (in press).

Nephrology and transplantation medicine

New insights into the progression of chronic renal failure

Meguid El Nahas, Mohsen El Kossi and Hamdy Abo Zenah

An increasing number of patients in the UK require renal replacement therapy every year. This reflects the rise in the incidence of end-stage renal failure (ESRF) in the UK by about 50% over the last decade. The average annual incidence in the early 1990s of 50 new patients per million population has now increased to an estimated 100 new cases per million population, with an anticipated steady annual increase of around 8% [1]. This mirrors the trend worldwide of increased incidence and prevalence of ESRF, and has been attributed both to the considerable rise in the referral of diabetic patients with progressive renal diseases and also to the increasing number of elderly patients with ESRF [1]. It is therefore imperative to improve our understanding of the risk factors associated with progressive renal failure as well as of the mechanisms underlying the progressive scarring of the kidneys.

☐ RISK FACTORS

Many factors have been implicated in the progression of chronic renal failure (CRF) including:

- ☐ old age

- ☐ male gender

- ☐ patient genotype [2].

    Other risk factors are more amenable to intervention, such as:

- ☐ systemic hypertension

- ☐ proteinuria

- ☐ dyslipidaemia

- ☐ smoking [3]

- ☐ hyperglycaemia (in diabetes).

    The identification of these risk factors has prompted the study of their effects on renal function and structure. This review will discuss some of these effects, and describe interventions based on their manipulation which are aimed at slowing the progression of CRF.

Systemic hypertension

There is little doubt that systemic hypertension, both systolic and diastolic, is associated with an accelerated rate of progression of CRF in patients with diabetic and non-diabetic nephropathies [2,3]. In the Multiple Risk Factor Intervention Trial (MRFIT) of men in the USA, systemic hypertension was associated with a proportional increase in the incidence of ESRF. The rate of decline of renal function in patients with non-diabetic nephropathies has been estimated to be twice as fast in those with diastolic blood pressure above 90–95 mmHg. Similar observations have been made in patients with diabetic nephropathies [4].

Systemic hypertension can affect both the development and the progression of glomerulosclerosis and tubulointerstitial fibrosis (TIF). The transmission of systemic hypertension to the glomeruli leads to a rise in intraglomerular pressure, which in turn initiates glomerular sclerosis. Intraglomerular hypertension leads to injury of the glomerular capillary endothelial lining. This initiates a process within the glomeruli analogous to that observed in large vessels during the course of atherosclerosis [5]. In particular, injured endothelial cells activate the release of pro-inflammatory and procoagulant factors by the glomerulus which attracts inflammatory cells (including monocytes) to the glomerular capillaries and favours microthrombus formation. Infiltration of the glomeruli by activated monocytes/macrophages and the formation of lipid-laden foam cells will initiate interactions between these cells and resident glomerular cells leading to the activation and proliferation of the latter. These interactions depend on cell-to-cell contact as well as the communication between cells through the release of a wide range of cytokines, chemokines and growth factors. Activation of mesangial and epithelial cells leads to phenotypic changes associated with increased synthesis of extracellular matrix (ECM) which contributes to glomerulosclerosis [5].

Systemic hypertension can also contribute to the initiation and progression of TIF, initially through glomerular injury and the spilling over into the tubular lumen of various pro-inflammatory, mitogenic and fibrogenic mediators from damaged glomeruli [6]. An alternative mechanism is that the proteinuria and lipiduria associated with glomerular injury could initiate proximal tubular activation and interstitial inflammation and fibrosis (see sections on proteinuria and dyslipidaemia).

Finally, prolonged systemic hypertension leads to glomerulosclerosis as well as arteriolosclerosis, resulting in tubulointerstitial ischaemia and hypoxia. A mounting body of evidence suggests that chronic renal ischaemia and hypoxia can lead to the activation of profibrotic mediators within the renal interstitium. In particular, hypoxia stimulates both the proliferation of interstitial fibroblasts and also tubular epithelial cells to produce excessive amounts of ECM, while reducing their release of collagenolytic enzymes (matrix metalloproteinases) [7]. This microenvironment would favour the development of interstitial fibrosis.

Proteinuria

It has long been recognised that the severity of proteinuria correlates closely with the rate of progression of CRF [2,3]. In addition, clinical evidence suggests an additive effect of proteinuria and systemic hypertension on the rate of decline of CRF [2]. More recently, it has been postulated that the proteinuria may contribute to the progression of renal scarring [8]. It has been suggested that the increased traffic of proteinaceous macromolecules within the glomeruli would overload the mesangial phagocytic and clearance capacity, thus leading to mesangiosclerosis and ultimately to glomerulosclerosis. Proximal tubular cells in the interstitium can be stimulated to release pro-inflammatory cytokines and chemokines by incubation with albumin [8]. This, in turn, initiates interstitial inflammation which often precedes and contributes to the development of renal interstitial fibrosis [6,8]. Incubation with albumin can also stimulate the release of profibrotic growth factors from the proximal tubular cells, and even their release of ECM components.

Undoubtedly, such activation of tubular cells by proteins would generate a microenvironment conducive to the development of interstitial renal fibrosis. In addition, overloading tubular cells with albumin has been shown in an experimental rat model of albumin overload nephropathy to cause marked tubular apoptosis and atrophy [6]. The combination of tubular atrophy and interstitial fibrosis would contribute to the progression of CRF.

Dyslipidaemia

CRF is associated with dyslipidaemia, characterised by a rise in low-density lipoproteins (LDL) and, in particular, in intermediate-density lipoproteins, reflecting increased synthesis but also decreased lipoprotein lipase activity. Such dyslipidaemia has previously been implicated in the pathogenesis of the cardiovascular complications of CRF. The more recent suggestion that it may play a role in the progression of CRF and the associated renal scarring [9] was substantiated by the observation that the circulating levels of LDL and the associated apolipoprotein B correlate with the rate of decline in glomerular filtration rate (GFR) [9]. In addition, an additive effect has been described whereby raised LDL and proteinuria lead to an acceleration of CRF. Similar observations have been made in patients with progressive diabetic nephropathy [4].

Dyslipidaemia is likely to affect the pathogenesis of both glomerulosclerosis and TIF. Within the scarred glomerulus, the accumulation of LDL and oxidised LDL contributes to the formation of foam cells and to the overload and activation of mesangial cells. Consequently, lipid accumulation within scarred glomerular capillaries would have the same detrimental effect as is observed within atherosclerotic vessel walls. In the tubulointerstitium, tubular uptake of lipids and fatty acids in particular is thought to activate tubular cells to release chemokines, cytokines and growth factors [6]. Further, it has been suggested that the potential toxicity of albumin on tubular cells may depend on their fatty acid content. Consequently, lipiduria would initiate interstitial microinflammatory changes and contribute to the progression of tubulointerstitial scarring.

Smoking

The effects of smoking on the progression of CRF have been long overlooked. It has only recently come to the attention of nephrologists and diabetologists that heavy smoking may be detrimental to proteinuria and kidney function. In diabetic nephropathy, clinical evidence suggests that smoking exacerbates microalbuminuria and the progression of diabetic nephropathy [10]. In non-diabetic nephropathies, the incidence of ESRF appears to be proportional to the amount of cigarettes smoked [10]. In addition, heavy smoking may also have poor prognostic implications for the morbidity and mortality of patients on dialysis and recipients of a transplanted kidney.

It is likely that heavy smoking affects the kidneys in more than one way, including through an increase in systemic hypertension, proteinuria and dyslipidaemia.

☐ CLINICAL INTERVENTIONS

With the rise in the number of patients with CRF and ESRF, a clearer idea of the incriminated risk factors enables physicians and nephrologists to target them in an attempt to slow the progression of CRF (Table 1).

Table 1 Chronic renal failure intervention targets and recommendations.

Intervention target	Recommendation
Blood pressure	• <140/90 mmHg in patients with no or mild (<1 g/day) proteinuria
	• <130/80 mmHg in patients with moderate to severe proteinuria, including those with diabetic nephropathy
Proteinuria	• Reduce to <1 g/day. ACE inhibitors can be used in young individuals, those with mild to moderate renal insufficiency and those not at risk of renovascular disease. Dietary salt restriction may potentiate the antihypertensive and antiproteinuric effect of ACE inhibition
	• ACE inhibitors should be used with extreme care and close monitoring of serum creatinine and renal function in patients with serum creatinine levels >300 μmol/l, in the elderly and those at risk of renovascular disease
Dyslipidaemia	• Serum total cholesterol level should be reduced to <5 mmol/l
	• Triglycerides should be reduced to <4 mmol/l
Smoking	• Stopping smoking should be encouraged

ACE = angiotensin-converting enzyme.

Systemic hypertension and proteinuria

The first risk factor to target is systemic hypertension. There is little doubt that control of systemic hypertension slows the progression of diabetic and non-diabetic nephropathies [2–4,11]. However, recent clinical observations have raised questions about both the type of antihypertensive agents used in patients with progressive nephropathies and the target blood pressure. It is becoming increasingly evident that the control of hypertension alone without a concomitant reduction in the associated proteinuria may not be enough to slow progression [2]. Therefore, interventions should target both these factors.

With this in mind, and supported by animal experimentation, angiotensin-converting enzyme (ACE) inhibitors have been proposed as the antihypertensive agents of choice in patients with progressive CRF [11,12]. Clinical trials have shown them to be effective in controlling hypertension and reducing proteinuria, and it has been suggested that ACE inhibitors may have a therapeutic advantage over other antihypertensive agents in slowing the progression of CRF in diabetic and non-diabetic nephropathies [12]. This latter advantage is likely to be apparent at higher levels of blood pressure (mean arterial blood pressure (MAP) >100 mmHg; >140/90 mmHg) in proteinuric patients. At lower blood pressure levels, other antihypertensive agents would achieve the same results on both proteinuria and progression of CRF [12]; in other words, if blood pressure can be reduced to levels around 120/70–130/80 mmHg in patients with progressive diabetic and non-diabetic nephropathies, there will be a slowing of the decline in GFR regardless of the antihypertensive agent(s) used. Such target blood pressure levels are all the more relevant since the progression of CRF depends on the severity of proteinuria. Patients with heavy proteinuria (>3 g/day) require a more marked reduction in their blood pressure (MAP <92 mmHg; ca 120/70 mmHg) to achieve the same level of slow decline in renal function observed in non-proteinuric patients.

Dyslipidaemia

As with the control of hypertension, control of dyslipidaemia has a dual advantage in that it slows the progression of CRF and alleviates the severity of the cardiovascular complications that plague patients with ESRF. Although clinical trials on control of dyslipidaemia and CRF progression have not so far been conclusive, it is reasonable to adopt an interventionist approach in these patients at major risk of ischaemic heart disease who suffer a high cardiovascular morbidity and mortality. Dietary and pharmacological interventions should aim at controlling dyslipidaemia and also reducing total serum cholesterol levels to <5 mmol/l and triglycerides to <4 mmol/l.

Smoking

Patients with progressive CRF should be encouraged to stop smoking.

☐ RECOMMENDATIONS FOR THE MANAGEMENT OF PATIENTS WITH PROGRESSIVE CHRONIC RENAL FAILURE

Based on the above review, the following recommendations can be made:

1   All patients with serum creatinine above 150 μmol/l should be brought to the attention of a nephrologist.

2   Early detection of hypertension is warranted. This may justify 24-hour ambulatory blood pressure measurements to detect early changes and initiate therapy before there is end-organ damage. Early intervention would be more justifiable in patients with progressive nephropathies and/or proteinuria.

3   Measurement of 24-hour urinary protein excretion is warranted in all patients with impaired renal function. This would identify those with moderate (>1 g/day) or severe (>3 g/day) proteinuria who are at risk of progressive renal insufficiency, and allow their targeting for more zealous blood pressure control and interventions aimed at reducing proteinuria to less than 1g/day.

4   Lipid levels should be checked in patients with CRF. Early intervention minimises the long-term lipid-related cardiovascular complications and may be beneficial in reducing proteinuria and the progression of CRF.

5   Patients with CRF who smoke should be encouraged to stop.

REFERENCES

1   Roderick PJ, Ferris G, Feest TG. The provision of renal replacement therapy in adults in England and Wales: recent trends and future directions. *QJM* 1998; **91**: 581–7.

2   Locatelli F, Del Vecchio L. Natural history and factors affecting progression of human renal diseases. In: El Nahas AM (ed). *Mechanisms and Clinical Management of Chronic Renal Failure.* Oxford: Oxford University Press, 2000: 20–79.

3   El Nahas AM, Tamimi N. The progression of chronic renal failure: a harmful quarter. *QJM* 1999; **92**: 421–4.

4   Mogensen C-E. Diabetic nephropathy: natural history and management. In: El Nahas AM (ed). *Mechanisms and Clinical Management of Chronic Renal Failure.* Oxford: Oxford University Press, 2000: 211–40.

5   Dworkin LD, Weir MR. Hypertension in parenchymal renal disease: role in progression. In: El Nahas AM (ed). *Mechanisms and Clinical Management of Chronic Renal Failure.* Oxford: Oxford University Press, 2000: 173–210.

6   Jernigan SM, Eddy AA. Experimental insights into the mechanisms of tubulointerstitial scarring. In: El Nahas AM (ed). *Mechanisms and Clinical Management of Chronic Renal Failure.* Oxford: Oxford University Press, 2000: 104–45.

7   Norman JT, Clark IM, Garcia PL. Hypoxia promotes fibrogenesis in human renal fibroblasts. *Kidney Int* 2000; **58**: 2351–66.

8   Harris KPG. Proteinuria: implications for progression and management. In: El Nahas AM (ed). *Mechanisms and Clinical Management of Chronic Renal Failure.* Oxford: Oxford University Press, 2000: 146–72.

9   Attman PO. Progression of renal failure and lipids – is there evidence for a link in humans? *Nephrol Dial Transplant* 1998; **13**: 545–7.

10   Orth SR, Stockmann A, Conradt C, Ritz E, *et al.* Smoking as a risk factor for end-stage renal failure in men with primary renal disease. *Kidney Int* 1998; **54**: 926–31.

11   Coles GA, El Nahas AM. Clinical interventions in chronic renal failure. In: El Nahas AM (ed). *Mechanisms and Clinical Management of Chronic Renal Failure.* Oxford: Oxford University Press, 2000: 401–23.

12   Tamimi N, El Nahas AM. Angiotensin-converting enzyme inhibition: facts and fiction. Review. *Nephron* 2000; **84**: 299–304.

☐ SELF-ASSESSMENT QUESTIONS

1   The annual incidence of end-stage renal failure (ESRF) in the UK is currently around:
    (a) 10 per million population (pmp)
    (b) 40 pmp
    (c) 60 pmp
    (d) 100 pmp

2   The most common cause of ESRF in the UK is:
    (a) Diabetic nephropathy
    (b) Small kidneys of unknown aetiology
    (c) Polycystic kidney disease
    (d) Chronic glomerulonephritis
    (e) Essential hypertension

3   The following risk factors are associated with progressive chronic renal failure (CRF):
    (a) Female gender
    (b) Old age
    (c) Hypertriglyceridaemia
    (d) Smoking
    (e) Systemic hypertension

4   The management of CRF involves:
    (a) Control of systemic hypertension
    (b) Reduction of proteinuria
    (c) A high protein diet
    (d) Correction of metabolic acidosis
    (e) Correction of hypocalcaemia

5   The effect of angiotensin II on the kidney involves:
    (a) Haemodynamic effects
    (b) Trophic effects
    (c) A profibrotic influence
    (d) A kaliuretic effect
    (e) Proteinuric effects

ANSWERS

1a False	2a False	3a False	4a True	5a True
b False	b False	b True	b True	b True
c False	c False	c False	c False	c True
d True	d True	d True	d True	d False
	e False	e True	e True	e True

Renal vasculitis

David Jayne

□ INTRODUCTION

The hallmark of renal vasculitis is a focal necrotising glomerulonephritis usually associated with crescent formation and renal impairment. This pattern occurs in the context of primary and secondary vasculitic syndromes, of which those associated with anti-neutrophil cytoplasm autoantibodies (ANCA) are the most frequent. Renal vasculitis has an annual incidence of 10–15 per million and accounts for 5% of the cases of end-stage renal failure (ESRF). There is an approximately equal sex distribution and the incidence rises with age (it is most common in those over 60 years). It has a two-year mortality of 25%, and frequent chronic morbidity and incapacity due to ESRF, relapsing vasculitis or the adverse effects of therapy. These outcomes are partly preventable because immunosuppressive therapy is effective in controlling vasculitis, but results have been impeded by confusion over classification, diagnostic delay, a lack of an evidence base for therapeutic decisions and the relative rarity of this disease.

□ CLASSIFICATION

The histological definition of vasculitis requires leukocyte infiltration and fibrinoid necrosis of the vessel wall, accompanied by thrombotic occlusion of the vessel lumen with distal infarction. The glomerulus is a differentiated capillary bed. Capillaritis with focal infarction is the typical vasculitic lesion, but there may also be extraglomerular involvement of larger vessels.

Primary vasculitis syndromes are defined according to the predominant size of vessel involved and the association of the syndrome with circulating ANCA (Table 1) [1,2]. The histological appearance, response to treatment and outcome of renal vasculitis in syndromes predominantly involving small vessels usually associated with ANCA are similar. These syndromes have been grouped under the term 'ANCA-associated vasculitis'.

Most cases of *rapidly progressive glomerulonephritis* can be attributed to one of the syndromes associated with renal vasculitis (Table 2). The light microscopic appearance of the glomerulus in the different vasculitic syndromes is often similar, but patients may be classified according to the immunofluorescence and serological findings which reflect the underlying pathogenesis (Table 3). Polyarteritis nodosa, giant cell arteritis and Takayasu's arteritis may involve the renal arteries or segmental branches, causing hypertension and renal infarction, but glomerular lesions are absent and ANCA is negative [1].

Table 1 Classification of primary vasculitic syndromes.

Size of predominant vessel involvement	'ANCA-associated'*	'ANCA-negative'
Small 'microscopic'	Wegener's granulomatosis Microscopic polyangiitis (renal-limited vasculitis)	Henoch-Schönlein purpura Cryoglobulinaemic vasculitis Anti-glomerular basement membrane disease
Medium (muscular arteries)	Churg-Strauss angiitis	Polyarteritis nodosa Kawasaki disease
Large		Giant cell arteritis Takayasu's arteritis

*Usually ANCA-positive.

Table 2 Clinico-pathological syndromes associated with renal vasculitis in the London audit 1995–2000.

Vasculitis subclassification	No.	%
Primary, systemic, small vessel, pauci-immune:	(256)	(82)
Wegener's granulomatosis	92	29
Microscopic polyangiitis	120	38
Renal-limited vasculitis	33	11
Churg-Strauss angiitis	11	4
Primary, systemic, small vessel, immune-complex:	(50)	(16)
Henoch-Schönlein purpura	25	8
Cryoglobulinaemia	7	2
Anti-glomerular basement membrane disease	18	6
Primary, systemic, medium vessel vasculitis:		
Polyarteritis nodosa	17	6
Total	*313*	*100*

Table 3 Classification of rapidly progressive glomerulonephritis according to renal immunofluorescence and serology.

Type	Renal immunofluorescence	Serology	Diagnosis
I	Linear	anti-GBM	anti-GBM disease
II	Granular	ANA Low C3, C4	SLE, HSP Post-infectious cryoglobulinaemia
III	Pauci-immune	ANCA	Vasculitis

ANA = anti-nuclear antibodies; ANCA = anti-neutrophil cytoplasm autoantibodies; GBM = glomerular basement membrane; HSP = Henoch-Schönlein purpura; SLE = systemic lupus erythematosus.

☐ PATHOGENESIS

No consistent major histocompatibility complex associations have been found in primary small vessel vasculitides. α1-anti-trypsin deficient phenotypes are associated with more aggressive proteinase 3 (PR3)-ANCA-associated vasculitis and weaker associations with Fc and complement alleles have been reported [3]. A mouse strain with a high incidence of spontaneous myeloperoxidase (MPO)-ANCA-associated renal vasculitis has been developed, and it is possible that stronger genetic linkages await discovery.

These syndromes are rarely associated with malignancy, chronic infections (including endocarditis and bronchiectasis) and drugs (hydralazine, propyl thiouracil and penicillamine). A role of ANCA in the pathogenesis of renal and pulmonary capillaritis is supported by their close association with circulating ANCA and weaker associations with ANCA isotype and titre. ANCA induce degranulation of tumour necrosis factor (TNF)-primed neutrophils *in vitro* and promote neutrophil-dependent endothelial cytotoxicity. Experimental renal vasculitis also occurs in animals immunised with ANCA antigens [4,5]. Other vasculitic manifestations, in particular upper respiratory tract involvement in Wegener's granulomatosis, often occur in the absence of ANCA. T cell clones derived from Wegener's biopsies express a T helper 1 cytokine phenotype and disease activity is related to soluble interleukin (IL)-2 receptor levels. Treatments targeting T cells, including cyclosporin and anti-thymocyte globulin, are effective.

The macrophage is a dominant cell type in the glomerulus in renal vasculitis and macrophage proliferation contributes to crescent formation. Levels of urinary macrophage-derived chemokines, such as monocyte chemotactic peptide-1, correlate with disease activity. Macrophages also contain ANCA antigens, but the extent to which macrophage activation is ANCA-dependent has not been determined.

☐ DIAGNOSIS

The onset of renal vasculitis is insidious, with no specific features pointing to renal involvement. Patients have typically been unwell with constitutional symptoms, fatigue, malaise, fevers, weight loss and polymyalgia for several months before renal vasculitis is diagnosed. Common signs of extrarenal vasculitis include flitting arthritis, a purpuric rash, upper respiratory tract disease, sinusitis, deafness, epistaxis and episcleritis. Cough with haemoptysis points to pulmonary involvement. Microscopic haematuria is always present and red cell casts are a strong pointer to a severe glomerulonephritis. Proteinuria has little diagnostic significance in pauci-immune renal vasculitis but may be a presenting feature in Henoch-Schönlein purpura and cryoglobulinaemia. ANCA are present in over 90% of renal vasculitis occurring in the context of a pauci-immune, primary, systemic small vessel vasculitis, but the absence of ANCA does not exclude the diagnosis [6]. The specificity of the ANCA indirect immunofluorescence assay is enhanced by PR3-ANCA and MPO-ANCA enzyme-linked immunoadsorbent assays (ELISAs). Positive results are classified as cytoplasmic (C)-ANCA or peri-nuclear (P)-ANCA.

The combination of C-ANCA/PR3-ANCA or P-ANCA/MPO-ANCA positivity has a 95% specificity for renal vasculitis in the appropriate clinical setting [6].

A renal biopsy remains fundamental to the diagnosis, although this should not delay the onset of treatment – in fact, some have argued it is unnecessary if the ANCA is positive. Histology gives some prognostic information, the proportion of normal glomeruli being most strongly correlated with outcome [7].

☐ TREATMENT

Systemic vasculitis with renal involvement was fatal before the availability of dialysis and immunosuppressive therapy. Survival was improved by corticosteroids in the 1950s, but full control of vasculitis required the addition of cytotoxic agents. Cyclophosphamide has become the most popular of these. However, the long-term use of cyclophosphamide has led to a high incidence of bladder and lympho-proliferative malignancies necessitating alternative approaches. A collaborative group, the European Vasculitis Study (EUVAS) Group, reviewed treatment protocols during the 1990s and found a wide variation in the dosing and duration of both cyclophosphamide and corticosteroids [2]. EUVAS developed the following strategy towards rational therapy of vasculitis (Table 4):

1   Subgrouping of patients at diagnosis according to disease extent and severity.

2   High-dose therapy for induction remission and long-term low-dose therapy to maintain remission.

3   Consensus agreement on 'gold standard' regimens.

4   Randomised trials designed to test the best alternative to the standard regimens.

Early systemic vasculitis

For patients with early systemic disease, methotrexate was compared to cyclo-phosphamide for remission induction in the NOn-Renal wegener's Alternative treatment with Methotrexate (NORAM) trial [2]. Preliminary results showed similar remission rates for both limbs at three months (60%) and six months (85%). In view of its relative safety, methotrexate appears a better induction agent for this subgroup, but further data from the NORAM trial on subsequent relapse rates are awaited.

Generalised vasculitis

The generalised subgroup was defined by threatened vital organ function, usually renal, and cyclophosphamide was considered an essential component of initial therapy. The CYClophosphamide or AZAthioprine for REMission (CYCAZAREM) trial in 145 such patients compared a standard regimen of oral cyclophosphamide daily for 12 months with switching to azathioprine at the time of

Table 4 Subgrouping of primary systemic vasculitis at presentation, consensus standard and alternative regimens, and randomised trials designed by the European Vasculitis Study Group (EUVAS).

Clinical subgroup	Constitutional symptoms	Typical ANCA status	Threatened vital organ function	Serum creatinine (µmol/l)	Therapy		
					Standard	Alternative	EUVAS trial
Localised	No	Negative	No	<120			
Early systemic	Yes	Positive or negative	No	<120	CYC + PRED	MTX + PRED	NORAM
Generalised	Yes	Positive	Yes	<500	CYC + PRED 12 months	Switch to AZA at remission	CYCAZAREM
Severe	Yes	Positive	Organ failure	>500	iv methyl prednisolone	Plasma exchange	MEPEX
Refractory	Yes	Positive or negative	Yes	Any level			

Trials: CYCAZAREM = CYClophosphamide or AZAthioprine for REMission; MEPEX = MEthylprednisolone or Plasma EXchange; NORAM = NOn-Renal wegener's Alternative treatment with Methotrexate.

(ANCA = anti-neutrophil cytoplasm autoantibodies; AZA = azathioprine; CYC = cyclophosphamide; iv = intravenous; MTX = methotrexate; PRED = prednisolone).

remission. This trial showed that the primary end-point (relapse rate) was the same in both limbs (Fig. 1) [2]. Remission was achieved in 93% by six months, only 2% progressed to ESRF during the 18 months of the trial, and the overall mortality was 7%. However, there were severe adverse effects in more than 25% of the patients, infection associated with neutropenia being most frequent. Although effective at suppressing vasculitis activity, patient morbidity, as assessed by the Short Form 36 questionnaire, was considerable during the remission phase of the trial.

Contributory factors to chronic morbidity in vasculitis include:

☐   subclinical disease activity

☐   the accumulation of non-healing scars due to the disease or its treatment

☐   adverse effects of ongoing treatment.

Severe renal disease

Up to 50% of patients with renal vasculitis present with a creatinine above 500 μmol/l in imminent need of dialysis. Additional therapy aims to arrest vasculitis

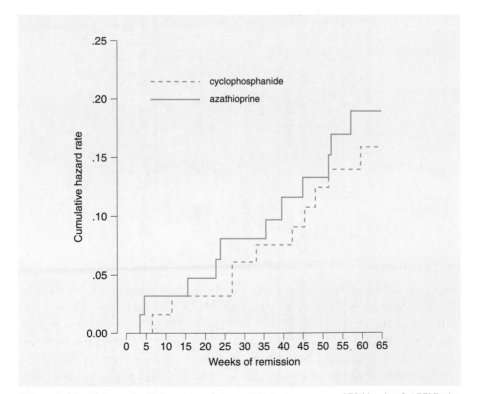

Fig. 1 Cumulative hazard rate for relapse in the CYClophosphamide or AZAthioprine for REMission (CYCAZAREM) trial for remission therapy with cyclophosphamide or azathioprine (reproduced, with permission, from [2]).

more quickly and optimise the chances of renal recovery. The ongoing Methylprednisolone or Plasma Exchange (MEPEX) trial is comparing the rate of renal recovery with either the addition of 3 g of intravenous (iv) methyl prednisolone or seven plasma exchanges [2].

A rationale for plasma exchange developed from the treatment of anti-glomerular basement membrane disease and, with the discovery of ANCA, has demanded renewed attention. Existing literature is weak but points to a possible benefit of plasma exchange for this subgroup (Table 5). A further potential indication for plasma exchange in vasculitis is in diffuse pulmonary haemorrhage, the pulmonary renal syndrome, where the histology is an alveolar capillaritis analogous to the glomerular lesion, and also closely associated with ANCA. It carries a high mortality, and survival depends on rapid control of alveolar haemorrhage.

Table 5 Comparison of renal recovery with and without plasma exchange in patients with primary, systemic, pauci-immune, small vessel vasculitis and renal failure: published studies and unpublished experience (Jayne).

| Ref. | No. of patients | Plasma exchange | |
		Received	Not received
8	12	5/8	3/4
9	19	10/11	3/8
10	11	3/4	2/7
11	20	9/11	5/9
12	8	4/6	1/2
13	22	6/12	2/10
Jayne*	26	9/16	4/10
Total	88	46/68 (67%)	20/50 (40%)

* unpublished data.

Remission therapy

Relapse occurs in up to 50% of patients and is more common in patients with Wegener's granulomatosis and with PR3-ANCA positivity. In addition to methotrexate and azathioprine, other drugs used for the maintenance of remission include mycophenolate mofetil, cyclosporin, tacrolimus and leflunomide. The antibiotic sulfamethoxazole/trimethoprim reduces relapse rates in Wegener's granulomatosis, probably by reducing the frequency of respiratory tract infections which promote relapse. Nasal carriage of *Staphylococcus aureus* is associated with relapse, and the role of bacterial eradication with topical mupirocin is the subject of a current study [14].

The optimal duration of remission therapy after renal vasculitis has not been determined. A further EUVAS trial is comparing withdrawal of azathioprine and prednisolone at 24 months versus continuing for 48 months [14].

Serological monitoring during remission includes erythrocyte sedimentation rate, C-reactive protein and ANCA levels. The first two markers are non-specific, being influenced by infection and other factors, while there is a complex relationship between ANCA and disease activity. The conversion of a negative to a positive ANCA during remission or sustained rises in ANCA are associated with subsequent disease relapse in about 75% of cases. Published reports show conflicting results because of variation in immunosuppressive therapies, patient subgroups and type of ANCA assay. Also, the interassay variability of ANCA assays is high, making interpretation of minor changes in titre or binding level difficult. Treatment should not be dictated by ANCA, but *changes* in ANCA should encourage investigation for signs of vasculitis activity and closer supervision. It is not clear whether or not treatment should be withdrawn in the face of a positive ANCA.

Alternative treatments

Administration of cyclophosphamide by iv pulses as opposed to daily oral therapy has been the focus of three randomised trials, summarised in a recent meta-analysis [15]. There was equal efficacy in terms of remission and prevention of renal failure. Although neutropenia and infections were less with the iv route, there was a higher relapse rate.

Immunomodulation with iv immunoglobulin (Ig) has been effective in certain cases because it interacts with ANCA to inhibit binding to ANCA antigens and prevent ANCA-induced neutrophil activation. A placebo-controlled trial demonstrated an improvement in vasculitic activity in 15 of 17 cases of refractory vasculitis [16]. The use of iv Ig is complicated by expense and nephrotoxicity. Lymphocyte depletion, either with anti-thymocyte globulin or CAMPATH-1H (anti-CD52), has led to sustained treatment-free remissions. There has also been recent experience with autologous stem cell transplantation [17].

Dialysis and transplantation

Prevention of the relapses that occur on dialysis is complicated by the increased infective risk of immunosuppression in this subgroup. Renal transplantation reduces the vasculitic relapse rate, presumably due to the concurrent anti-rejection therapy, and recurrence of vasculitis in the graft is rare. ANCA positivity at the time of transplantation is not a barrier to a successful outcome.

☐ CONCLUSIONS

The discovery of ANCA and the international consensus on vasculitis classification have been major advances both to the researcher and the clinician. In the future, determination of the aetiology will require revision of the classification system, and diagnostic criteria need to be developed and tested.

Recent collaborative studies have developed tools for the assessment of disease activity and damage which have improved the quality of prospective trials [18]. A European consensus on treatment regimens is developing with the availability of the results of large-scale trials. These indicate the high efficacy of remission induction protocols, but also their toxicity and the frequency of relapse when immunosuppressive doses are reduced.

These issues have been highlighted by the results of an audit of renal vasculitis in London which found important determinants of survival to be:

☐   age over 60 years

☐   presenting creatinine level

☐   ESRF

☐   neutropenia-associated sepsis.

During the five-year follow-up of this audit, 50% of surviving patients relapsed. The challenge of future research is to design safer induction regimens and to improve renal function rescue. Newer biological drugs, including TNF and IL-1 blockade, have exciting potential in this area. Of equal importance is the need for patients to be referred early, before renal failure develops, when the outcomes are generally favourable.

REFERENCES

1   Jennette JC, Falk RJ, Andrassy K, Bacon PA, *et al.* Nomenclature of systemic vasculitides. Proposal of an international consensus conference. Review. *Arthritis Rheum* 1994; **37**: 187–92.

2   European therapeutic trials in ANCA-associated systemic vasculitis: disease scoring, consensus regimens and proposed clinical trials. Review. European Community Study Group on Clinical Trials in Systemic Vasculitis ECSYSVASTRIAL. *Clin Exp Immunol* 1995; **101**(Suppl 1): 29–34.

3   Griffith ME, Lovegrove JU, Gaskin G, Whitehouse DB, Pusey CD. C-antineutrophil cytoplasmic antibody positivity in vasculitis patients is associated with the Z allele of alpha-1-antitrypsin, and P-antineutrophil cytoplasmic antibody positivity with the S allele. *Nephrol Dial Transplant* 1996; **11**: 438–43.

4   Brouwer E, Huitema MG, Klok PA, de Weerd H, *et al.* Antimyeloperoxidase-associated proliferative glomerulonephritis: an animal model. *J Exp Med* 1993; **177**: 905–14.

5   Harper L, Savage CO. Pathogenesis of ANCA-associated systemic vasculitis. Review. *J Pathol* 2000; **190**: 349–59.

6   Hagen EC, Daha MR, Hermans J, Andrassy K, *et al.* Diagnostic value of standardized assays for anti-neutrophil cytoplasmic antibodies in idiopathic systemic vasculitis. EC/BCR Project for ANCA Assay Standardization. *Kidney Int* 1998; **53**: 743–53.

7   Hogan SL, Nachman PH, Wilkman AS, Jennette JC, Falk RJ. Prognostic markers in patients with antineutrophil cytoplasmic autoantibody-associated microscopic polyangiitis and glomerulonephritis. *J Am Soc Nephrol* 1996; **7**: 23–32.

8   Glockner WM, Sieberth HG, Wichmann HE, Backes E, *et al.* Plasma exchange and immunosuppression in rapidly progressive glomerulonephritis: a controlled, multi-center study. *Clin Nephrol* 1988; **29**: 1–8.

9   Pusey CD, Rees AJ, Evans DJ, Peters DK, Lockwood CM. Plasma exchange in focal necrotizing glomerulonephritis without anti-GBM antibodies. *Kidney Int* 1991; **40**: 757–63.

10   Cole E, Cattran D, Magil A, Greenwood C, *et al.* A prospective randomized trial of plasma exchange as additive therapy in idiopathic crescentic glomerulonephritis. The Canadian Apheresis Study Group. *Am J Kidney Dis* 1992; 20: 261-9.

11   Levy JB, Winearls CG. Rapidly progressive glomerulonephritis: what should be first-line therapy? Review. *Nephron* 1994; 67: 402-7.

12   Guillevin L, Cevallos R, Durand-Gasselin B, Lhote F, *et al.* Treatment of glomerulonephritis in microscopic polyangiitis and Churg-Strauss syndrome. Indications of plasma exchanges, meta-analysis of 2 randomized studies on 140 patients, 32 with glomerulonephritis. *Ann Med Interne (Paris)* 1997; 148: 198–204.

13   Haubitz M, Schellong S, Gobel U, Schurek HJ, *et al.* Intravenous pulse administration of cyclophosphamide versus daily oral treatment in patients with antineutrophil cytoplasmic antibody-associated vasculitis and renal involvement: a prospective, randomized study. *Arthritis Rheum* 1998; 41: 1835–44.

14   Jayne DR, Rasmussen N. Treatment of antineutrophil cytoplasm autoantibody-associated systemic vasculitis: initiatives of the European Community Systemic Vasculitis Clinical Trials Study Group. Review. *Mayo Clin Proc* 1997; 72: 737–47.

15   Groot KD, Adu D, Savage CO. The value of pulse cyclophosphamide in ANCA-associated vasculitis: meta-analysis and critical review. *Nephrol Dial Transplant* 2001; 16: 2018–27.

16   Jayne DR, Chapel H, Adu D, Misbah S, *et al.* Intravenous immunoglobulin for ANCA-associated systemic vasculitis with persistent disease activity. *QJM* 2000; 93: 433–9.

17   Lockwood CM, Thiru S, Isaacs JD, Hale G, Waldmann H. Long-term remission of intractable systemic vasculitis with monoclonal antibody therapy. *Lancet* 1993; 341: 1620–2.

18   Luqmani RA, Exley AR, Kitas GD, Bacon PA. Disease assessment and management of the vasculitides. Review. *Baillières Clin Rheumatol* 1997; 11: 423–46.

☐ SELF ASSESSMENT QUESTIONS

1   Concerning serological tests for vasculitis:
   (a) A negative test for anti-neutrophil cytoplasm autoantibodies (ANCA) excludes the diagnosis of vasculitis
   (b) ANCA are usually associated with immune complex deposition in the kidney
   (c) Monitoring ANCA levels is of value during the remission phase of vasculitis
   (d) ANCA levels are unaffected by immunosuppressive therapy
   (e) Myeloperoxidase (MPO)-ANCA can occur in Wegener's granulomatosis

2   In the histological evaluation of renal vasculitis:
   (a) Diagnosis requires the presence of extraglomerular vasculitis
   (b) Renal vasculitis is subclassified according to light microscopic findings
   (c) Linear deposition of immunoglobulin G is found in Henoch-Schönlein purpura
   (d) Glomerular lesions are frequent in polyarteritis nodosa
   (e) Foci of fibrinoid necrosis are the most common glomerular abnormalities

3   The prognosis of renal vasculitis:
   (a) Is related to age at diagnosis
   (b) The development of end-stage renal failure (ESRF) is unrelated to serum creatinine at diagnosis
   (c) Immunosuppressive therapy has improved rates of patient survival
   (d) Mortality at two years is approximately 25%
   (e) Proteinase 3-ANCA has a higher rate of ESRF than MPO-ANCA

4   Concerning immunosuppressive therapy in vasculitis:
(a) Intravenous pulse cyclophosphamide (CYC) is clearly superior to daily oral administration
(b) CYC can be safely withdrawn at the time of remission
(c) The optimal duration of remission therapy with azathioprine is unknown
(d) Methotrexate is ineffective in primary systemic vasculitis
(e) Plasma exchange has no place in the management of renal vasculitis associated with ANCA

5   Concerning the toxicity of immunosuppressive therapy in vasculitis:
(a) CYC is associated with both bladder and lymphoproliferative malignancies
(b) Azathioprine has no effect on the rate of subsequent malignancy
(c) Drug toxicity contributes to the mortality of vasculitis
(d) An important aim of CYC therapy is to induce neutropenia
(e) Corticosteroid side effects are no longer a problem with current regimens

ANSWERS

1a False	2a False	3a True	4a False	5a True
b False	b False	b False	b True	b False
c True	c False	c True	c True	c True
d False	d False	d True	d False	d False
e True	e True	e False	e False	e False

Strategies for increasing kidney transplantation using non-heart beating and living donors

Michael Nicholson

□ INTRODUCTION

Kidney transplant programmes around the world continue to be limited by a shortage of suitable donor organs. At the time of writing, more than 5,000 patients are awaiting a kidney transplant in the UK and Ireland. As the transplant rate has stabilised between 1,500 and 1,700 transplants a year, this waiting list increases annually. Powerful and sustained demographic changes underlie these statistics. The annual death rate from both road traffic accidents and intracerebral haemorrhage has decreased significantly over the last 20 years due to improvements in road safety and the treatment of hypertension, respectively. This has led to a contraction of the available pool of brain-stem dead, heart-beating donors (HBDs) from intensive care units (ICUs), a trend unlikely to change significantly in the coming years. Whilst current efforts to maintain the transplant rate from brain-stem dead HBDs should continue, it is important that the transplant community looks to develop transplantation from other donor sources. The two currently available additional sources of transplant kidneys are non-heart beating donors (NHBD) and living donors (LD).

This chapter will first examine the use of NHBD kidneys for transplantation [1] and then explore the potential role of laparoscopic donor nephrectomy, the most recent innovation in LD kidney transplantation [2]. The Leicester experience of these techniques will be used to illustrate the opportunities and challenges they provide.

□ NON-HEART BEATING DONOR TRANSPLANTATION

Suitable patients who die suddenly as a result of irreversible cardiorespiratory arrest can be considered as potential NHBDs (for criteria of eligibility see below). In this situation, death is diagnosed using cardiac criteria rather than the brain-stem criteria used in ICU-based HBDs. Kidney transplantation using organs taken from NHBDs is feasible because the human kidney can recover function following a considerable period of warm ischaemic anoxic damage. The exact limits of recoverable renal damage following warm ischaemia are not known in man, but it is clear from NHBD data that human kidneys can be successfully transplanted after periods of up to 40 minutes of warm ischaemia.

Technical aspects

The ischaemic damage suffered by NHBD kidneys is limited by performing a rapid *in situ* cooling of the kidneys. This may be achieved by a number of techniques, the simplest being the use of a double balloon, triple lumen catheter placed into the aorta via a femoral artery cut down in the groin. If the catheter is placed correctly, with the lower balloon jammed at the aortic bifurcation and the upper balloon positioned above the renal arteries, the renal circulation is effectively isolated and the kidneys can be flushed with preservation fluid held at 4°C. The blood is vented through a catheter placed in the inferior vena cava via the femoral vein in the groin.

This method of *in situ* perfusion has three important effects:

1   It washes the blood out of the kidneys, thus preventing intrarenal thrombosis.

2   The kidneys are cooled rapidly to a temperature (<10°C) at which the Na+K+ pump is inhibited and renal tubular oxygen consumption is dramatically decreased.

3   The interstitial spaces of the kidney are filled with hypertonic preservation fluid, which prevents cell death caused by intracellular swelling.

A plain X-ray can be used to check the position of the intra-aortic catheter if the balloons are filled with contrast medium. A total of 10–20 litres of preservation fluid is commonly used to maintain *in situ* renal perfusion prior to organ retrieval.

Other methods of *in situ* renal cooling include the use of intraperitoneal catheters and extracorporeal total body cooling using a simple cardiopulmonary bypass circuit.

After obtaining consent from relatives, the NHBD can be moved to an operating theatre and a bilateral donor nephrectomy performed using standard techniques. The retrieved kidneys can be held in simple static ice storage prior to transplantation. However, accumulating evidence suggests that better results are obtained after preservation by pulsatile machine perfusion, and many centres are adopting this method.

NHBD kidneys are transplanted using standard surgical techniques. A number of immunosuppressive strategies have been employed. It has been common practice to limit early exposure to the nephrotoxic calcineurin inhibitors by using either antibody induction therapy (avoiding calcineurin inhibitors altogether) or low doses of these drugs in triple therapy combinations. In Leicester, the currently favoured protocol is low-dose tacrolimus plus mycophenolate mofetil and prednisolone.

Results

The Leicester transplant programme employs NHBD, HBD and LD kidneys, allowing a comparison of the results obtained with these three different types of donor [3]. The NHBD programme began in 1992. Over the subsequent eight-year period, 350 kidney transplants were performed, 77 (22%) of which used kidneys from NHBDs, 224 (64%) from HBDs and 49 (14%) from LDs (Fig. 1).

Source of kidneys

The majority of the NHBDs came from uncontrolled donors in whom there was a sudden and unexpected cardiac arrest. The main source was patients dying of cardiorespiratory arrest immediately before or shortly after admission to the accident and emergency department. A small number of patients who died in the general medical wards as a result of catastrophic intracranial haemorrhage eventually became NHBDs.

Criteria for acceptability

The criteria for acceptable NHBD in Leicester includes an upper age limit of 60 years and a warm ischaemic time limit of 40 minutes. This warm time refers only to the period of absolute circulatory arrest and excludes periods during which external

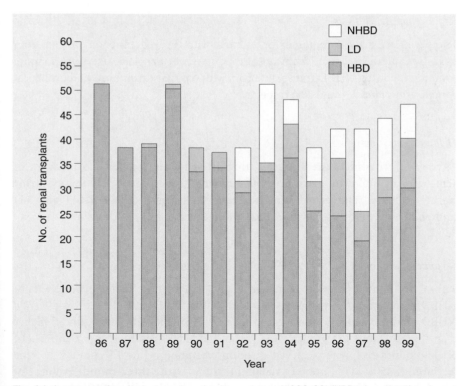

Fig. 1 Leicester renal transplant numbers by donor source (1986–99) (HBD= heart-beating donor; LD = living donor; NHBD = non-heart beating donor).

cardiac massage is being performed. In view of the uncontrolled nature of the donation, the average time of ischaemic damage prior to *in situ* cooling was 25 minutes (range 5–53 min). The detrimental nature of this initial ischaemic insult is reflected in the early results of NHBD transplantation with significantly higher levels of both primary non-function and delayed graft function in comparison to HBD and LD kidneys (Table 1).

Table 1 Early graft function rates.

	NHBD (n=77)		HBD (n=224)		LD (n=49)	
	No.	%	No.	%	No.	%
Primary non-function	7	9	6	3	1	2
Delayed graft function	65	84	47	21	2	4
Initial function	5	7	171	76	46	94

HBD= heart-beating donor; LD = living donor; NHBD = non-heart beating donor.

Requirement for dialysis

The period of dialysis required for kidneys with delayed function ranged from 4–52 days (mean 19 days). Technical complications of transplantation were no more common following NHBD transplantation, with vascular thrombosis and urological complication rates 1% and 3%, respectively.

Delayed graft function

Although there is literature to suggest that delayed graft function is a predictor of acute rejection following renal transplantation, this does not appear to be true for NHBD kidneys. The acute rejection rates following NHBD, HBD and LD transplantation were 29%, 33% and 47%, respectively.

Serum creatinine

Serum creatinine levels were consistently and significantly higher in recipients of NHBD kidneys than in recipients of kidneys from HBD and LD sources. Overall, NHBD kidneys yielded serum creatinine levels approximately 30–50 μmol/l higher than the HBD and LD groups. Analysis of individual results shows that 55% of NHBD kidney recipients achieved a serum creatinine below 150 μmol/l, but the remaining 45% had poorer renal function with three-month values of 200–330 μmol/l. This suggests that, whilst they are viable, some NHBD kidneys are transplanted with a limited number of functioning glomeruli.

Allograft survival rates

Perhaps surprisingly, the decrement in early renal function seen with NHBD kidney transplants does not seem to be reflected in poor allograft survival rates. Allograft survival following NHBD transplantation has been demonstrated in a number of notable studies to be similar to that achieved with conventional HBD cadaveric kidneys [4–6]. This finding is supported by the Leicester analysis (Fig. 2) in which the NHBD kidney five-year survival results are even as good as those from LD. In view of such findings, it is difficult to support the fairly widespread belief that the vast majority of NHBDs provide organs of poor quality – an argument that has fuelled the reluctance to accept NHBD kidney transplantation.

Summary

NHBD kidneys can make a significant contribution to the total number of renal transplants performed. In Leicester, NHBD kidneys account for more than 20% of the transplant programme, and similar levels of activity have been described in the Netherlands [7]. Projections by Terasaki's group [8] suggest that the potential pool

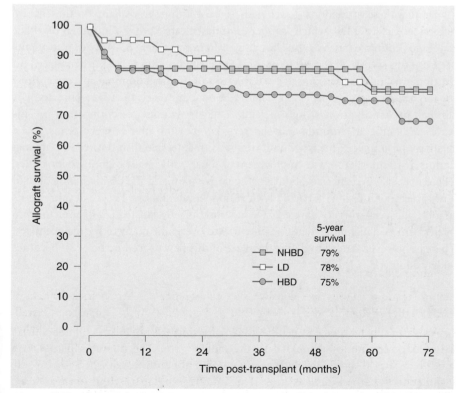

Fig. 2 Graft survival of kidney transplants from heart-beating (HBD), non-heart beating (NHBD) and live donors (LD).

of NHBDs is so large that maximal exploitation of this donor source could bridge the gap between supply and demand in renal transplantation.

It is becoming increasingly clear that NHBD kidney transplants can yield acceptable results, at least in the medium term. Nevertheless, this donor source has not been extensively used in the UK and Ireland where it has tended to be supported by only a small number of enthusiasts. The establishment and maintenance of a successful NHBD programme is highly labour intensive for transplant co-ordinators and surgeons [9], which is likely to be an important factor in preventing this form of transplantation becoming more widely accepted. The solution is to provide more resources to establish a number of pilot programmes to see if the good results obtained by some groups can be achieved more generally.

☐ LAPAROSCOPIC LIVE NEPHRECTOMY FOR RENAL TRANSPLANTATION

Kidney transplantation from LDs has many advantages, including:

- ☐ short ischaemic times
- ☐ excellent initial graft function
- ☐ the best long-term graft survival data.

Despite these attractions, fewer than 15% of kidney transplants in the UK are performed using LDs, which compares unfavourably with a number of other developed countries such as the USA and Scandinavia where 35–45% of transplants are from this source. The difficulty with LD transplantation is the burden placed on the donor, who must be exposed to all the risks of major abdominal surgery entirely for the benefit of another person. The traditional approach for LD nephrectomy is through an extraperitoneal loin incision, with or without resection of a rib. This leaves a significant wound, and the recovery period after surgery tends to be relatively prolonged. This is without doubt a considerable disincentive to potential donors, particularly those in employment or those with a young family to look after. There may also be concerns about postoperative pain and the cosmetic outcome of a nephrectomy incision, particularly in young female donors. Recent developments in minimal access surgery have enabled laparoscopically assisted LD nephrectomy to be performed, a technique with the potential to overcome many of the disincentives. There is, however, a need to define the place of this new procedure before it becomes widely adopted.

Laparoscopic nephrectomy: the operation

Laparoscopically assisted LD nephrectomy is performed under general anaesthesia using a transperitoneal approach to the kidney [10]. The donor is placed in a modified lateral position and a pneumoperitoneum established by needle insufflation of carbon dioxide. In general, four 12-mm laparoscopic ports are used to introduce the video-laparoscope and the various dissection instruments into the abdomen. After mobilising the colon away from the kidney and opening Gerota's fascia, the renal artery and vein are dissected free from their surrounding attachments. The ureter is mobilised with a generous amount of surrounding tissue to maintain its blood supply and is then clipped or stapled and divided at the pelvic brim. Once the kidney has been mobilised from its bed and is attached only by its vascular pedicle, a small retrieval incision is made in the abdomen. This needs to be approximately 8 cm in length and can be made transversely above the pubis or in the midline around the umbilicus. The renal artery and vein are divided after being secured with either simple metal clips or a laparoscopic stapling device.

The kidney can be removed either by placing it in a plastic retrieval bag and pulling this through a small retrieval incision or directly by placing the hand into the abdomen through a slightly larger retrieval incision.

It is usual to remove the left kidney as it has longer blood vessels, but right nephrectomy is also possible with the laparoscopic assisted technique. If the right kidney is chosen, a retrieval incision is made transversely in the right upper quadrant of the abdomen following laparoscopic dissection, and the renal vein and artery can then be clamped directly rather than using laparoscopic techniques. This allows safe division of the relatively short right renal vein flush with the inferior vena cava. With all these techniques, it takes only a few minutes to remove the kidney from the abdomen once the vessels have been cross-clamped so there is therefore a short warm ischaemic interval.

Problems with laparoscopic donor nephrectomy

Technical challenges

Since the first performance of laparoscopic donor nephrectomy at the Johns Hopkins Bayview Medical Centre, Baltimore, USA, in 1995 [10] many centres in the USA and a few in Europe have adopted the technique. A small number of published series have demonstrated a high technical success rate, but the operation is technically challenging and requires advanced laparoscopic skills. This may limit its wide application as it is unusual for surgeons to be trained in both transplant and laparoscopic methods. An innovation which may broaden the application of laparoscopic assisted nephrectomy is the use of so-called 'handoscopy'. In this technique, a pneumoperitoneum is created as before, then the surgeon introduces one hand into the abdominal cavity through a specially designed air-tight sleeve but uses laparoscopic instruments to dissect the kidney. The introduction of a hand allows an improved tactile sense which may facilitate the dissection of important structures such as the renal vessels and possibly reduces the total operating time [11].

Difficulty of access

The lack of direct access during laparoscopic dissection makes it much more difficult to control inadvertent haemorrhage caused, for example, by the avulsion of small branches of the renal vein. Pre-operative imaging by spiral computed tomographic angiography has proved invaluable in planning operations. Careful study of the computerised 3D reconstructions of the kidney and its vascular anatomy provides the surgeon with a unique knowledge of the relevant anatomy prior to embarking on the surgery: for example, the surgeon is able to use this pre-operative imaging to identify difficult tributaries arising from the posterior aspect of the renal vein and develop a plan to deal with these before encountering them.

Comparative results of open versus laparoscopic live donor nephrectomy

There have not so far been any randomised trials of open versus laparoscopic LD nephrectomy [12] but there are a number of good studies comparing the outcome of the newer technique with historical controls [13–16]. All these studies have suggested that, compared with traditional open nephrectomy, the laparoscopic technique is associated with:

☐   a shorter hospital stay

☐   less requirement for postoperative analgesia

☐   improved donor recovery times.

The Leicester results

In Leicester, the results of an initial series of 18 laparoscopically assisted operations have been compared with a historical control group of 34 open nephrectomies, the latter performed via a retroperitoneal approach to the kidney with resection of the 12th rib. This comparison showed that the laparoscopic operation was associated with a shorter donor inpatient stay (from approximately six days to four days) and a significantly lower postoperative parenteral narcotic requirement. Laparoscopic donors started driving their cars and resumed exercise more quickly than patients undergoing traditional open donor nephrectomy. They also returned to work, on average, five weeks after the operation compared with 12 weeks in the open operation group (Table 2).

On the negative side, the operating time was longer in the laparoscopic group (mean 225 min vs 135 min) and kidneys removed by this new technique were exposed to longer initial warm times (mean ca 5 min vs ca 2 min).

Concerns about laparoscopic donor nephrecetomy

The reported results suggest that laparoscopic donor nephrectomy has a number of advantages over the conventional open operation to the donor, but the outcome in the recipient must also be considered. There are a number of concerns:

1   A legitimate concern that the more limited laparoscopic approach could lead to the kidney being damaged during retrieval, with the result that the morbidity of the procedure is simply transferred from the donor to the recipient.

2   It has been noticed that transplant kidneys removed laparoscopically are associated with a slower fall in recipient serum creatinine over the first two

Table 2 Intra-operative and early postoperative outcome for open donor nephrectomy (ODN) and laparoscopic donor nephrectomy (LDN).

	ODN (n=34)		LDN (n=18)		
	Mean ± SD	Range	Mean ± SD	Range	**p**
Time in operating theatre (min)	135 ± 22	85–200	225 ± 41	180–325	<0.0001
First warm ischaemic time (min)	1.6 ± 1.7	1–9	4.5 ± 1.3	3–7	<0.0001
Resumption of oral fluids (days)	1.4 ± 0.9	1–5	1.3 ± 0.5	1–2	NS
Resumption of diet (days)	3.1 ± 1.3	1–6	2.2 ± 0.7	1–3	0.0258
Inpatient stay (days)	6.0 ± 1.8	4–11	4.1 ± 1.0	2–6	0.0002

SD = standard deviation.

weeks post-transplant [5,15]. This may be a consequence of the pneumoperitoneum exposing the kidney to a prolonged period of elevated intra-abdominal pressure, leading to a reduction in renal blood flow and urine output [17].

3   There are reports of a higher incidence of ureteral complications following the early experience of the laparoscopic operation [16]. The ureteric blood supply of a transplanted kidney is provided exclusively by a small branch of the renal artery which runs a variable course downwards from the hilum of the kidney. This blood vessel may be more at risk of damage during blunt laparoscopic dissection.

4   Ureteric ischaemia may also occur at a lower level if the surrounding connective tissue is stripped too closely. One way of avoiding this is to dissect the ureter and gonadal vessels together. It has been suggested that the incidence of ureteric complications after laparoscopic retrieval can be reduced with this technical modification and increasing experience [16,18].

Effect of laparoscopic nephrectomy on live donations

Two groups in Baltimore have recorded a significant increase in the number of live donations since the introduction of the laparoscopic operation and attribute this directly to the perceived advantages of this technique [14,19]. However, it is common in the USA for patients to travel thousands of miles to undergo surgery in specialist centres, and some of the local increases in living donation described may simply reflect a redistribution of activity.

☐ CONCLUSION

The early experience of laparoscopic assisted LD nephrectomy clearly suggests that this technique has the potential to become a major advance in renal transplantation.

Enthusiasm for laparoscopic nephrectomy is increasing around the world, but there is currently insufficient evidence to support its widespread introduction. It is timely, therefore, to consider performing a prospective, randomised, multicentre clinical trial comparing open and laparoscopic donor nephrectomy. Such a trial would need to address both donor recovery times and the outcome of transplants in the recipient.

REFERENCES

1   Nicholson ML. Renal transplantation from non heart-beating donors: opportunities and challenges. *Transplant Rev* 2000; 14: 1–17.

2   Nicholson ML, Veitch PS. Laparoscopic live-donor nephrectomy. *Nephrol Dial Transplant* 2000; 15: 1124–6.

3   Nicholson ML, Metcalfe MS, White SA, Doughman TM, *et al.* A comparison of the results of renal transplantation from non-heart-beating conventional cadaveric, and living donors. *Kidney Int* 2000; 58: 2585–91.

4   Wijnen RM, Booster MH, Stubenitsky BM, De Boer J, *et al.* Outcome of transplantation of non-heart-beating donor kidneys. *Lancet* 1995; 345: 1067–70.

5   Andrews PA, Denton MD, Compton F, Koffman CG. Outcome of transplantation of non-heart-beating donor kidneys. *Lancet* 1995; 346: 53.

6   Cho YW, Terasaki PI, Cecka JM, Gjertson DW. Transplantation of kidneys from donors whose hearts have stopped beating. *N Engl J Med* 1998; 338: 221–5.

7   Kootstra G, Wijnen R, van Hooff JP. Twenty percent more kidneys through a non heart beating programme. *Transplant Proc* 1991; 23: 910.

8   Terasaki PI, Cho W, Cecka JM. Strategy for eliminating the kidney shortage. *Clin Transpl* 1997: 265–7.

9   Nicholson ML, Dunlop P, Doughman TM, Wheatley TJ, *et al.* Work-load generated by the establishment of a non-heart beating kidney transplant programme. *Transpl Int* 1996; 9: 603–6.

10 Ratner LE, Ciseck LJ, Moore RG, Cigarroa FG, *et al.* Laparoscopic live donor nephrectomy. *Transplantation* 1995; 60: 1047–9.

11 Slakey DP, Wood JC, Hender D, Thomas R, Cheng S. Laparoscopic living donor nephrectomy: advantages of the hand-assisted method. *Transplantation* 1999; 68: 581–3.

12 Merlin TL, Scott DF, Rao MM, Wall DR, *et al.* The safety and efficacy of laparoscopic live donor nephrectomy: a systematic review. *Transplantation* 2000; 70: 1659–66.

13 Ratner LR, Montgomery RA, Kavoussi LR. Laparoscopic live donor nephrectomy: the four year Johns Hopkins University experience. Review. *Nephrol Dial Transplant* 1999; 14: 2090–3.

14 Flowers JL, Jacobs S, Cho E, Morton A, *et al.* Comparison of open and laparoscopic live donor nephrectomy. *Ann Surg* 1997; 226: 483–9; discussion 489–90.

15 Nogueira JM, Cangro CB, Fink JC, Schweitzer E, *et al.* A comparison of recipient renal outcomes with laparoscopic versus open live donor nephrectomy. *Transplantation* 1999; 67: 722–8.

16 Philosophe B, Kuo PC, Schweitzer EJ, Farney AC, *et al.* Laparoscopic versus open donor nephrectomy. *Transplantation* 1999; 68: 497–502.

17 Kirsch AJ, Hensle TW, Chang DT, Kayton ML, *et al.* Renal effects of CO_2 insufflation: oliguria and acute renal dysfunction in a rat pneumoperitoneum model. *Urology* 1994; 43: 453–9.

18 Sasaki T, Finelli F, Barhyte D, Trollinger J, Light J. Is laparoscopic donor nephrectomy here to stay? *Am J Surg* 1999; 177: 368–70.

19 Ratner LE, Kavoussi LR, Sroka M, Hiller J, *et al.* Laparoscopic assisted live donor nephrectomy – a comparison with the open approach. *Transplantation* 1997; 63: 229–33.

□ SELF ASSESSMENT QUESTIONS

1 The following donor criteria would exclude non-heart beating organ donation (NHBD):
(a) Donor age over 60 years
(b) Total circulatory arrest for a period of 30 minutes
(c) Death on a medical ward rather than in the accident department
(d) Death from a solid organ malignancy
(e) Death outside hospital

2 NHBD kidney transplants in Leicester:
(a) Have five-year graft survival rates similar to live donor transplants
(b) Account for 10% of the total transplant programme
(c) Have a delayed graft function rate of over 80%
(d) Are associated with higher rejection rates than transplants from heart-beating donors
(e) Have a higher rate of thrombosis than conventional transplants

3 Live kidney donation:
(a) Accounts for 25% of transplants in the UK
(b) Is associated with excellent recipient graft function
(c) Has traditionally required a large loin incision often with resection of a rib
(d) Has no significant risks for the donor
(e) Has been used more widely in the USA than in the UK

4 Laparoscopic live donor nephrectomy:
(a) Is a simple laparoscopic procedure
(b) Is facilitated by pre-operative spiral computed tomography angiography
(c) Is not a suitable technique when the right kidney is being donated
(d) Has not yet been widely utilised in the USA since its introduction in 1995
(e) Leads to a slight increase in the renal warm ischaemic time

5 When compared with traditional open operations, laparoscopic donor nephrectomy is associated with:
(a) A shorter hospital inpatient stay
(b) Similar requirement for postoperative analgesia
(c) Shorter operating times
(d) A quicker postoperative fall in recipient serum creatinine
(e) A quicker return to work for the donor

ANSWERS

1a True	2a True	3a False	4a False	5a True
b False	b False	b True	b True	b False
c False	c True	c True	c False	c False
d True	d False	d False	d False	d False
e False	e False	e True	e True	e True

Erythropoietin in the treatment of renal anaemia

Iain Macdougall

☐ INTRODUCTION

The availability of recombinant human erythropoietin (r-HuEPO) is without doubt the most significant development in the management of patients with chronic renal failure (CRF) in the last decade. The need for EPO supplementation to treat the anaemia of CRF was first recognised in the 1960s, but the technology required to produce this substance in sufficient quantities for therapeutic use proved elusive until the 1980s. The first major breakthrough was the purification and isolation of the structure of HuEPO in 1977 [1] and the cloning and expression of the gene for EPO was finally achieved in 1983 [2]. Remarkably, clinical trials of r-HuEPO began as early as 1985 on both sides of the Atlantic and it was licensed as a therapeutic agent in the UK in 1990.

The management of renal anaemia was most unsatisfactory prior to this development. Despite attempts to minimise blood losses, and the use of pharmacological dosages of parenteral iron, oral folic acid and androgens, many patients still required regular blood transfusions. These caused several additional problems:

- ☐ increased susceptibility to infections (particularly viral)

- ☐ iron overload

- ☐ suppression of endogenous EPO production, and

- ☐ sensitisation to HLA antigens (thereby rendering successful renal transplantation more difficult).

Now, some 10 years later, millions of patients worldwide have benefited from r-HuEPO therapy. Recently, a second-generation EPO analogue was launched which is also manufactured using recombinant DNA technology.

☐ BIOCHEMISTRY AND PHYSIOLOGY OF ERYTHROPOIETIN

The major reason for the success of r-HuEPO therapy in the treatment of renal anaemia is because this anaemia is largely caused by inappropriately low circulating EPO levels (Fig. 1) [3]. EPO is synthesised in the peritubular cells of the kidney (Fig. 2). With progressive renal damage, these cells die and EPO production is

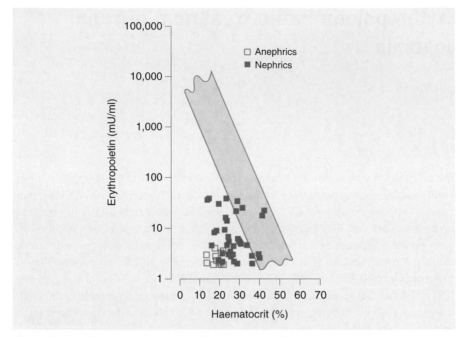

Fig. 1 Relationship between haematocrit and serum erythropoietin levels in non-uraemic and uraemic individuals. The hatched area shows the normal relationship between these two parameters derived from normal healthy controls and patients with iron deficiency anaemia. The open and closed squares represent anephric and nephric patients with chronic renal failure.

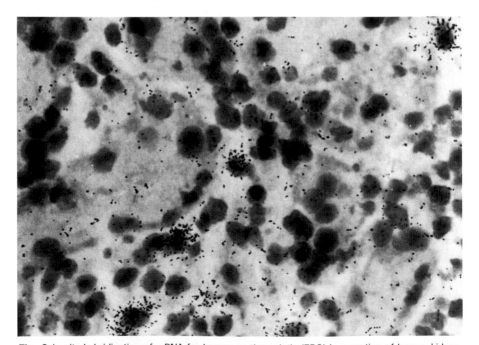

Fig. 2 *In situ* hybridisation of mRNA for human erythropoietin (EPO) in a section of human kidney. The black dots represent EPO mRNA and are sited in the peritubular fibroblasts.

diminished. Adequate levels of EPO are required both to maintain a healthy haemoglobin concentration and to control the massively proliferative process of red cell production (turnover rate 2 million new cells per second).

The anaemia of renal failure can therefore be regarded as a hormone-deficient state, similar to that seen in diabetes mellitus in which the pancreas fails to secrete adequate amounts of insulin. As with diabetes, the logical treatment is to replace the deficiency with supplemental hormone. Many other factors can contribute towards the development of renal anaemia but are of considerably less importance than the EPO deficiency. They include:

☐   shortened red cell survival as a result of haemolysis or hypersplenism

☐   'uraemic inhibitors' of erythropoiesis

☐   hyperparathyroidism with marrow fibrosis

☐   aluminium toxicity

☐   iron and folate deficiency, and

☐   excessive blood loss.

EPO is a glycoprotein hormone containing 165 amino acids with a molecular weight of about 34 kDa. It is heavily dependent on its carbohydrate side chains for maintaining viability *in vivo*. Removal of the sialic acid residues on these chains causes the hormone to be cleared rapidly via the liver. EPO acts on specific transmembrane receptors found on a variety of cell types, notably erythroid progenitor cells in which it promotes proliferation and differentiation (Fig. 3). It also has an anti-apoptotic action, prolonging the survival of these cells.

The intracellular action of EPO is beginning to be understood (Fig. 4). Once bound, EPO causes its receptor to dimerise. This action stimulates the JAK-2 kinase enzyme which in turn causes tyrosine phosphorylation of a number of intracellular proteins, including the EPO receptor itself. Various intracellular signalling molecules have been found to be important for the action of EPO, particularly STAT-5 which is the major transcription factor. There is also a negative influence on this intracellular chain of events, mediated via haematopoietic cell phosphatase (HCP), which dephosphorylates and thereby inactivates the JAK-2 kinase enzyme. EPO receptors are also present on other cell types, for example endothelial cells and neuronal tissue, but the physiological role (if any) of EPO in these tissues remains unclear.

☐ INITIAL CLINICAL STUDIES WITH RECOMBINANT HUMAN ERYTHROPOIETIN

The first two clinical studies of r-HuEPO therapy in the treatment of renal anaemia were initiated in Seattle and in London and Oxford in late 1985 to early 1986 [4,5]. Both studies were in haemodialysis patients in whom the EPO was injected intravenously three times a week, coinciding with the dialysis sessions. There was a dose-dependent increase in haemoglobin concentration, thus confirming for the first time the efficacy of this new and exciting agent.

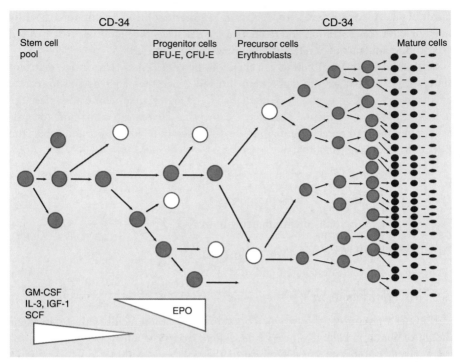

Fig. 3 Diagrammatic representation of erythroid progenitor cell development indicating the stage at which erythropoietin (EPO) acts. The action of EPO is predominantly on BFU-E and CFU-E progenitor cells (GM-CSF = granulocyte-macrophage colony stimulating factor; IGF = insulin-like growth factor; IL = interleukin; SCF = stem cell factor).

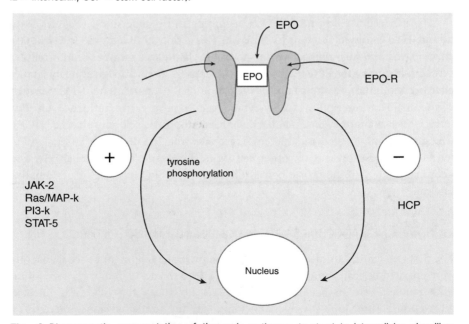

Fig. 4 Diagrammatic representation of the main pathways involved in intracellular signalling following activation of the erythropoietin receptor (EPO-R) (HCP = haematopoietic cell phosphatase).

There has been considerable change in the approach to r-HuEPO therapy over the 10 years since it became available, with a gradual move towards increasing the use of the subcutaneous route of administration, analogous to insulin therapy in diabetes, for several reasons:

1   The pharmacokinetics and pharmacodynamics of subcutaneously-administered r-HuEPO more closely resemble the physiological production of EPO in normal healthy individuals.

2   It is impractical to use the intravenous route in peritoneal dialysis patients and in patients with CRF not yet requiring dialysis.

3   There are studies suggesting that lower doses of r-HuEPO may be required if the drug is given by the subcutaneous route [6].

The most commonly used starting dose of EPO in renal failure patients is 2,000 units two or three times a week.

☐ RESPONSE TO RECOMBINANT HUMAN ERYTHROPOIETIN THERAPY

Most CRF patients (90–95%) respond to r-HuEPO therapy with a slow, but progressive dose-dependent rise in haemoglobin concentration. The aim is to increase the haemoglobin by approximately 0.25 g/dl per week (or 1 g/dl per month). Rises in haemoglobin in excess of this will require a dose reduction of r-HuEPO and vice versa.

Reasons for poor response

Even with increasing doses of r-HuEPO, some patients still show a suboptimal response, for which many causes have now been recognised (Table 1). The most important reason for poor response is iron deficiency, which was found in even the early clinical trials. Iron deficiency may be *absolute*, where the total body iron stores

Table 1 Causes of poor response to erythropoietin.

Major	Minor
Iron deficiency	Blood loss
Infection/Inflammation	Hyperparathyroidism
Underdialysis	Aluminium toxicity
	Vitamin B12/Folate deficiency
	Haemolysis
	Marrow disorders, eg MDS
	Haemoglobinopathies
	ACE inhibitors
	Carnitine deficiency
	Anti-EPO antibodies

ACE = angiotensin-converting inhibitor; EPO = erythropoietin; MDS = myelodysplastic syndrome.

are exhausted (manifest by a low serum ferritin level) or *functional*, where there are adequate body iron stores but a failure to mobilise iron rapidly enough to satisfy the demands of the bone marrow for erythropoiesis. Both these types of iron deficiency are treated with iron supplementation. Unfortunately, replacement by oral iron has been disappointing, almost certainly due to poor compliance and poor absorption from the gastrointestinal tract. As a result, intravenous iron has been widely used in patients receiving r-HuEPO therapy, in whom it has not only been shown to enhance the response to EPO therapy but also to reduce dosage requirements [7]. Other major causes of a poor response to r-HuEPO include infection or inflammation, and underdialysis.

☐ TARGET HAEMOGLOBIN AND STRATEGIES FOR TREATING RENAL ANAEMIA

The most controversial aspect of renal anaemia management over the last decade has been the target haemoglobin for which to aim. The initial clinical trials of r-HuEPO used a target haemoglobin of around 11 g/dl (ie subnormal correction of anaemia). This habit has persisted, driven by concerns that complete normalisation of haemoglobin concentration may have adverse consequences for the patient. The additional amount of r-HuEPO (and hence cost) required for full correction of the anaemia has also limited the widespread adoption of this strategy.

Clinical trials

The controversy about the target haemoglobin formed the basis of a large randomised prospective clinical trial in the USA in 1,233 haemodialysis patients [8]. Half the patients were randomised to aim for a haematocrit of about 42% (haemoglobin ca 14 g/dl) and the other half targeted a 'conventional' haematocrit of about 30% (haemoglobin ca 10 g/dl). Primary end-points in this study were all-cause mortality and first non-fatal myocardial infarction. The study was prematurely aborted after 29 months because of a slight increase in mortality in the high haemoglobin group which was approaching statistical significance (Fig. 5) [8]. However, this study was conducted in high risk patients who had pre-existing cardiac disease. Several subsequent similar 'normalisation of haemoglobin' studies have failed to confirm any increase in mortality with full correction of anaemia.

Early correction or prevention of renal anaemia

More recently, the focus has shifted towards the earlier correction of renal anaemia, even before the patient reaches the stage of needing dialysis. Several large multicentre clinical trials investigating this issue are in progress in the UK, Canada and Australia, and a worldwide study, Cardiovascular Reduction Early Anaemia Treatment with Epoeitin Beta (CREATE), has recently been launched to examine the potential benefits of preventing renal anaemia ever developing. It is too early to know what these studies will show, but the hypothesis is that the benefits of early correction of renal anaemia may be even greater if there has not been time for the

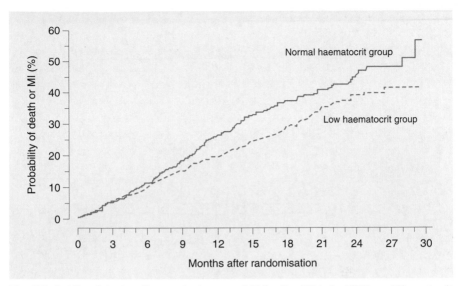

Fig. 5 Probability of death or first non-fatal myocardial infarction (MI) in the US Normal Haematocrit Cardiac Trial (reproduced, with permission, from [8]).

patient to develop the adverse pathophysiological (particularly cardiac) consequences of long-standing chronic anaemia.

□ BENEFITS OF TREATING RENAL ANAEMIA WITH RECOMBINANT HUMAN ERYTHROPOIETIN

In addition to providing a more physiological means of correcting renal anaemia and avoiding the need for regular blood transfusions, it has become apparent that r-HuEPO therapy has produced significant secondary clinical benefits for the patients. There is a plethora of literature on this topic, and the most significant of these benefits are:

□ improved quality of life

□ increased exercise capacity, and

□ improved cardiac function.

In addition, the patient often reports an improvement in anaemic symptoms, notably lethargy, muscle fatigue, poor energy levels, and breathlessness on exertion. However, perhaps the most significant clinical benefit associated with correction of anaemia by r-HuEPO therapy is regression of left ventricular hypertrophy (LVH) seen after six months of treatment (Fig. 6) [9]. It has since become apparent that the two major factors influencing LVH in CRF are hypertension and anaemia. Furthermore, LVH has also been shown to be an independent predictor of mortality in this patient population. The hypothesis, therefore, is that r-HuEPO therapy will cause an improvement in survival in renal failure patients, for which there is some preliminary supporting evidence.

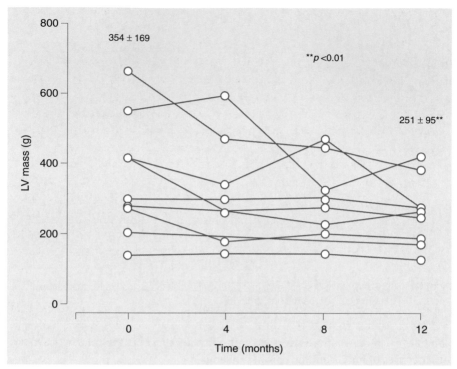

Fig. 6 Effect of recombinant human erythropoietin therapy on left ventricular (LV) mass in a small cohort of haemodialysis patients (reproduced, with permission, from [9]).

The bleeding tendency of uraemia caused by platelet dysfunction is also improved by r-HuEPO therapy, as are both sexual and endocrine functions. There are also improvements in immune function, including such effects as enhanced phagocytic killing of bacteria by polymorphonuclear leukocytes and enhanced seroconversion to vaccines such as hepatitis B vaccine.

The most important benefits are listed in Table 2 which, taken as a whole, illustrate that r-HuEPO therapy has considerably enhanced *quality* of life and may even increase *quantity* of life.

Table 2 Benefits from correction of renal anaemia.

Increased/improved	Decreased:
• quality of life	• cardiac output
• exercise capacity	• angina
• brain/cognitive function	• left ventricular hypertrophy
• sleep patterns	• bleeding tendency
• sexual function	• depression
• endocrine function	• hospitalisations
• immune function	• transfusions
• muscle metabolism	
• nutrition	

□ ADVERSE EFFECTS OF RECOMBINANT HUMAN ERYTHROPOIETIN THERAPY

Hypertension

There are few adverse consequences of r-HuEPO and they are generally easy to manage. About 20–30% of renal failure patients receiving the drug develop a worsening of hypertension, possibly requiring additional antihypertensive medication. The cause is still not fully explained but it may be mediated via increased peripheral vascular resistance secondary to reversal of hypoxic vasodilatation, increased endothelin vasoconstrictor tone, a rise in blood viscosity, and possibly a direct vasoconstrictor action of EPO on endothelial cells. Interestingly, development of hypertension has not been seen in other patient populations (eg with rheumatoid arthritis or malignancy) treated with much higher doses of r-HuEPO. The severe hypertension found in the early clinical trials of r-HuEPO which resulted in encephalopathy and seizures is no longer seen, possibly due to more cautious correction of anaemia and less use of intravenous administration of r-HuEPO.

Vascular access thrombosis

The use of r-HuEPO therapy has also been associated with an increased risk of vascular access thrombosis. This again may be mediated via enhanced coagulation or blood viscosity, but this is not a problem in most patients with a good arteriovenous fistula or polytetrafluoroethylene graft.

Minor side effects

Minor side effects include:

- □ skin irritation around the site of the injection
- □ reduced dialyser efficiency in some patients causing decreased solute clearance, and
- □ myalgia/influenza-like symptoms associated with the first few injections.

Antibodies to r-HuEPO causing red cell aplasia have been described but are vanishingly rare given the millions of patients who have received this treatment worldwide.

□ NEW ERYTHROPOIETIC AGENTS

As with most therapeutic agents, particularly successful ones, much research has been directed towards synthesising and developing new erythropoietic substances. The first of these, which was licensed recently, is novel erythropoiesis stimulating protein (NESP, darbepoetin alfa, Aranesp™). This is a hyperglycosylated analogue of EPO that differs from native and recombinant human EPO by the substitution of five amino acids and the addition of two extra N-linked sialic acid-containing carbohydrate side chains (Fig. 7) [10]. These changes make the molecule more stable *in vivo* but it has the same mechanism of action as r-HuEPO, namely via activation of the EPO receptor.

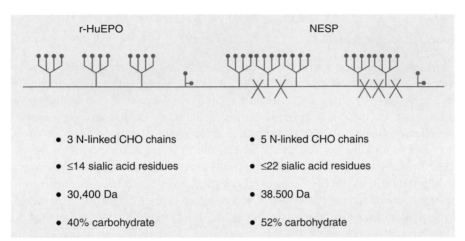

Fig. 7 Comparison of the biochemical structure of novel erythropoiesis stimulating protein (NESP) and recombinant human erythropoietin (r-HuEPO) (CHO = carbohydrate).

Small molecule EPO-mimetic peptides demonstrate an EPO-like action both *in vitro* and *in vivo*. They have been shown to activate the EPO receptor, inducing the proliferation of erythroid progenitor cells. Although not orally active themselves, they may form the template by which a non-peptide, orally active EPO mimetic can be designed in the future [11].

As stated previously, HCP is an intracellular molecule that negatively regulates the action of EPO. Inhibitors of HCP have been synthesised. These allow erythroid progenitor cells to become more responsive to EPO.

Finally, when EPO gene therapy was tested in animals there was enhanced erythropoietic activity. However, as with other types of gene therapy, there are many hurdles to overcome and it will be many years before this could become a viable therapeutic option.

☐ CONCLUSIONS

r-HuEPO therapy has been the most exciting development in the management of CRF patients in the last decade. It is highly effective, the vast majority of patients respond, and there are considerable benefits for the patient, including improved quality of life, increased exercise capacity and improved cardiac function. In most instances, the drug is injected subcutaneously two or three times a week and regular monitoring of the haemoglobin concentration, iron status and blood pressure is required. Most patients will need intravenous iron supplementation to maximise their response to r-HuEPO, and a small proportion may require the introduction or intensification of antihypertensive therapy.

There has been much debate about the appropriate target haemoglobin concentration to aim for in this patient population, and increasing interest in starting treatment earlier in the course of the disease. Newer pharmacological agents to stimulate erythropoiesis are being researched, and further developments in this exciting area of medicine are expected over the next decade.

Acknowledgement

I am grateful to my secretary, Christine Mitchell, for help in the preparation of this manuscript.

REFERENCES

1 Miyake T, Kung CK, Goldwasser E. Purification of human erythropoietin. *J Biol Chem* 1977; **252**: 5558–64.

2 Lin FK, Suggs S, Lin CH, Browne JK, *et al.* Cloning and expression of the human erythropoietin gene. *Proc Natl Acad Sci USA* 1985; **82**: 7580–4.

3 Caro J, Brown S, Miller O, Murray T, Erslev AJ. Erythropoietin levels in uremic nephric and anephric patients. *J Lab Clin Med* 1979; **93**: 449–58.

4 Winearls CG, Oliver DO, Pippard MJ, Reid C, *et al.* Effect of human erythropoietin derived from recombinant DNA on the anaemia of patients maintained by chronic haemodialysis. *Lancet* 1986; ii: 1175–8.

5 Eschbach JW, Egrie JC, Downing MR, Browne JK, Adamson JW. Correction of the anemia of end-stage renal disease with recombinant human erythropoietin. Results of a combined phase I and II clinical trial. *N Engl J Med* 1987; **316**: 73–8.

6 Kaufman JS, Reda DJ, Fye CL, Goldfarb DS, *et al.* Subcutaneous compared with intravenous epoetin in patients receiving hemodialysis. Department of Veterans Affairs Cooperative Study Group on Erythropoietin in Hemodialysis Patients. *N Engl J Med* 1998; **339**: 578–83.

7 Fishbane S, Frei GL, Maesaka J. Reduction in recombinant human erythropoietin doses by the use of chronic intravenous iron supplementation. *Am J Kidney Dis* 1995; **26**: 41–6.

8 Besarab A, Bolton WK, Browne JK, Egrie JC, *et al.* The effects of normal as compared with low hematocrit values in patients with cardiac disease who are receiving hemodialysis and epoetin. *N Engl J Med* 1998; **339**: 584–90.

9 Macdougall IC, Lewis NP, Saunders MJ, Cochlin DL, *et al.* Long-term cardiorespiratory effects of amelioration of renal anaemia by erythropoietin. *Lancet* 1990; **335**: 489–93.

10 Macdougall IC. Novel erythropoiesis stimulating protein. Review. *Semin Nephrol* 2000; **20**: 375–81.

11 Johnson DL, Jolliffe LK. Erythropoietin mimetic peptides and the future. Review. *Nephrol Dial Transplant* 2000; **15**: 1274–7.

☐ SELF ASSESSMENT QUESTIONS

1 Erythropoietin:
   (a) Is a glycoprotein containing 245 amino acids
   (b) Is synthesised in the tubular epithelial cells of the kidney
   (c) Prevents apoptosis of erythroid progenitor cells
   (d) Controls red cell production with a turnover rate of two million new cells per second
   (e) Stimulates an intracellular signalling mechanism involving the transcription factor STAT-1

2 Major causes of a poor response to recombinant human erythropoietin (r-HuEPO) therapy include:
   (a) Hyperparathyroidism
   (b) Underdialysis
   (c) Haemolysis

(d) Vitamin B12 or folate deficiency
(e) Iron deficiency

3   EPO therapy in the treatment of renal anaemia:
(a) Is usually commenced at a dose of 2,000 units two or three times a week
(b) Is effective in 90–95% of patients
(c) Improves the bleeding tendency of uraemia caused by platelet dysfunction
(d) Is associated with the development of hypertension in 40–50% of patients treated
(e) May reduce the response to vaccines such as hepatitis B vaccine

4   Patients on EPO therapy should have regular monitoring of:
(a) Liver function tests
(b) Creatine kinase levels
(c) Blood pressure
(d) Pulse rate
(e) Iron status

5   Novel erythropoiesis stimulating protein:
(a) Is a new EPO agent containing five additional amino acids compared with native EPO or r-HuEPO
(b) Contains two extra N-linked carbohydrate side chains compared with r-HuEPO
(c) Has a molecular weight of 30,400 Da
(d) Is metabolically more stable *in vivo* than r-HuEPO
(e) Has the same mechanism of action as r-HuEPO

ANSWERS

1a False	2a False	3a True	4a False	5a False
b False	b True	b True	b False	b True
c True	c True	c True	c True	c False
d True	d False	d False	d False	d True
e False	e True	e False	e True	e True

Diabetes:
increasing life expectancy

Is there anything new about insulin therapy?

Stephanie Amiel

☐ WHAT IS WRONG WITH CURRENT THERAPY?

Diabetes mellitus is common. Its prevalence is set to double by the year 2010 (Fig. 1) [1] when three million people in Britain will have the disease. The economic, social and personal costs of the long-term complications of diabetes are immense as diabetes causes most of Britain's blindness, renal failure and non-traumatic amputations, as well as premature cardiovascular disease. The risk of complications of diabetes falls significantly as diabetes control, estimated by measuring glycated haemoglobin (HbA1c) concentrations, is improved [2,3]. However, in most studies and clinics, a lowering of HbA1c is accompanied by a near-linear increase in risk of severe hypoglycaemia. For example, in the American Diabetes Control and Complications Trial (DCCT) lowering HbA1c reduced risk of progression of early retinopathy by up to 76%, but a 1% fall in HbA1c was associated with a 38% increase in risk of a severe hypoglycaemic episode [2]. Less dramatic, but similar, associations were seen in type 2 diabetic patients intensively treated in the UK Prospective Diabetes Study, where a 1% reduction in HbA1c was estimated to reduce risk of microvascular disease by about 35%, but again was associated with increased risk of severe hypoglycaemia, especially with insulin therapy [3].

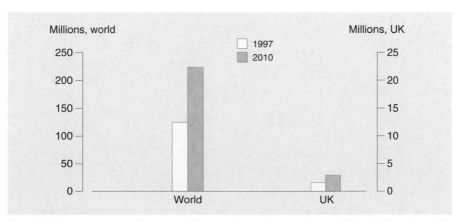

Fig. 1 Rising prevalence of diabetes mellitus, worldwide (left) and for the UK (right) (data from [1], with permission).

The problems with current insulin therapies stem from their inability to mimic physiology. The main problems relate to the pharmacokinetics, the route of administration and the lack of feedback control of plasma insulin levels. The cartoon in Fig. 2 represents the plasma insulin levels of a commonly used insulin regimen, a mixed insulin injection taken before breakfast and before the evening meal, superimposed on the insulin profiles of a healthy person eating three meals a day. Note the low, but persistent, background insulin and the large, but transient, prandial peaks for the healthy person. Conventional soluble insulin is too slow in onset, insufficiently peaked and much too long in duration to replace the prandial bursts, while intermediate acting insulins are too peaked and too short in duration adequately to replace background control, especially overnight – particularly if the evening meal (and dose) is taken early and the rising is late! Even the most common regimen for intensified therapy, which involves moving the evening intermediate acting insulin to bedtime, and replacing the morning intermediate acting insulin (taken at breakfast for lunch 6 hours later) with a lunchtime injection of soluble insulin, fails to replicate endogenous insulin (Fig. 3).

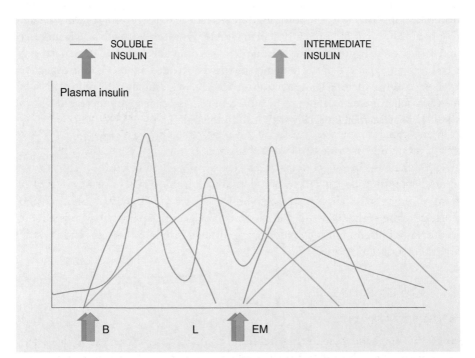

Fig. 2 Cartoon of plasma insulin profiles from injection of mixed insulins before breakfast (B) and before evening meal (EM) compared with the insulin profile from a healthy person eating three meals a day (B, lunch (L) and EM) (red line). The blue arrows and blue lines show the injection time and subsequent blood insulin profile from soluble insulin; the green arrows and green lines show those from intermediate acting insulin. Where the sum of the blue plus green lines is higher than the red line, the patient is at risk from hypoglycaemia. The exogenous insulins tend not to last through the night, leaving the patient at risk from morning hyperglycaemia.

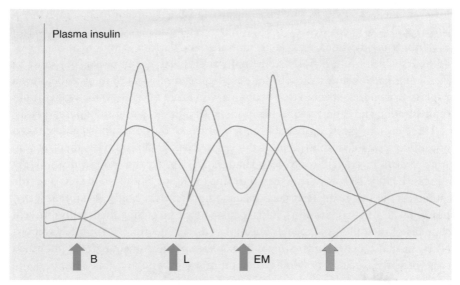

Fig. 3 A more physiological insulin replacement regimen comprises a soluble insulin injected before each meal and an intermediate acting insulin at bedtime. More flexibility might be achieved if the intermediate acting insulin was administered before breakfast and before bed, to provide a flattish basal insulin replacement, on which meal related doses of soluble insulin could be superimposed more or less at will (key as for Fig. 2).

☐ THE HISTORY OF INSULIN THERAPY

The first soluble insulins were isolated from pancreata of cows and pigs. Between 1936 and 1951 the intermediate and long acting insulins were developed as extra zinc or protamine was added to retard absorption of the insulin into the circulation. In 1972, the insulin preparations were cleaned of other pancreatic products by chromatography, producing the mono-component insulins. These insulins were less immunogenic than their predecessors and the action profiles became sharper and shorter. In the early 1980s, the development of genetic engineering allowed the production of insulin molecules identical to human insulin by bacteria and yeast in large commercial quantities.

☐ DESIGNER INSULINS

Fast acting analogues

Soluble insulin forms hexamers in solution and it is the need for these to dissociate into monomers for absorption from the subcutaneous depot that slows the onset and prolongs the action of the insulin *in vivo*. Manipulation of the human insulin gene allowed the production of insulins which did not associate, and monomeric insulins (the rapid acting insulin analogues) were born. The first of these had a long residence time on the insulin receptor and may have stimulated trophic rather than metabolic pathways within the cells – it caused breast cancer in a susceptible mouse model [4].

However, the next two, B28lys29pro (lispro insulin, Humalog) [5] and B28Asp (NovoRapid) [6] were free of this problem. These insulins start to act within 15 minutes of injection, peak at 50 minutes and have a duration of action of 3–5 hours which is much closer to the natural prandial insulin peak. They must be taken *immediately* before a carbohydrate containing meal – *not* 30 minutes before – a property that endears them to many patients who either find the gap between insulin administration and eating inconvenient or feel significant guilt for not observing it.

These insulins give demonstrably better control of the postprandial glucose than conventional soluble insulins, but in the large Phase III clinical trials there was no improvement in overall control as changes in HbA1c did not seem clinically impressive [7,8]. This was almost certainly due to 'escape' of the blood glucose as the insulin ran out before the next meal-related injection (Fig. 4) [9]. As more is learnt about how to use these insulins, in particular how to combine them with different regimens of multiple basal insulin injections (usually neutral protamine Hagedorn (NPH) insulins), better control might be expected. A meta-analysis of the published trials with lispro insulin showed a reduction in severe hypoglycaemia rates [10].

The fast acting analogues have unequivocal benefit in the reduction of nocturnal hypoglycaemia (Fig. 5) [11], but this is likely to be associated with a significant period of hyperglycaemia in the earlier part of the night [12] unless appropriate basal insulin replacement or injection timing is included. It follows that these fast acting analogues may best confer benefit in continuous subcutaneous insulin therapy (insulin pump therapy), where the fast acting analogue is delivered steadily at a pre-set rate through an indwelling subcutaneous catheter over 24 hours by a

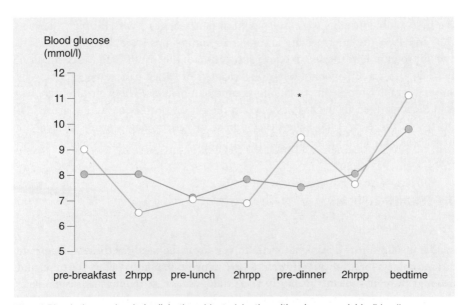

Fig. 4 Blood glucose levels in diabetic subjects injecting either human soluble (blue lines, orange circles) or a very fast acting insulin analogue (green lines, yellow circles) before meals. Postprandial hyperglycaemia is better controlled with the latter, but there is a tendency for glucose to rise further before the next meal (hrpp = hours postprandial) (redrawn, with permission, from [9]).

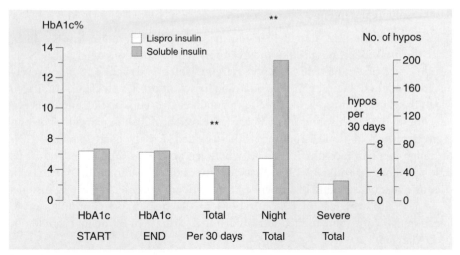

Fig. 5 Glycated haemoglobin (HbA1c) and hypoglycaemia (hypos) rates during a trial of lispro insulin (Humalog) versus human soluble insulin, with a bedtime intermediate acting insulin as overnight basal replacement. Overall glycaemic control (left) was not much improved, but in these well controlled patients there was a marked reduction in nocturnal hypoglycaemia (right) (**significant) (data from [11], with permission).

small portable pump [13]. The pump can be activated to deliver a bolus of insulin at meal times which is no different from any pre-prandial subcutaneous injection. The basal delivery of insulin removes the problem of insulin exhaustion between meals.

Pump therapy with fast acting insulin analogues

Pump therapy is also the only way adequately to treat a vigorous dawn phenomenon (the normal rise in insulin requirement from about 3-8 am), as the pumps allow a number of different basal settings over a 24-hour period. Pump therapy with fast acting insulin analogues offers significant advantages in terms of basal insulin replacement and regimen flexibility, but these devices are relatively expensive and some patients find them psychologically unacceptable. The literature suggests that patients on intensified therapy can obtain modest further improvement with less risk of hypoglycaemia using pumps, and the main current evidence base shows a significant benefit for patients with recurrent severe hypoglycaemia [14].

Historically, insulin pumps carried an increased risk of diabetic ketoacidosis as any failure of insulin delivery (eg air in the infusion set) leaves the patient insulin deficient extremely rapidly. The improved safety features of the current generation of pumps, and the increased understanding of people involved in their use, have much improved the situation. However, pump therapy is effective – and safe – only in the hands of well-motivated patients prepared to measure blood glucose four times daily as a routine. In such hands, it can be extremely effective.

Basal insulin replacement

It follows that the next 'designer' insulin needed is a background insulin which lacks the peaked action profile and relatively short duration of classical NPH insulins. The first candidate is insulin glargine which is designed to be relatively insoluble at physiological pH, thus retarding its action profile. In clamp studies, in which the glucose infusions required to maintain euglycaemia after a subcutaneous injection of the test insulins are compared, the action of insulin glargine shows an impressive lack of peak associated with sustained activity over 24 hours [15]. Although its pharmacokinetics can vary between people, within an individual its action is more reproducible than that of conventional insulins. The difficulty in attaining adequate mixing of suspended conventional intermediate acting insulins to achieve uniform insulin concentrations in the insulin preparation prior to injection may contribute to their intra-individual variance in action and should not affect glargine.

In early, short trials, glargine insulin appeared to offer better control of fasting blood glucose with less nocturnal hypoglycaemia than conventional intermediate acting insulin, although the overall effects were not quite as impressive in 16-week trials [16,17]. However, there is evidence of better control of fasting blood glucose levels. Glargine has a greater affinity for the human insulin-like growth factor receptor than human insulin, but the clinical significance of this is uncertain. The place of insulin glargine in routine therapy remains to be determined, but there is no doubt of the need for an insulin that exhibits this sort of pharmacodynamics.

Inhaled insulin

Outside the diabetic clinic, the fear of injections *per se* is seen as one of the barriers to good glycaemic control. In fact, although a number (unquantified) of patients have a needle phobia, modern insulin injections are much less painful than the less-regarded pain of home blood glucose monitoring. Nevertheless, injections are not fun. What patients really hate is the need for constant vigilance – the loss of spontaneity in lifestyle – that good glycaemic control seems to require.

The most recent in a line of endeavours to avoid injections in diabetes is the introduction of insulins designed to be taken by inhalation through the lung alveolar surface [18]. Preliminary 'proof of concept' trials have demonstrated that inhaled insulins deliver equivalent control to conventional subcutaneous insulin injection, probably with an action profile akin to that of a fast acting analogue. However, the only published trial to date compares an intensified insulin therapy (basal insulin with inhalations at each meal) with non-intensified therapy (twice daily mixed insulins), which makes it difficult to attribute more than proof of efficacy. Inhaled insulin doses are recorded in milligrams, not units, and the bioavailability is 10% – so it is not a cheap option. Inhaled insulin may have a niche market for patients with needle phobia, but in this author's opinion it will be a significant step forward only if it can be shown to promote earlier transfer of inadequately controlled type 2 patients on to the insulin they need or an increased take-up of flexible multiple daily insulin administration regimens with better control and quality of life in type 1 disease. The other absolute requirement for an inhaled insulin is a clear demonstration of an absence of adverse effects on the lung with chronic administration.

Meanwhile, as Edwin Gale pointed out, worldwide, children are dying from lack of insulin, provision of which would cost 'about 1% of the development costs of each new luxury insulin' [19]. Nevertheless, the burden of living with diabetes is such that it would not be appropriate to deny patients less stressful management options if these prove to be efficacious.

☐ HEPATIC DELIVERY OF EXOGENOUS INSULIN

The major acute problem of exogenous insulin therapy is the risk of hypoglycaemia. Most of this risk is because exogenous insulin is not responsive to the great variation in insulin requirements experienced over a 24-hour period, but there is evidence that the relative peripheral hyperinsulinaemia of subcutaneously injected insulin may also contribute to hypoglycaemia risk. Fewer hypoglycaemic episodes appear to occur in patients with equivalent diabetes control treated with intraperitoneal insulin infusion therapy [20]. However, very few centres are experienced with this form of therapy and a hepatoselective insulin might be expected to have similar benefit. Pro-insulin was one such compound, but trials were discontinued early when an excess of cardiovascular disease occurred in the test group. A recent description of a large insulin molecule, complexed to an analogue of thyroxine, which first leaves the circulation in the sinusoids of the liver shows some promise [21].

☐ ISLET TRANSPLANTATION

Finally, the recent report by Shapiro and colleagues in Edmonton, Canada [22] of the most consistent success in achieving insulin independence by intra-portal infusion of isolated donated human islets in type 1 diabetic patients offers the hope of a glucose-responsive insulin therapy in diabetes. The Edmonton protocol should be reproducible elsewhere as its success is explained on the basis of:

- ☐ excellent islet separation procedures, eschewing animal proteins in the process

- ☐ the avoidance of insulin-resistant steroids in the post-transplant immunosuppressive regimen, and

- ☐ the use of multiple donors per patient.

However, until the problems of the paucity of pancreas donors and the potential toxicity of the immunosuppression have been resolved by further research this procedure will be available to type 1 patients only when conventional therapies fail in some significant way – most commonly, recurrent severe hypoglycaemia, but also progressive *early* microvascular complications despite optimised therapies.

Table 1 Comparison of severe hypoglycaemia (SH) rates between intensified and conventional insulin therapy in type 1 diabetic subjects in the Diabetes Control and Complications Trial (DCCT) and the Dusseldorf programme.

	Insulin regimen	Episodes SH/100 patients/year
DCCT	Conventional	18.7
	Intensified	61.2
Dusseldorf	Conventional	28.0
	Intensified	17.0

□ CONCLUSIONS

While awaiting resolution of these problems insulin therapy can do better than at present. A five-day inpatient training programme for type 1 diabetic patients has been in use in Germany over about the last decade [23]. It relies upon twice daily NPH insulin for basal replacement, with variable meal-related injections of conventional soluble insulins for meals, in doses determined by the patients to cover the meal they plan to eat. This regimen appears to deliver, for at least six years, the lower HbA1c suggested by the evidence base as necessary to reduce long-term complications, but uniquely without increased incidence of severe hypoglycaemia. Table 1 shows a comparison of type 1 diabetic subjects in DCCT and the Dusseldorf programme. Although the difference in absolute rates may be due to different definitions used in the two programmes, the relative change in hypoglycaemia rate with intensification of therapy is probably genuine. The major benefits to patients are in restoring their ability to eat flexibly and the avoidance of adding prescriptive diets to the need for multiple daily insulin injections.

New insulins may offer real benefit in terms of patient convenience and diabetic control, but we could also be doing a lot better with those we already have available.

REFERENCES

1 Amos AF, McCarty DJ, Zimmet P. The rising global burden of diabetes and its complications: estimates and projections to the year 2010. *Diabet Med* 1997; 14(Suppl 5): S1–85.

2 The effect of intensive treatment of diabetes on the development and progression of long-term complications in insulin-dependent diabetes mellitus. The Diabetes Control and Complications Trial Research Group. *N Engl J Med* 1993; 329: 977–86.

3 Intensive blood-glucose control with sulphonylureas or insulin compared with conventional therapy and risk of complications in patients with type 2 diabetes (UKPDS 33). UK Prospective Diabetes Study (UKPDS) Group. *Lancet* 1998; 352: 837–53.

4 Hamel FG, Siford GL, Fawcett J, Chance RE, *et al.* Differences in the cellular processing of AspB10 human insulin compared with human insulin and LysB28ProB29 human insulin. *Metabolism* 1999; 48: 611–7.

5 Howey DC, Bowsher RR, Brunelle RL, Rowe HM, *et al.* [Lys(B28), Pro(B29)]-human insulin: effect of injection time on postprandial glycemia. *Clin Pharmacol Ther* 1995; 58: 459–69.

6 Mudaliar SR, Lindberg FA, Joyce M, Beerdsen P, *et al.* Insulin aspart (B28 asp-insulin): a fast-acting analog of human insulin: absorption kinetics and action profile compared with regular human insulin in healthy nondiabetic subjects. *Diabetes Care* 1999; 22: 1501–6.

7   Anderson JH Jr, Brunelle RL, Koivisto VA, Trautmann ME, *et al.* Improved mealtime treatment of diabetes mellitus using an insulin analogue. Multicenter Insulin Lispro Study Group. *Clin Ther* 1997; **19**: 62–72.

8   Lindholm A, McEwen J, Riis AP. Improved postprandial glycemic control with insulin aspart. A randomized double-blind cross-over trial in type 1 diabetes. *Diabetes Care* 1999; **22**: 801–5.

9   Ciofetta M, Lalli C, Del Sindaco P, Torlone E, *et al.* Contribution of postprandial versus interprandial blood glucose to HbA1c in type 1 diabetes on physiologic intensive therapy with lispro insulin at mealtime. *Diabetes Care* 1999; **22**: 795–800.

10 Brunelle BL, Llewelyn J, Anderson JH Jr, Gale EA, Koivisto VA. Meta-analysis of the effect of insulin lispro on severe hypoglycemia in patients with type 1 diabetes. *Diabetes Care* 1998; **21**: 1726–31.

11 Heller SR, Amiel SA, Mansell P. Effect of the fast-acting insulin analog lispro on the risk of nocturnal hypoglycemia during intensified insulin therapy. U.K. Lispro Study Group. *Diabetes Care* 1999; **22**: 1607–11.

12 Ahmed AB, Home PD. The effect of the insulin analog lispro on nighttime blood glucose control in type 1 diabetic patients. *Diabetes Care* 1998; **21**: 32–7.

13 Zinman B, Tildesley H, Chiasson JL, Tsui E, Strack T. Insulin lispro in CSII: results of a double-blind crossover study. *Diabetes* 1997; **46**: 440–3.

14 Bode BW, Steed RD, Davidson PC. Reduction in severe hypoglycemia with long-term continuous subcutaneous insulin infusion in type I diabetes. *Diabetes Care* 1996; **19**: 324–7.

15 Lepore M, Pampanelli S, Fanelli C, Porcellati F, *et al.* Pharmacokinetics and pharmaco-dynamics of subcutaneous injection of long-acting human insulin analog glargine, NPH insulin, and ultralente human insulin and continuous subcutaneous infusion of insulin lispro. *Diabetes* 2000; **49**: 2142–8.

16 Raskin P, Klaff L, Bergenstal R, Halle JP, *et al.* A 16-week comparison of the novel insulin analog insulin glargine (HOE 901) and NPH human insulin used with insulin lispro in patients with type 1 diabetes. *Diabetes Care* 2000; **23**: 1666–71.

17 Rosenstock J, Park G, Zimmerman J. Basal insulin glargine (HOE 901) versus NPH insulin in patients with type 1 diabetes on multiple daily insulin regimens. U.S. Insulin Glargine (HOE 901) Type 1 Diabetes Investigator Group. *Diabetes Care* 2000; **23**: 1137–42.

18 Laube BL, Benedict GW, Dobs AS. The lung as an alternative route of delivery for insulin in controlling postprandial glucose levels in patients with diabetes. *Chest* 1998; **114**: 1734–9.

19 Gale EA. Two cheers for inhaled insulin. *Lancet* 2001; **357**: 324–5.

20 Jeandidier N, Selam JL, Renard E, Guerci B, *et al.* Decreased severe hypoglycemia frequency during intraperitoneal insulin infusion using programmable implantable pumps. Evadiac Study Group. *Diabetes Care* 1996; **19**: 780–7.

21 Shojaee-Moradie F, Powrie JK, Sundermann E, Spring MW, *et al.* Novel hepatoselective insulin analog: studies with a covalently linked thyroxyl-insulin complex in humans. *Diabetes Care* 2000; **23**: 1124–9.

22 Shapiro AM, Lakey JR, Ryan EA, Korbutt GS, *et al.* Islet transplantation in seven patients with type 1 diabetes mellitus using a glucocorticoid-free immunosuppressive regimen. *N Engl J Med* 2000; **343**: 230–8.

23 Muller UA, Femerling M, Reinauer KM, Risse A, *et al.* Intensified treatment and education of type 1 diabetes as clinical routine. A nationwide quality-circle experience in Germany. ASD (the Working Group on Structured Diabetes Therapy of the German Diabetes Association). *Diabetes Care* 1999; **22**(Suppl 2): B29–34.

□ SELF ASSESSMENT QUESTIONS

1   There is a firm evidence base to support the conversion to rapid acting insulin analogues:

(a) To improve control in patients with a high glycated haemoglobin (HbA1c)

(b) To reduce risk of nocturnal hypoglycaemia

(c) To lower fasting blood glucose levels in type 1 diabetic patients

(d) To reduce the number of injections needed to control blood glucose in patients with type 1 diabetes

(e) In continuous subcutaneous insulin infusion therapy

2   The novel long acting insulin analogue glargine insulin:
(a) Is less readily mixed in the vial than conventional intermediate acting insulin
(b) Shows less binding to the insulin-like growth factor receptor than conventional human insulin
(c) Is visually indistinguishable from a soluble (regular) insulin
(d) Is relatively insoluble at physiological pH
(e) Has a longer duration of action than Human Insulatard

3   The current indications for human islet transplantation include:
(a) Recurrent severe hypoglycaemia
(b) Recurrent diabetic ketoacidosis (DKA) because of psychological problems with compliance with insulin therapies
(c) Poor control because of insulin resistance
(d) Steroid therapy for other illness
(e) Willingness to undertake lifelong immunosuppression

4   A type 1 diabetic patient:
(a) Will commonly achieve near normoglycaemia on twice daily mixed insulins, providing insulin peaks for three meals and overnight control
(b) May experience nocturnal hypoglycaemia secondary to the pre-evening meal conventional soluble insulin
(c) Should be advised to aim for the lowest HbA1c achievable
(d) Is likely to achieve better control of the morning (pre-breakfast) insulin if the evening dose of intermediate acting insulin is given as late as possible
(e) Needs to mix the conventional soluble insulin thoroughly before administration

5   Insulin pump therapy:
(a) Is supported by a good evidence base showing its efficacy in patients with recurrent severe hypoglycaemia
(b) Is the treatment of choice for patients with a marked dawn phenomenon
(c) Is a safe option in patients reluctant to monitor their own blood glucose
(d) Carries less risk of DKA now than when introduced 20 years ago
(e) Gives best results if used with a human intermediate acting insulin

ANSWERS

1a False	2a False	3a True	4a False	5a True
b True	b False	b False	b True	b True
c False	c True	c False	c True	c False
d False	d True	d False	d True	d True
e True	e True	e True	e False	e False

Thiazolidinediones: increasing insulin sensitivity

Philip Home

☐ INTRODUCTION

Thiazolidinediones are members of a class of drugs which bind to a group of nuclear receptors, the peroxisome proliferator-activated receptors (PPAR) [1]. Other drugs with similar insulin sensitising effects also bind to these receptors, most notably to the PPARγ. This chapter will discuss PPARγ-agonists, some of which are thiazolidinediones.

It is now well recognised that insulin insensitivity ('resistance') and the metabolic syndrome surrounding it are related to our modern lack of exercise and high fat and high calorie diet (Fig. 1) [2]. This is coupled, of course, with genetic factors which are not appropriate for our kind of lifestyle, but which were honed to suit our foraging ancestors thousands of generations ago. Our large burden of cardiovascular disease is probably related to this background of insulin insensitivity, not just in diabetes but also in the more general population.

However, not everybody who is overweight develops diabetes. There are other factors which lead to defects in insulin secretion, probably mainly genetic and possibly partly also concerned with the development of the pancreas [3]. In the

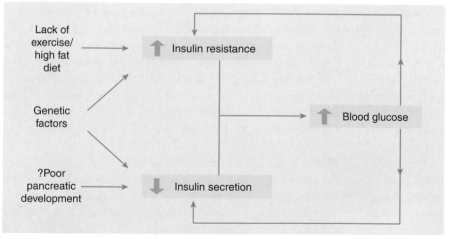

Fig. 1 Pathogenesis of type 2 diabetes [2].

context of insulin insensitivity, deficient insulin secretion leads to elevation of blood glucose concentrations. The interaction between insulin resistance and deficient secretion is probably not enough on its own to account for the degree of hyperglycaemia commonly seen in people with diabetes. However, hyperglycaemia has a feedback effect, in that it increases insulin insensitivity and decreases insulin secretion further ('glucose toxicity'), thus precipitating people into diabetes.

It follows that therapy for diabetes can be approached by:

☐   increasing insulin secretion

☐   exogenous insulin delivery, or

☐   improving insulin sensitivity.

In diabetes care we are currently witnessing an explosion of interest in new drugs and insulins and in the physiological regulatory processes in which they exert their effects. Many of the interactions between the liver, adipose tissue and muscle during the cycle of alternating feeding and fasting are incompletely understood. The opportunities for understanding the origins of insulin insensitivity have never been greater, partly because of the advances which have come from studies of PPARγ-agonists and their receptor [4]. One of the actions of PPARγ-agonists is to increase glucose uptake into fat cells, but this is probably only one of the mechanisms by which they improve insulin insensitivity in the body. A full understanding of this area will have to await major advances in our understanding of biochemical physiology over the next 10 years.

☐ PEROXISOME PROLIFERATOR-ACTIVATED RECEPTORS

PPARs are members of the nuclear receptor superfamily of transcription factors. When these receptors bind their ligand, they act on the gene to promote gene transcription [4]. PPARs bind to the DNA of the gene as heterodimers with the retinoid X receptor. Drugs targeted at the latter would be expected to give synergistic effects. The natural ligands (possibly fatty acids), the transcription product and the way it affects cellular enzymes are not known. It is known that these drugs switch on or off production of a number of different enzymes in adipose tissue, muscle and the liver in a physiologically coherent pattern. One of the effects of PPARγ-agonist drugs is to lower fatty acids in the blood, a mechanism which enhances insulin sensitivity to some extent.

The fibrate drugs bind to a related receptor, the PPARα. Indeed, it was while looking for a new fibrate that a Japanese company accidentally hit on the thiazolidinediones and discovered that they lower blood glucose. Some of the drugs discussed in this chapter bind to more than one PPAR and there is some interest in pan-PPAR-agonists. Furthermore, many of these drugs lower serum triglycerides, a feature shared with the fibrates. The three-dimensional structure and binding site of the PPAR family are now well understood and some newer drugs such as farglitazar have been designed to fit neatly into the binding site. A number of new drugs in this class are expected over the next few years.

The three classes (α, γ, δ) of PPARs are differently distributed in different tissues. PPARγ is predominantly expressed in fat cells but is also found on monocytes and in the epithelium of the large intestine. PPARα (fibrate) is more generally distributed (liver, kidney, heart and muscle) and the δ receptor is found in nearly all tissues.

☐ PEROXISOME PROLIFERATOR-ACTIVATED RECEPTOR γ-AGONISTS

Liver toxicity

The first thiazolidinedione drug to reach the market was troglitazone, an agent of relatively low potency and low efficacy. There is also a thiazolidinedione moiety on both pioglitazone and rosiglitazone, each now licensed. The newer agents tend to be much more potent in terms of receptor binding than the old ones (Fig. 2), but the binding ratios do not match the ratios of clinical efficacy, although replacing numerical position with categorical position retains the order.

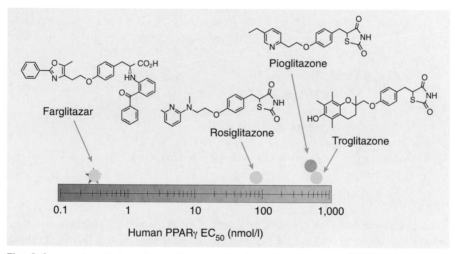

Fig. 2 Comparative binding of peroxisome proliferator-activated receptor (PPARγ-agonists (data reproduced, with permission, from Timothy M Willson, SmithKline Beecham).

Troglitazone

Following the introduction of troglitazone in the US, there were 17 fatal events due to hepatic necrosis in its first year of use in an exposure of about one million people. A Food and Drug Administration hearing reviewed the data, but troglitazone remained on the market with restricted conditions. The main reason was that, although it had caused 17 deaths, the best estimates of its efficacy were that it was saving about 20 times as many cardiovascular deaths (estimates range from five to 200). After pioglitazone and rosiglitazone became available, and their hepatic toxicity was established as negligible, there was no reason to continue with troglitazone which was withdrawn. Interestingly, both the regulatory authorities and the pharmaceutical industry missed the toxicity of troglitazone. Looking back at the data, it seems evident that major rises in alanine aminotransferase (ALT) in the trials were about three times as common in patients on active therapy as in patients on placebo.

Rosiglitazone and pioglitazone

There is no elevation of ALT in relation to placebo with either rosiglitazone or pioglitazone. US exposure to these drugs since May 1999 has been in well over one million people. Inevitably, some hepatocellular injury events have been recorded in such a large population of people on therapy, but these have been in complicated cases, and there have no deaths or liver failure (Fig. 3) [5]. The European licence conditions for regular monitoring of liver function now seem obsolete, but it is probably wise to check liver function texts before starting these drugs.

Raised ALT >3 x upper normal limit (clinical trials)
Troglitazone: 1.9% (placebo 0.6%)
Rosiglitazone: 0.2% (placebo 0.2%)

US exposure since May 1999
$>4 \times 10^6$ prescriptions, $>1 \times 10^6$ people
4 reports of hepatocellular injury – all complicated
No deaths/liver failure

Fig. 3 Rosiglitazone and hepatotoxicity (ALT = alanine aminotransferase) [5].

Glucose-lowering efficacy

Efficacy studies tend to be reported from people with typical type 2 diabetes, with an average age about 60 years and body mass index (BMI) 30–32 kg/m². In these studies, glycated haemoglobin (HbA1c), the primary outcome measure, was usually disgracefully poor at baseline.

Monotherapy

As monotherapy, a typical study is that of Aronoff and colleagues with pioglitazone (Fig. 4) [6]. Clear improvements in blood glucose control were found with increasing dosage of pioglitazone, with a gain approaching 2.0% in HbA1c at a dose of 45 mg, particularly after adjustment for change in the placebo group. This is a large effect for a clinical study compared with the older studies of sulphonylureas and metformin. Many similar trials were reviewed in the health technology assessments prepared for the National Institute for Clinical Excellence (NICE), without any particular criticisms of them being made. There is little doubt that these agents are effective in lowering blood glucose.

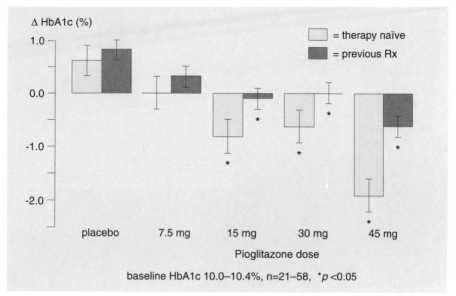

Fig. 4 Effect of pioglitazone on glycated haemoglobin (HbA1c) in people with type 2 diabetes (R_x = treatment) [6].

Combination therapy

Clearly however, we are not interested only in monotherapy – indeed, because of the poor cost-effectiveness of these expensive drugs, perhaps not at all. The availability of long-established glucose-lowering drugs has determined that in Europe (in contrast to the US) rosiglitazone and pioglitazone are not licensed for use except in combination with those drugs. In a study of combination therapy, Wolffenbuttel and colleagues compared the combination of rosiglitazone 1 mg and 2 mg twice daily (4 mg is now the recommended starting dose) with a sulphonylurea against placebo (Fig. 5) [7]. There was a placebo-adjusted change of HbA1c from baseline of about 1.0%. This is a useful effect in people with diabetes, which should reduce their cardiovascular and retinopathy risks by about 15% and 30–40%, respectively. Rosiglitazone is therefore effective in combination with a sulphonylurea. Equivalent efficacy has been shown in combination with metformin.

A question which arises here is whether these effects are persistent. None of the studies published to date is for longer than 26 weeks' treatment, so we have to rely on observational data for what happens over longer periods. From the SmithKline data on rosiglitazone [5], at least in combination with metformin (Fig. 6) [8], it appears that the efficacy continues unchanged, at least out to two years. There are also some data from the US with troglitazone suggesting good effects over longer periods. Thus, the effect of these agents is not a short-term effect which subsequently disappears.

One point of use in routine clinical practice is that there is a relationship between BMI and the efficacy of these drugs. This might not seem surprising because insulin resistance is higher in people who are more obese. The changes in HbA1c for people with a BMI less than 25.0 kg/m² ('normal weight') compared with those who are

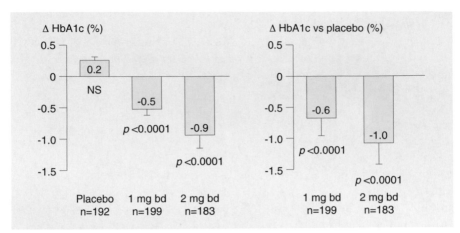

Fig. 5 Rosiglitazone in combination with a sulphonylurea (26-week study) (HbA1c = glycated haemoglobin; NS = not significant) [7].

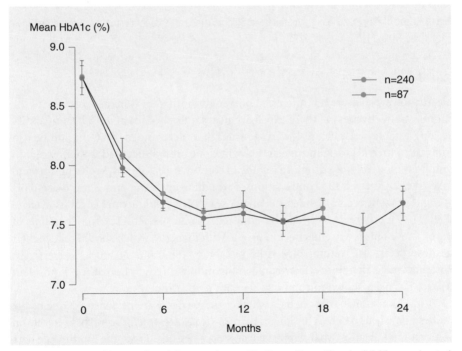

Fig. 6 Long-term efficacy of rosiglitazone in combination with metformin (HbA1c = glycated haemoglobin) [8].

overweight or obese show that the effects of rosiglitazone in combination with metformin are greater in the latter. Not much change in HbA1c should therefore be expected in those people who are really insulin-*deficient* rather than insulin-*resistant* – which of course fits in with the perception of how these drugs work.

Other aspects of the metabolic syndrome

It is not only glucose lowering that is of interest in the management of people with type 2 diabetes, but also treatment of other aspects of the metabolic syndrome including raised triglycerides, low high-density lipoprotein (HDL), hypertension and microalbuminuria. The lipid lowering profiles of the drugs tested to date differ (Table 1). This is becoming an area of controversy, no doubt fuelled by rival claims from some of the drug manufacturers.

Serum low-density lipoprotein (LDL) cholesterol level seemed to rise with troglitazone, and possibly rather more so with rosiglitazone. There is an interpretation trap here, in that it appears that the *quality* of the LDL improves with these agents: that is, the LDL particle size is larger, and the LDL is probably not as atherogenic as occurs naturally in people with type 2 diabetes. These findings may therefore not be as adverse as they seem. Pioglitazone and farglitazar appear to have no effect on LDL concentration, while HDL is more consistently raised by these drugs, notably by farglitazar which seems to raise it by 20%.

Serum triglycerides are variably decreased by these drugs. Reductions of 15% or greater with some of the newer agents (eg farglitazar) are potentially extremely valuable in terms of risk prevention, if this finding can be extrapolated from studies of fibrates in people with type 2 diabetes as in the Veterans Affairs High-Density Lipoprotein Cholesterol Intervention Trial [9].

Table 1 Peroxisome proliferator-activated receptor (PPARγ-agonists: effect on blood lipid profiles.

	Cholesterol		Triglycerides
	HDL	LDL	
Troglitazone	↑2–3	↑10	↓15
Rosiglitazone	↑?12	↑10	↓0
Pioglitazone	↔	↑10	↓15
Farglitazar	↔	↑20	↓30

HDL = high-density lipoprotein; LDL = low-density lipoprotein.

Different doses of farglitazar show a reduction in urinary albumin:creatinine ratio compared with placebo in a phase II drug study completed in 2000, with statistically significant reductions (40–50%) in albumin excretion rate. However, we have to wait for the cardiovascular outcome trial results in 5–6 years' time (for pioglitazone and rosiglitazone) to know whether these changes in cardiovascular risk factors can be translated into improved cardiovascular outcome.

These drugs also tend to lower blood pressure, troglitazone by perhaps 3 mmHg, and farglitazar at high doses by a quite useful 6 mmHg systolic. Hopefully, some of the newer agents will target this broad-spectrum approach to risk factor reduction in the future.

Safety concerns

The reduction in blood pressure may, however, be related to some of the safety concerns with this group of agents. There is no doubt that they all cause some degree of haemodilution, perhaps 5–10%. This is not associated with a change in red cell mass or red cell turnover, so the HbA1c data seem secure. The reason for this effect is not clear. Anaemia is recorded with a frequency of 2% in the trials but, in terms of a population of people shifting downwards through haemodilution, this is just the lower tail shifting across the threshold of the definition of anaemia.

Peripheral oedema is a common side effect – about 5% in rosiglitazone studies [5]. It is less of a problem in combination with sulphonylureas and metformin than with insulin. The reason for this effect is unclear, but may be related to the vasodilatation that is also associated with the blood pressure lowering effect. The problem of peripheral oedema and fluid retention in association with insulin led the European regulatory authorities not to allow its use. Rosiglitazone and pioglitazone are specifically contraindicated in the data sheets for use with insulin therapy in Europe, although paradoxically pioglitazone is licensed for use in combination with insulin in the US, and physicians use rosiglitazone in that way.

The concern over fluid retention is whether it can induce cardiac failure in susceptible individuals. In some of the rosiglitazone studies cardiac failure was recorded as an adverse event, but in phase III drug trials peripheral oedema will be overdiagnosed as cardiac failure, as indeed it is in ordinary clinical practice [10]. Echocardiographic studies with rosiglitazone show no change in either ejection fraction or left ventricular mass but, since the number of subjects in those studies was often only about 100, the question remains whether there will be any cases of induced cardiac failure as a result of what seems to be peripheral fluid retention.

Clinical use

Only rosiglitazone and pioglitazone are currently licensed and marketed in Europe. The licenses are for combination therapy with metformin or sulphonylurea, and not for monotherapy or for combination therapy with insulin. The two drugs are not cost-effective as monotherapy, and it can certainly be assumed that NICE would not have approved them in that role had the license allowed them to be so considered. There is no evidence of improved late outcomes in contrast to surrogate measures such as risk factors for late complications compared with sulphonylurea and metformin. Of course, these last two drugs have been around for 30–50 years and are very cheap, so in economic terms they are 'dominant' (cheaper and assumed to be at least as effective).

The NICE guidance now is that rosiglitazone and pioglitazone should be used in people on a sulphonylurea with poor glucose control who are unable to take metformin either because of intolerance or because it is contraindicated, or for people on metformin and a sulphonylurea with inadequate blood glucose control, the kind of people who might be coming to insulin therapy (Table 2) [11,12]. The overall cost of the glitazones has been estimated to be about two-thirds or less that of insulin therapy, so again in cost-effectiveness terms they dominate insulin therapy (there is no evidence that one or the other is more effective).

One difficulty, however, is whether the newly prescribed glitazone should be added to the sulphonylurea and metformin or substituted for one of them. NICE recommended the latter, taking a purist line because of the lack of evidence (absence of studies) of effectiveness of triple therapy. In their development programme, neither manufacturer could conceive that a licence would not be granted to cover triple combination therapy if their drug was shown to be effective both in combination with sulphonylurea and metformin separately. However, the Committee for Proprietary Medicinal Products failed to agree that use for either drug. This matters, as the PPARγ-agonists can take 1.5–3 months to be fully effective, while withdrawal of the sulphonylurea will cause deterioration in days. Accordingly, and rationally, in clinical practice this part of the guidance is being ignored for the most part.

Table 2 Use of peroxisome proliferator-activated receptor (PPAR)γ-agonists.

- Only rosiglitazone and pioglitazone available
- Current licence only for combination therapy with metformin or sulphonylurea
- Not cost-effective as monotherapy
- Contraindicated with insulin therapy
- NICE guidance:
    - people on a sulphonylurea who are unable to take metformin
    - people on metformin and a sulphonylurea with inadequate blood glucose control

NICE = National Institute for Clinical Excellence.

□ THE FUTURE

PPARγ-agonists may have other useful effects. Buchanan studied Spanish women in Los Angeles with a history of gestational diabetes which had gone into remission after pregnancy [13]. When followed on troglitazone for over two years there was a notable increase in insulin sensitivity, and their relative risk of developing diabetes was about half that of a population not so treated. The safety of these agents in pregnancy has not been established. However, the study shows that there may be a role for these agents much earlier in the disease process, provided that the £400 per annum which this kind of therapy currently costs can be afforded.

Acknowledgement

PDH, on behalf of the University of Newcastle upon Tyne, has been a consultant to, and received research support from, the companies that now constitute GlaxoSmithKline.

REFERENCES

1   Kersten S, Desvergne B, Wahli W. Roles of PPARs in health and disease. Review. *Nature* 2000; **405**: 421–4.
2   Stern MP. The insulin resistance syndrome. In: Alberti KGMM, Zimmet P, DeFronzo RA (eds). *International Textbook of Diabetes Mellitus*, 2nd edn. Chichester: John Wiley, 1997: 255–83.

3   Yki-Järvinen H. Pathogenesis of non-insulin-dependent diabetes mellitus. Review. *Lancet* 1994; **343**: 91–5.

4   Schoonjans K, Auwerx J. Thiazolidinediones: an update. *Lancet* 2000; **355**: 1008–10.

5   SmithKline Beecham. *Rosiglitazone: a clinician's resource file.* Welwyn Garden City: SmithKline Beecham, 1999.

6   Aronoff S, Rosenblatt S, Braithwaite S, Egan JW, *et al.* Pioglitazone hydrochloride monotherapy improves glycemic control in the treatment of patients with type 2 diabetes: a 6-month randomized placebo-controlled dose-response study. The Pioglitazone 001 Study Group. *Diabetes Care* 2000; **23**: 1605–11.

7   Wolffenbuttel BH, Gomis R, Squatrito S, Jones NP, Patwardhan RN. Addition of low-dose rosiglitazone to sulphonylurea therapy improves glycaemic control in type 2 diabetic patients. *Diabet Med* 2000; **17**: 40–7.

8   SmithKline Beecham Pharmaceuticals. *Avandia — taking control of type 2 diabetes.* Welwyn Garden City: SmithKline Beecham, 2000.

9   Rubins HB, Robins SJ, Collins D, Fye CL, *et al.* Gemfibrozil for the secondary prevention of coronary heart disease in men with low levels of high-density lipoprotein cholesterol. Veterans Affairs High-Density Lipoprotein Cholesterol Intervention Trial Study Group. *N Engl J Med* 1999; **341**: 410–8.

10   Caruana L, Petrie MC, Davie AP, McMurray JJ. Do patients with suspected heart failure and preserved left ventricular systolic function suffer from 'diastolic heart failure' or from misdiagnosis? A prospective descriptive study. *Br Med J* 2000; **321**: 215–8.

11   National Institute for Clinical Excellence. *Guidance on the use of rosiglitazone for Type 2 diabetes mellitus.* Technology Appraisal Guidance No. 9. London: NICE, 2000. (www.nice.org.uk)

12   National Institute for Clinical Excellence. *Guidance on the use of pioglitazone for Type 2 diabetes mellitus.* Technology Appraisal Guidance No. 21. London: NICE, 2001. (www.nice.org.uk)

13   Buchanan TA, Xiang AH, Peters RK, Kjoŝ SL, *et al.* Response of pancreatic beta-cells to improved insulin sensitivity in women at high risk for type 2 diabetes. *Diabetes* 2000; **49**: 782–8.

HOPE and other recent trials of antihypertensive therapy in type 2 diabetes

Rudy Bilous

☐ INTRODUCTION

Hypertension and diabetes have been called the 'bad companions' because of their additive and multiplicative effects on cardiovascular (CV) risk. Analysis of a Finnish cohort of diabetic and non-diabetic men revealed that the seven-year risk for a CV event was the same for diabetic patients without a history of previous myocardial infarction (MI) as for non-diabetic subjects with a history of MI [1]. This risk was effectively doubled for any given blood pressure level in diabetic compared with non-diabetic men in the MRFIT study [2] (see end of text for explanation of studies). The UKPDS found that about one-third of newly diagnosed type 2 diabetic patients had hypertension, defined as being on previous antihypertensive therapy or having a blood pressure higher than 160/90 mmHg [3]. It has been estimated that blood pressure will be higher than 140/90 mmHg, the current treatment threshold recommended by the Joint British Societies [4], in over 80% of diabetic patients in their lifetime. Finally, patients with essential hypertension have a 2.5-fold risk of developing diabetes compared with their age- and sex-matched normotensive counterparts (blood pressure <140/90 mmHg) [5].

Given these appalling statistics, it is hardly surprising that there has been a series of large studies of antihypertensive therapy in diabetic subjects – although the diabetic group usually comprised a subset of the total study population. This review will consider seven trials (HOPE [6,7], HOT [8], SYST-EUR [9], CAPPP [10], STOP-2 [11], NORDIL [12] and INSIGHT [13]). It is not a meta-analysis, but an attempt to outline the studies, condense their results and draw attention to any potential caveats.

☐ HOPE AND MICRO-HOPE

The HOPE and MICRO-HOPE studies (Table 1) [6,7] investigated the effects on the primary outcome of a composite of MI, stroke or CV death of an angiotensin-converting enzyme (ACE) inhibitor, ramipril, 10 mg/day, vitamin E 400 IU/day, or both or placebo in a 2 × 2 factorial design. The 9,297 patients included in the study had a previous history of CV disease or diabetes plus one other CV risk factor:

☐ hypertension: blood pressure above 160/90 mmHg or on antihypertensive therapy

Table 1 MICRO-HOPE at a glance: ramipril versus placebo [6,7].

Duration of study	4.5 years
Mean age	65.4 years
No. with diabetes	3,496
% of total cohort with diabetes	39
% of patients with diabetes and:	
hypertension	56 (>160/90 mmHg or on treatment)
raised cholesterol	66
microalbuminuria	32 (ACR >2 mg/mmol)
previous cardiovascular disease	68
Smokers (%)	15
Primary end-points	MI
	Stroke
	Cardiovascular death
Event rate/1,000 patient-years	34: ramipril 10 mg/day
(diabetic cohort)	44: placebo

ACR = urinary albumin: creatinine ratio; MI = myocardial infarction.

☐   serum total cholesterol: above 5.2 mmol/l

☐   high-density lipoprotein cholesterol: above 0.9 mmol/l

☐   smoking

☐   microalbuminuria: urinary albumin:creatinine ratio (ACR) above 2 mg/mmol.

Patients were excluded if they were taking ACE inhibitors or vitamin E, or if they had:

☐   suffered an MI or stroke within the previous four weeks

☐   heart failure and/or ejection fraction less than 40%

☐   overt proteinuria: ACR above 36 mg/mmol

☐   uncontrolled hypertension (blood pressure not specified).

The study was originally designed to last 3.5 years; it was then extended to five years, but was prematurely stopped at 4.5 years.

There were 3,577 patients (39%) with diabetes, of whom 3,496 (98%) had type 2 disease; 1,996 (57%) of this subset had a previous history of hypertension, 2,335 (67%) an elevated total cholesterol and 1,140 (33%) microalbuminuria, while 15% were active smokers. Baseline glycaemia is hard to estimate, but the glycated haemoglobin (DCCT standardised) was probably about 7.6%.

Results

Vitamin E had no effect, but ramipril reduced the combined primary outcome by 25% (95% confidence intervals (CI) 12–36%, $p = 0.0004$). This magnitude of effect was also seen for each individual end-point: relative risk (RR) reduction 22% (95% CI 6–36%) for MI, 33% (95% CI 10–50%) for stroke and 37% (95% CI 21–51%) for CV death. The overall CV event rate was 19.8% over 4.5 years, similar to the rate reported in UK diabetic populations.

Event rates per 1,000 person-years were not reported but have been estimated from the results in order to compare them with other studies. Assuming an average follow-up of 4.5 years, there were 8,136 and 7,961 patient-years' treatment for the ramipril and placebo groups, respectively, giving event rates of 34 and 44 per 1,000 patient-years for the primary end-points in the two groups, respectively. For specific diabetes end-points, there was a significant reduction of 24% (95% CI 3–40%) in overt nephropathy (ACR >36 mg/mmol) and a non-significant reduction of 22% (CI –9 to 28%) in the need for laser photocoagulation. To prevent one primary end-point event, 22 patients would need to be treated with ramipril for 4.5 years and 28 to prevent one CV death.

The results for the diabetic cohort were similar to the total study group, but there was a greater benefit in those with pre-existing CV disease (18.7% vs 10.2% reduction in the primary end-point). Newly diagnosed diabetes was less frequent in the ramipril group. This finding is difficult to interpret because diagnosis depended upon opportunistic detection and there were more events in the placebo group (and presumably more opportunity for detection) than in the ramipril group.

Caveats

These impressive results would seem to imply that most type 2 patients should be on an ACE inhibitor. It is estimated that 78% of the non-proteinuric hospital clinic population with type 2 diabetes in Middlesbrough would satisfy the entry criteria for the study. However, there are some concerns.

1   About one-third of patients stopped the study medication. The reason is not stated in most cases. It is also unknown whether these patients could be assessed at the end of the study and/or whether a 'last result carried forward analysis' was used for missing data.

2   There was a small, but statistically significant, reduction in blood pressure (2/1 mmHg) in the ramipril group. In some ways, it is surprising this was not greater as over half the patients were hypertensive at baseline. Such a small drop in blood pressure almost certainly cannot explain the magnitude of effect, but *post hoc* analysis of the UKPDS blood pressure cohort suggests more observed benefit from antihypertensive therapy than might be predicted from blood pressure reduction alone [14].

3   The most important consideration is the balance of patients in the placebo and ramipril treated groups with and without a previous history of CV disease at baseline: 47 more patients had previous coronary artery disease in the placebo group, and ramipril treatment prevented 44 MIs; 26 more patients had had a previous stroke, 32 were prevented by ramipril; 89 fewer patients in the ramipril group had no previous CV disease and 74 combined end-points were prevented.

As previously mentioned, event rates were much lower in patients with a previous history of cardiovascular disease. Although the test for interaction between presence and absence of CV disease at baseline and results of therapy was non-significant, there must be a small cause for concern.

4   The nephroprotective results in the microalbuminuric patients are significant only if the ACR values are analysed. They are non-significant in terms of the more precise timed urine collections. It is also notable that ACR values increased throughout the study in the ramipril treated patients despite a less steep initial change during the first year.

Conclusions

The HOPE and MICRO-HOPE studies have provided evidence of a specific benefit of ACE inhibition in diabetic and non-diabetic patients at increased CV risk, which in practice includes most of those with type 2 diabetes. These patients usually also have blood pressures above the current recommended treatment thresholds, so there seems little doubt that ACE inhibitors should now be used as first-line therapy for blood pressure control in diabetes. Despite the caveats, this therapy should probably be extended to normotensive patients who have a high CV risk.

☐ HOT

HOT [8] was a large trial in 26 countries in which 18,790 patients (1,501 with diabetes) with baseline diastolic blood pressures of 100–115 mmHg were randomised to three target levels: less than 90 mmHg, 85 mmHg and 80 mmHg. Therapy was initially based upon the dihydropyridine calcium-channel blocker (CCB) felodipine. Patients were also randomly assigned to 75 mg aspirin or placebo. Mean follow-up was 3.8 years. Patient details and results are listed in Table 2.

Table 2 HOT at a glance: calcium-channel blocker and other drugs to target diastolic blood pressures less than 90 mmHg, 85 mmHg and 80 mmHg [8].

Duration of study	3.8 years
Mean age	61.5 years
No. with diabetes	1,501
% of total cohort with diabetes	8
% of patients with:	
hypertension	100 (diastolic >100 mmHg)
raised cholesterol	–
microalbuminuria	–
previous cardiovascular disease	8.7
Smokers (%)	15
Primary end-points	Non-fatal MI
	Stroke
	Cardiovascular death
Event rate/1,000 patient-years	24.4: diastolic <90mm Hg
(diabetic cohort)	11.9: diastolic <80mm Hg

MI = myocardial infarction.

Results

Achieved blood pressures were 144/85 mmHg, 141/83 mmHg and 140/81 mmHg for the three target groups, respectively; 12%, 7% and 6% of patients in these groups had diastolic pressures above 90 mmHg. There was no significant effect of the lower diastolic blood pressure for the group as a whole, but a highly significant reduction from 24.4 to 11.9 events per 1,000 patient-years in the diabetic cohort – a lower event rate than in the HOPE study, although there was no effect on MI and stroke separately. Aspirin prevented 53 major CV events, but was associated with an excess 59 major non-fatal bleeds. The reduction in MI rate per 1,000 patient-years was 2.5 and 1.5 in diabetic and non-diabetic subjects.

Conclusions

Low risk patients with primarily diastolic hypertension do not show benefit from blood pressure reduction unless they also have diabetes. There does not appear to be a deleterious effect of diastolic blood pressure reduction below 80 mmHg. Aspirin use for primary prevention of MI is effective, but the benefit is outweighed by excess risk of gastrointestinal haemorrhage.

☐ SYST-EUR

The main SYST-EUR trial in 4,695 elderly patients (≥60 years) with blood pressure 160–219/95 mmHg was reported in 1997. A *post hoc* analysis was undertaken of the 492 (10.5%) type 2 diabetic patients (Table 3) [9]. Patients were randomised either to the CCB nitrendipine or placebo, with options to combine or replace with enalapril or hydrochlorothiazide, or both, in order to achieve a systolic blood

Table 3 SYST-EUR at a glance: calcium-channel blocker or placebo alone or with enalapril/diuretics [9].

Duration of study	Median 2 years
Mean age	76.2 years
No. with diabetes	492
% of total cohort with diabetes	10.5
% of patients with diabetes and:	
hypertension	100 (systolic >160 mmHg)
raised cholesterol	–
proteinuria	15.5
previous cardiovascular disease	35
Smokers (%)	6.3
Primary end-points	Fatal and non-fatal MI
	Stroke
	Cardiovascular death
Event rate/1,000 patient-years	57.6: placebo (BP fall 14/3 mmHg)
(diabetic cohort)	22: nitrendipine (BP fall 22/7 mmHg)

BP = blood pressure; MI = myocardial infarction.

pressure below 150 mmHg. Prior to enrolment, 62% of the diabetic cohort were on antihypertensive therapy, 35% had had previous CV disease, 15.5% were proteinuric and 6.3% were current smokers. The median follow-up was two years, with a primary end-point of fatal and non-fatal stroke.

Results

Blood pressure fell by a mean of 14/3 mmHg and 22/7 mm Hg in the placebo and nitrendipine groups, respectively. ACE inhibitors were given to 60% of patients in the placebo group and 43% in the nitrendipine group. Event rates were high, at 57.6 per 1,000 patient-years for fatal and non-fatal MI, stroke and CV death combined on placebo, with a significant reduction of 62% (95% CI 19–80%) to 22 per 1,000 patient-years in the nitrendipine group.

Conclusions

Despite the small numbers, the *post hoc* analysis in high risk type 2 diabetic patients showed impressive benefit in terms of systolic blood pressure reduction. The dihydropyridine CCB nitrendipine was as effective as monotherapy as in combination with an ACE inhibitor.

☐ CAPPP

CAPPP was another large trial in 10,985 low risk patients, most of whom had previously untreated diastolic hypertension (>100 mmHg) (Table 4) [10]. Only 329 (3%) had a previous history of ischaemic heart disease, MI or stroke and 527 (5%) had diabetes. Patients were randomised to captopril 50 mg/day in one or two doses, or to beta-blockers (atenolol/metoprolol) 50–100 mg once daily and diuretics (hydrochlorothiazide 25 mg/bendrofluazide 2.5 mg). The primary end-point was non-fatal MI and stroke and CV death, with a mean follow-up of 6.1 years.

Results

The event rate was about 11 per 1,000 patient-years – much lower than in HOPE and HOT. There was no difference between treatment groups except for non-fatal stroke which, curiously, was significantly increased in the captopril group. However, mean achieved blood pressure was consistently lower in the beta-blocker/thiazide group. Randomisation was incomplete, with more diabetic subjects and a higher baseline blood pressure in the captopril arm. Fewer new cases of diabetes occurred in those treated with captopril. Again, the diabetic cohort showed a positive benefit of captopril for the primary end-point (RR reduction 41%, 95% CI 9–62%, $p = 0.019$).

Table 4 CAPPP at a glance: captopril versus beta-blockers/diuretics [10].

Duration of study	Mean 6.1 years
Mean age	52.6 years
No. with diabetes	527
% of total cohort with diabetes	5.3
% of patients with diabetes and:	
hypertension	100 (diastolic >100 mmHg)
raised cholesterol	–
microalbuminuria	–
previous cardiovascular disease	9
Smokers (%)	22
Primary end-points	Non-fatal MI
	Stroke
	Cardiovascular death
Event rate/1,000 patient-years (whole group)	11 for all groups (41% RR reduction for captopril in diabetic cohort, $p = 0.019$)

MI = myocardial infarction; RR = relative risk.

Conclusions

This study suffers from poor baseline comparability and a less than ideal (once daily) dose of captopril. The observed excess in stroke on captopril in this trial is an isolated finding, almost certainly a result of study design.

☐ STOP-2

The STOP-2 trial was another attempt to test some of the new antihypertensive drugs against beta-blockers and diuretics (Table 5) [11]. A total of 6,614 patients, aged 70–84 years, with blood pressure above 180 mmHg systolic or above 105 mmHg diastolic, or both, of whom 721 (11%) had diabetes were randomised to a beta-blocker/thiazide, ACE inhibitor or CCB-based regimen. The minimum duration of treatment was four years and the primary end-point was CV death due to MI or stroke.

Results

About 60% of patients were still on their assigned medication at the end of the study. The three treatment regimens were similarly effective at blood pressure reduction (average 161/82 mmHg). The observed CV death rate was about 33 per 1,000 patient-years for all groups. The event rate was 43 per 1,000 years for the same major CV end-points as in the HOT and HOPE studies. Treatment effects were the same in the three groups, and the diabetic cohort showed no variation from the overall group. Fatal and non-fatal MI (RR reduction 23%, 95% CI 4–39%) and heart failure (RR reduction 22%, CI 3–34%) were less frequent on the ACE inhibitor than in the CCB group.

Conclusions

The results of the STOP-2 study demonstrate that similar reductions in blood pressure produce similar reductions in CV mortality. There were no specific benefits

Table 5 STOP-2 at a glance: angiotensin-converting enzyme inhibitor versus calcium-channel blocker versus beta-blockers/diuretics [11].

Duration of study	>4 years
Mean age	76 years
No. with diabetes	721
% of total cohort with diabetes	10.9
% of patients with diabetes and:	
hypertension	100 (>180/105 mmHg)
raised cholesterol	–
microalbuminuria	–
previous cardiovascular disease	24.1
Smokers (%)	7
Primary end-points	MI
	Stroke
	Cardiovascular death
Event rate/1,000 patient-years (whole cohort)	43 for all groups

MI = myocardial infarction.

for diabetic patients in this elderly population, probably because background event rates are already high in this age group.

☐ NORDIL

The NORDIL study was designed to test a non-dihydropyridine CCB against diuretics and beta-blockers (Table 6) [12]. A total of 10,881 patients, 727 (7%) with diabetes, aged 50–74 years (mean 60.4 years), with untreated diastolic hypertension (>100 mmHg) were enrolled; 22.5% were smokers and about 7% had a previous history of ischaemic heart disease or cerebrovascular disease. They were randomised to diltiazem 180–360 mg/day or to a beta-blocker or thiazide. The target diastolic blood pressure was below 90 mmHg. Other agents could be added in a stepwise fashion, with an ACE inhibitor at step 2 for the diltiazem group and step 3 for the

Table 6 NORDIL at a glance: diltiazem versus beta-blockers/diuretics [12].

Duration of study	4.5 years
Mean age	60.4 years
No. with diabetes	727
% of total cohort with diabetes	6.7
% of patients with:	
hypertension	100 (diastolic >100 mmHg)
raised cholesterol	–
microalbuminuria	–
previous cardiovascular disease	7
Smokers (%)	22.5
Primary end-points	MI
	Stroke
	Cardiovascular death
Event rate/1,000 patient-years	29: diabetic cohort
	16: whole group (no effect between therapies)

MI = myocardial infarction.

beta-blocker/thiazide patients. The primary end-points were fatal and non-fatal MI and stroke and CV death. Mean follow-up was 4.5 years, with 48,992 patient-years accumulated.

Results

Mean achieved blood pressure was 155/89 mmHg and 152/89 mmHg in the diltiazem and beta-blocker/thiazide groups, respectively. Only 77% of the diltiazem patients remained on their assigned therapy compared with 93% in the other group and about 50% of the patients in both groups were on additional therapy. Event rates were almost identical in the two groups and slightly lower than for HOPE.

Conclusions

The impact of the two treatments was the same, but fewer patients remained on diltiazem alone, thus more in this group must have been on ACE inhibitors because of the stepwise study design. No differences between treatments were observed in the small diabetic cohort.

□ INSIGHT

Once-daily nifedipine was compared with a diuretic in the INSIGHT trial which included 6,321 patients (1,302 with type 1 and 2 diabetes) (Table 7) [13] aged 55–80 years, with blood pressure above 150/95 mmHg or isolated systolic pressure above 160 mmHg plus another cardiovascular risk factor (plasma cholesterol above 6.43 mmol/l, smoking, family history of premature (<50 years) MI in parent or sibling, left ventricular hypertrophy, stable ischaemic heart disease, peripheral vascular disease or proteinuria 500 mg/day). Target blood pressure was a fall of 20/10 mmHg or below 140/90 mmHg. Patients were studied for a minimum of three years.

Table 7 INSIGHT at a glance: nifedipine LA versus diuretics [13].

Duration of study	>3 years
Mean age	65 years
No. with diabetes (mixed type 1 & type 2)	1,302
% of total cohort with diabetes	20.6
% of patients with:	
hypertension	100 (>150/95 mmHg)
raised cholesterol	52
proteinuria	2.5
previous cardiovascular disease	18
Smokers (%)	28.4
Primary end-points	MI
	Stroke
	Cardiovascular death
Event rate/1,000 patient-years	15.8: nifedipine (whole cohort)
	15.4: diuretic (whole cohort)
	1.47: hazard ratio for diabetes

MI = myocardial infarction.

Results

Blood pressure levels achieved were almost identical (138/82 mmHg at 3 years). Approximately two-thirds of the patients had remained on assigned monotherapy and 56–57% in both groups had reached the target blood pressure. Adverse events were more frequent in the nifedipine group, mainly due to symptomatic oedema in 28%. The overall composite event rate of CV death and non-fatal MI and stroke was 15.8 and 15.4 per 1,000 patient-years in the nifedipine and diuretic groups, respectively, with higher rates in the diabetic patients (hazard ratio for diabetes 1.47 (CI 1.16–1.86)).

Conclusions

There was no significant difference between the groups in terms of CV outcome but oedema was a problem in the nifedipine group. There was no specific diabetes benefit, but more metabolic problems (hyperglycaemia, hyperuricaemia, hyponatraemia, hypokalaemia, hyperlipidaemia) in the diabetic patients on thiazides.

☐ OVERALL CONCLUSIONS

It is important to reduce both systolic and diastolic blood pressure in diabetic patients, with possibly more benefit than for non-diabetic individuals. A target blood pressure of <140/80 mmHg, as recommended by the Joint British Societies [4], is firmly evidence-based. ACE inhibitors are probably first choice, based primarily on the HOPE study, but beta-blockers and diuretics are also effective. CCBs appear to offer no specific advantage, but neither do they have consistent disadvantages except for side effects such as oedema and headache. However, it is worth noting, first, that the studies were not powered to detect possibly important differences in MI rates (eg of the order of 10–15%) and, secondly, that CCBs are more expensive than some of the other alternatives.

☐ TRIAL ACRONYMS

CAPPP	Captopril Prevention Project
DCCT	Diabetes Control and Complications Trial
HOPE	Heart Outcomes Prevention Evaluation
HOT	Hypertension Optimal Treatment
INSIGHT	Intervention as a Goal in Hypertension Treatment
MRFIT	Multiple Risk Factor Intervention Trial
NORDIL	Nordic Diltiazem
STOP-2	Swedish Trial in Old Patients with Hypertension-2
SYST-EUR	Systolic Hypertension in Europe
UKPDS	UK Prospective Diabetes Study

REFERENCES

1   Haffner SM, Lehto S, Ronnemaa T, Pyorala K, Laakso M. Mortality from coronary heart disease in subjects with type 2 diabetes and in nondiabetic subjects with and without prior myocardial infarction. *N Engl J Med* 1998; **339**: 229–34.

2   Stamler J, Vaccaro O, Neaton JD, Wentworth D. Diabetes, other risk factors, and 12-yr cardiovascular mortality for men screened in the Multiple Risk Factor Intervention Trial. *Diabetes Care* 1993; **16**: 434–44.

3   Tight blood pressure control and risk of macrovascular and microvascular complications in type 2 diabetes: UKPDS 38. UK Prospective Diabetes Study Group. *Br Med J* 1998; **317**: 703–13.

4   Ramsay L, Williams B, Johnston GD, MacGregor G, *et al.* Guidelines for management of hypertension: report of the third working party of the British Hypertension Society. Review. *J Hum Hypertens* 1999; **13**: 569–92.

5   Gress TW, Nieto FJ, Shahar E, Wofford MR, Brancati FL. Hypertension and antihypertensive therapy as risk factors for type 2 diabetes mellitus. Atherosclerosis Risk in Communities Study. *N Engl J Med* 2000; **342**: 905–12.

6   Yusuf S, Sleight P, Pogue J, Bosch J, *et al.* Effects of an angiotensin-converting-enzyme inhibitor, ramipril, on cardiovascular events in high-risk patients. The Heart Outcomes Prevention Evaluation Study Investigators. *N Engl J Med* 2000; **342**: 145–53.

7   Effects of ramipril on cardiovascular and microvascular outcomes in people with diabetes Mellitus: results of the HOPE study and MICRO-HOPE substudy. Heart Outcomes Prevention Evaluation (HOPE) Study Investigators. *Lancet* 2000; **355**: 253–9.

8   Hansson L, Zanchetti A, Carruthers SG, Dahlof B, *et al.* Effects of intensive blood-pressure lowering and low-dose aspirin in patients with hypertension: principal results of the Hypertension Optimal Treatment (HOT) randomised trial. HOT Study Group. *Lancet* 1998; **351**: 1755–62.

9   Tuomilehto J, Rastenyte D, Birkenhager WH, Thijs L, *et al.* Effects of calcium-channel blockade in older patients with diabetes and systolic hypertension. Systolic Hypertension in Europe Trial Investigators. *N Engl J Med* 1999; **340**: 677–84.

10 Hansson L, Lindholm LH, Niskanen L, Lanke J, *et al.* Effect of angiotensin-converting-enzyme inhibition compared with conventional therapy on cardiovascular morbidity and mortality in hypertension: the Captopril Prevention Project (CAPPP) randomised trial. *Lancet* 1999; **353**: 611–6.

11 Hansson L, Lindholm LH, Ekbom T, Dahlof B, *et al.* Randomised trial of old and new antihypertensive drugs in elderly patients: cardiovascular mortality and morbidity. The Swedish Trial in Old Patients with Hypertension-2 study. *Lancet* 1999; **354**: 1751–6.

12 Hansson L, Hedner T, Lund-Johansen P, Kjeldsen SE, *et al.* Randomised trial of effects of calcium antagonists compared with diuretics and beta-blockers on cardiovascular morbidity and mortality in hypertension: the Nordic Diltiazem (NORDIL) study. *Lancet* 2000; **356**: 359–65.

13 Brown MJ, Palmer CR, Castaigne A, de Leeuw PW, *et al.* Morbidity and mortality in patients randomised to double-blind treatment with a long-acting calcium-channel blocker or diuretic in the International Nifedipine GITS Study: Intervention as a Goal in Hypertension Treatment (INSIGHT). *Lancet* 2000; **356**: 366–72.

14 Adler AI, Stratton IM, Neal HA, Yudkin JS, *et al.* Association of systolic blood pressure with macrovascular and microvascular complications of type 2 diabetes (UKPDS 36): prospective observational study. *Br Med J* 2000; **321**: 412–9.

☐ SELF ASSESSMENT QUESTIONS

1   Patients with type 2 diabetes:

(a) Have a lifetime risk of hypertension (>140/90 mmHg) of more than 80%

(b) Have the same 7-year risk of a cardiovascular (CV) event as non-diabetic patients with a previous history of myocardial infarction (MI)

(c) Over one-third have hypertension (>160/90 mmHg) at diagnosis

(d) Have hypertension unresponsive to beta-blockers

(e) Treated with vitamin E antioxidants have fewer CV events

2   The HOPE and MICRO-HOPE studies:
(a) Showed a relative risk reduction of 22% for MI in the ramipril group
(b) Revealed that one MI or stroke or CV death could be prevented for each
     100 patients treated with ramipril for a year
(c) Showed a stronger benefit of ramipril in preventing MI than thrombolysis
(d) Over 80% of patients remained on ramipril for the duration of the study
(e) Less than 50% of non-proteinuric type 2 diabetic patients in a typical UK
     hospital clinic population would meet the entry criteria for the studies

3   In the HOT study:
(a) 20% of patients had diabetes at baseline
(b) CV event rates were higher than in the MICRO-HOPE study
(c) A lower diastolic pressure was associated with more CV events
(d) Low-dose aspirin prevented over 50 major CV events
(e) Angiotensin-converting enzyme (ACE) inhibitors were superior to calcium-
     channel blockers (CCB)

4   In the SYST-EUR study:
(a) Older patients showed no CV benefit from treatment
(b) Achieved blood pressure levels were equal in the two arms of the study
(c) CCB were less effective as monotherapy than ACE inhibitors
(d) Lowering systolic blood pressure prevented approximately four major CV
     events per 100 patient-years
(e) Diuretic therapy was excluded

5   In comparative trials of newer versus older blood pressure treatments (CAPPP,
     NORDIL, INSIGHT, STOP-2):
(a) ACE inhibitors were associated with an increased risk of stroke in CAPPP
(b) The CCB nifedipine was associated with fewer side effects than its
     comparator
(c) Diltiazem therapy resulted in lower blood pressure levels than its
     comparator
(d) Patient compliance with diltiazem was better than with its comparator
(e) STOP-2 demonstrated that reductions in primary end-points were blood
     pressure and not therapy related

ANSWERS

1a True	2a True	3a False	4a False	5a True
b True	b True	b False	b False	b False
c True	c False	c False	c False	c False
d False	d False	d True	d True	d False
e False	e False	e False	e True	e True

Haematology

Molecular targeting as treatment for the chronic myeloid leukaemias

John Goldman and Nicholas Cross

☐ INTRODUCTION

The disease now designated chronic myeloid leukaemia (CML) was probably recognised for the first time in 1845. The first important clue to the underlying pathogenesis came more than 100 years later with the observation that leukaemic cells from CML patients had a consistent G group chromosomal abnormality, now universally referred to as the Philadelphia (Ph) chromosome. This was the first consistent chromosomal abnormality to be associated with malignancy. Its discovery has led in the last 15 years to the identification of the BCR-ABL fusion gene, now regarded as the immediate cause of the chronic phase of CML [1]. The detailed mechanisms by which the BCR-ABL oncoprotein causes the phenotypic features of CML have not yet been unravelled, but should be clarified before too long if the pace of research in CML in the last few years is any guide to the future.

About 90% of patients with a leukaemia classifiable on haematological grounds as CML have a Ph chromosome in their leukaemia cells. Approximately half the rest have a typical BCR-ABL fusion gene in association with a normal karyotype, with the gene usually located on a normal-appearing chromosome 22q but occasionally on chromosome 9q. The remaining patients lack BCR-ABL, but in some cases other fusion genes encoding tyrosine kinases have been identified (Fig. 1, Table 1) [1,2]. This chapter will briefly describe the clinical and haematological features of the CMLs with identified fusion genes and highlight molecular inhibitors that may prove useful in clinical practice.

☐ BCR-ABL POSITIVE CHRONIC MYELOID LEUKAEMIA

Ph-positive CML is one of the four major types of leukaemia, with an annual incidence of 1.0–1.4 per 100,000 population. Its incidence rises with age, so the disease is probably more common in the developed than the developing world. Classically, patients present with symptoms associated with anaemia, haemorrhage due to platelet dysfunction or with the effects of splenomegaly. Increasingly, patients are diagnosed before the onset of symptoms as a result of routine blood tests performed for unrelated reasons. The diagnosis is usually based on typical findings in the blood and marrow:

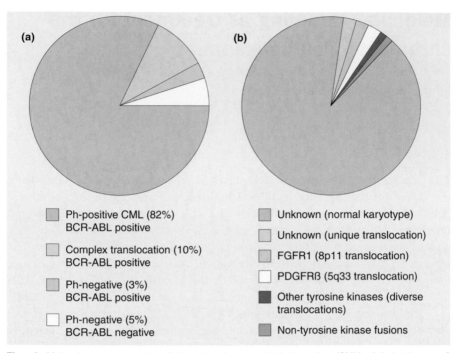

Ph-positive CML (82%)
BCR-ABL positive

Complex translocation (10%)
BCR-ABL positive

Ph-negative (3%)
BCR-ABL positive

Ph-negative (5%)
BCR-ABL negative

Unknown (normal karyotype)

Unknown (unique translocation)

FGFR1 (8p11 translocation)

PDGFRβ (5q33 translocation)

Other tyrosine kinases (diverse
translocations)

Non-tyrosine kinase fusions

Fig. 1 Molecular pathogenesis of the chronic myeloid leukaemias (CML): **(a)** incidence of Philadelphia (Ph) and BCR-ABL positivity in CML; **(b)** the molecular pathogenesis of myeloproliferative disorder/myelodysplastic syndromes (MPD/MDS), including BCR-ABL negative CML and atypical CML (FGFR = fibroblast growth factor receptor; PDGFR = platelet-derived growth factor receptor) (data from the Medical Research Council CML III trial reproduced, with permission, from [2]).

Table 1 Translocations involving tyrosine kinases in the chronic myeloid leukaemias (CML).

Disease	Translocation	Fusion gene
CML	t(9;22)(q34;q11)	BCR-ABL
EMS ·	t(8;13)(p11;q12)	ZNF198-FGFR1
	t(8;9)(p11;q33)	CEP110-FGFR1
	t(6;8)(q27;p12)	FOP-FGFR1
	t(8;22)(p11;q22)	BCR-FGFR1
aCML/CMML	t(5;12)(q33;p13)	ETV6-PDGFRβ
	t(5;10)(q33;q21)	H4-PDGFRβ
	t(5;7)(q33;q11)	HIP1-PDGFRβ
	t(5;17)(q33;p15)	RAB5-PDGFRβ
Other BCR-ABL	t(9;12)(q34;p13)	ETV6-ABL
negative CML	t(9;12)(p24;q13)	ETV6-JAK2
	t(9;22)(p24;q11)	BCR-JAK2

aCML = atypical chronic myeloid leukaemia; CMML = chronic myelomonocytic leukaemia; EMS = 8p11 myeloproliferative syndrome; FGFR = fibroblast growth factor receptor; PDGFR = platelet-derived growth factor receptor.

□   raised leukocyte count (20-300 x 10^9/l), with the differential showing a range of immature myeloid cells, including blasts, promyelocytes and myelocytes

□   the platelet count is often raised

□   there may be a variable degree of anaemia

□   the bone marrow aspirate is hypercellular with complete loss of normal fat spaces

□   cytogenetic analysis of dividing myeloid cells reveals a typical Ph chromosome [3].

Treatment

The standard immediate treatment for Ph-positive CML is hydroxyurea, which rapidly restores the leukocyte count to normal. Until recently, older patients (>50 years) have then been offered treatment with interferon (IFN)-α, alone or in conjunction with cytarabine, since IFN-α appears to prolong life in comparison with hydroxyurea, perhaps by 1–2 years. Allogeneic stem cell transplantation is currently the only approach that can cure CML, so younger patients with suitable stem cell donors (only about 20% of all patients) may be treated in this way. The risk of mortality from stem cell transplantation is appreciable, so the decision in a given patient whether to recommend a transplant or 'non-curative' treatment with IFN-α may be extremely difficult.

Tyrosine kinase inhibitors

The Ph translocation brings together portions of two normal genes, BCR on 22q and ABL on 9q, to generate the BCR-ABL fusion gene on the 22q-. In patients with a normal or ambiguous karyotype, BCR-ABL can be detected by molecular methods such as fluorescence *in situ* hybridisation or reverse-transcriptase polymerase chain reaction. The fusion gene is expressed as a p210[BCR-ABL] oncoprotein, with tyrosine kinase activity greatly enhanced in comparison with that of the normal ABL protein. BCR-ABL activates multiple signal transduction pathways and is thought to be the principal, possibly the sole, cause of the chronic phase of CML [1].

Theoretically, any agent able to block the kinase activity of the BCR-ABL protein or a relevant downstream signalling pathway could reverse the phenotype of CML. This reasoning led to preclinical studies which showed that the 2-phenylamino-pyrimidine molecule STI571, which occupies the ABL kinase adenosine triphosphate (ATP) binding site and inhibits tyrosine phosphorylation, could inhibit proliferation of CML cell lines and primary cells from CML patients [4,5]. As might be expected from its mode of action, STI571 is not completely specific for the ABL kinase and it has been found also to inhibit KIT and platelet-derived growth factor receptor (PDGFR) β. However, there is no evidence to suggest that these activities are relevant to its anti-leukaemia activity in Ph-positive CML.

STI571 (Glivec™). STI571 entered clinical trials in June 1998, and has now been tested extensively in patients with BCR-ABL positive CML in chronic phase, accelerated phase and blastic transformation [6]. It rapidly restores the leukocyte count to normal in patients previously treated with IFN-α and induces major cytogenetic responses in 40–50% of cases.

A prospective study has been launched in which previously untreated patients are randomly allocated to receive STI571 or IFN-α plus cytarabine. Preliminary data suggest that there may be about 60% complete cytogenetic responses – an impressive figure four or more times greater than can be achieved with IFN-α alone. The side effects include headaches, nausea, arthralgias and a variety of rashes, but they are in general manageable and much less disturbing to the patient than those associated with administration of IFN-α [5]. It is too early to predict the result of this prospective study, but there is a real possibility that STI571 may appreciably prolong life compared with IFN-α plus cytarabine.

As is common in pharmacology, acquired resistance to STI571 may limit its application as a single agent. Currently it is unclear the extent to which this resistance will prove a problem for patients on long-term treatment with this agent. Two mechanisms have been identified thus far:

1   Overexpression of BCR-ABL, usually as a result of gene amplification.

2   Mutations within the ATP binding domain that reduce the affinity of STI571 binding [7].

Resistance in cell lines may also result from overexpression of multidrug resistance proteins, but this has not been documented in patients so far.

Other agents. A variety of other agents have in the past been tested for their ability to block the kinase activity of the BCR-ABL protein, of which the most promising were the tyrphostins. However, they do not appear to have the specificity of STI571. The molecule designated PD180970 has activity similar to that of STI571 against the K562 CML cell line, but has not yet entered clinical practice. Other molecules are likely to follow in the near future.

Farnesyl transferase inhibitors

Any agent that inhibits farnesylation might interrupt the BCR-ABL derived signal for two reasons:

1   The BCR-ABL protein may act predominantly by activating the RAS pathway.

2   Activated RAS is functional only when attached to the inner surface of the plasma membrane by a prenyl group.

Several different farnesyl transferase inhibitors (FTIs) have been tested in preclinical work and one, SCH66366, has shown activity against a BCR-ABL transfected cell line in a murine model system [8], while another, R115777, is available for clinical use. Almost certainly the anti-leukaemic properties of FTIs are due to their effect on multiple, largely unknown, farnesylated targets and not only on RAS.

At least two FTIs have been tested in phase I/II studies in patients with a variety of malignancies including CML. Additional trials are planned. Given the fundamental role of RAS and other farnesylated proteins, it is somewhat surprising that these compounds appear to be well tolerated. Diverse tumours depend on RAS activation, so FTIs are likely to find wide application in the treatment of malignancy. Importantly, model systems have shown that FTIs may be active against cell lines that have acquired resistance to STI571, suggesting a possible role for them in future combination therapy.

Other compounds

No other compounds are currently available for targeted therapy in CML but several candidates are in development. Alternative methods to inhibit the activation of RAS have been explored, notably the development of molecules that block the recruitment of adapter molecules, such as Grb2, Crkl and Shc, which physically and functionally link BCR-ABL to RAS. Furthermore, analysis of BCR-ABL has indicated that its transforming function also depends on the PI3 kinase and signal transducer and activation of transcription (STAT) pathways (Fig. 2). Consequently, these are

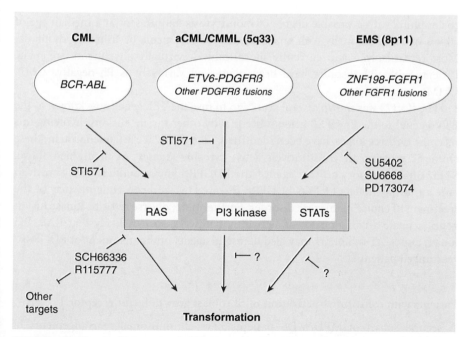

Fig. 2 Small molecules that may be useful for targeting deregulated tyrosine kinases or downstream signalling pathways in the chronic myeloid leukaemias (CML) (aCML = atypical CML; CMML = chronic myelomonocytic leukaemia; EMS = 8p11 myeloproliferative syndrome; FGFR = fibroblast growth factor receptor; PDGFR = platelet-derived growth factor receptor; STAT = signal transducer and activation of transcription).

also attractive targets for therapeutic intervention and it is likely that candidate inhibitors will become available in the near future.

☐ BCR-ABL NEGATIVE, CHRONIC MYELOID LEUKAEMIA-LIKE DISORDERS

As described above, roughly 5% of patients with a haematological picture of CML are negative for the BCR-ABL fusion gene on molecular analysis. These patients have typically been classified as either Ph-negative, BCR-ABL negative CML or atypical CML (aCML). More recently, BCR-ABL negative cases have been classified into a heterogeneous entity termed myeloproliferative disorder/myelodysplastic syndromes (MPD/MDS) that includes chronic myelomonocytic leukaemia (CMML), aCML and other related diseases, with the term 'CML' reserved for Ph- and/or BCR-ABL positive cases only [9,10]. The molecular pathogenesis of MPD/MDS is poorly understood, but a small subset of patients present with cytogenetic translocations that disrupt and constitutively activate protein tyrosine kinases, most commonly PDGFRβ or the fibroblast growth factor receptor (FGFR) 1 [11,12].

Patients with constitutive activation of platelet-derived growth factor receptor

A subset of patients with MPD/MDS present with a translocation that involves chromosome band 5q33, most commonly a t(5;12) but occasionally a t(5;10) or other variants. These patients have peripheral blood and/or bone marrow eosinophilia with a variable degree of monocytosis and present at a median age of 50–60 years, occasionally with anaemia, thrombocytopenia or trilineage dysplasia. Most remarkably – and currently inexplicably – virtually all patients are male. Patients with this disorder have been diagnosed variously as Ph-negative CML, CMML or aCML [10].

The t(5;12) was shown several years ago to fuse the TEL gene (now known as the ETV6 gene) to the PDGFRβ gene; subsequently other variant fusions involving this receptor tyrosine kinase have been identified. Like the BCR-ABL oncoprotein, these chimeric proteins are constitutively active tyrosine kinases. As mentioned above, STI571 has inhibitory activity against the PDGFRβ kinase and has been shown to cure a murine model of ETV6-PDGFRβ disease [13], and consequently may be the treatment of choice in this rare disorder. Furthermore, diverse tyrosine kinase fusion genes activate a common set of signalling pathways, so it is likely that RAS, PI3 kinase and STAT inhibitors may also be useful agents in the treatment of PDGFRβ-rearranged patients.

Patients with constitutive activation of fibroblast growth factor receptor 1

A second subset of MPD/MDS patients have chromosomal rearrangements of chromosome band 8p11, most commonly a t(8;13), but sometimes a t(6;8), t(8;9) or a less common variant. There is a wide age range at presentation, but the median is only 32 years. These individuals also have distinctive clinical features for which the term 8p11 myeloproliferative syndrome (EMS) has been suggested. Molecular analysis demonstrated that the translocations result in the fusion of several different partner genes (eg ZNF198, FOP, CEP110) to the receptor tyrosine kinase FGFR1 gene on 8p11. As with the BCR-ABL protein, these fusion proteins have constitutive enzymatic activity.

At presentation, the peripheral blood and bone marrow of patients with EMS have the appearance of a chronic MPD with prominent eosinophilia. In addition, there is a strikingly high incidence of non-Hodgkin's lymphoma that may be of either B cell or, more commonly, T cell phenotype. The disease is relatively aggressive and transforms into an acute leukaemia after a median interval of only six months. Where reported, the same clonal karyotypic abnormality is seen in both the lymphoma and myeloid cells, suggesting a common lymphoid/myeloid stem cell as the target for the original transforming event. Consistent with this hypothesis, the disease appears to be ineradicable by conventional chemotherapy, although some patients have apparently been cured by allogeneic bone marrow transplantation [12].

STI571 is inactive against FGFR1, and is therefore unlikely to benefit EMS patients. However, other compounds have been developed with anti-FGFR1 activity, for example SU5404, SU6668 and PD173074. Paralleling the effect of STI571 on the BCR-ABL protein, these compounds block the FGFR1 ATP binding site and are able to inhibit the growth of ZNF198-FGFR1 transformed cells. Although no patient with EMS has yet been treated with an FGFR1 inhibitor, the remarkable effects of STI571 in CML suggest that this approach may be beneficial. Preclinical data again suggest that targeting the downstream RAS, PI3 kinase and STAT pathways may also be effective in blocking the transforming activity of FGFR1 fusions.

☐ CONCLUSIONS

It has been anticipated for many years that a better understanding of the precise causes of malignancy would lead to rationally designed therapies targeted to neutralise the effects of specific pathogenetic lesions. It seems fitting that these aspirations should be first realised in CML, a disease which has served as a paradigm for our understanding of many aspects of malignancy. Although no patient has yet been cured by targeted therapy, there is considerable optimism that the disease might be controlled, or even eliminated, in the majority of patients who would hitherto have probably died as a result of overt leukaemia or treatment-related complications.

REFERENCES

1   Deininger MW, Goldman JM, Melo JV. The molecular biology of chronic myeloid leukemia. Review. *Blood* 2000; **96**: 3343–56.

2   Allan NC, Richards SM, Shepherd PC. UK Medical Research Council randomised, multicentre trial of interferon-alpha n1 for chronic myeloid leukaemia: improved survival irrespective of cytogenetic response. The UK Medical Research Council's Working Parties for Therapeutic Trials in Adult Leukaemia. *Lancet* 1995; **345**: 1392–7.

3   Savage DG, Szydlo RM, Goldman JM. Clinical features at diagnosis in 430 patients with chronic myeloid leukaemia seen at a referral centre over a 16-year period. *Br J Haematol* 1997; **96**: 111–6.

4   Deininger MW, Goldman JM, Lydon N, Melo JV. The tyrosine kinase inhibitor CGP57148B selectively inhibits the growth of BCR-ABL-positive cells. *Blood* 1997; **90**: 3691–8.

5   Druker BJ, Tamura S, Buchdunger E, Ohno S, *et al.* Effects of a selective inhibitor of the Abl tyrosine kinase on the growth of Bcr-Abl positive cells. *Nat Med* 1996; **2**: 561–6.

6   Druker BJ, Talpaz M, Resta DJ, Peng B, *et al.* Efficacy and safety of a specific inhibitor of the BCR-ABL tyrosine kinase in chronic myeloid leukemia. *N Engl J Med* 2001; **344**: 1031–7.

7   Mahon FX, Deininger MW, Schultheis B, Chabrol J, *et al.* Selection and characterization of BCR-ABL positive cell lines with differential sensitivity to the tyrosine kinase inhibitor STI571: diverse mechanisms of resistance. *Blood* 2000; **96**: 1070–9.

8   Peters DG, Hoover RR, Gerlach MJ, Koh EY, *et al.* Activity of the farnesyl protein transferase inhibitor SCH66336 against BCR/ABL-induced murine leukemia and primary cells from patients with chronic myeloid leukemia. *Blood* 2001; **97**: 1404–12.

9   Harris NL, Jaffe ES, Diebold J, Flandrin G, *et al.* World Health Organization classification of neoplastic diseases of the hematopoietic and lymphoid tissues: report of the Clinical Advisory Committee meeting – Airlie House, Virginia, November 1997. *J Clin Oncol* 1999; **17**: 3835–49.

10 Bain BJ. Eosinophilic leukaemias and the idiopathic hypereosinophilic syndrome. Review. *Br J Haematol* 1996; **95**: 2–9.

11 Kulkarni S, Heath C, Parker S, Chase A, *et al.* Fusion of H4/D10S170 to the platelet-derived growth factor receptor beta in BCR-ABL-negative myeloproliferative disorders with a t(5;10)(q33;q21). *Cancer Res* 2000; **60**: 3592–8.

12 Reiter A, Sohal J, Kulkarni S, Chase A, *et al.* Consistent fusion of ZNF198 to the fibroblast growth factor receptor-1 in the t(8;13)(p11;q12) myeloproliferative syndrome. *Blood* 1998; **92**: 1735–42.

13 Tomasson MH, Williams IR, Hasserjian R, Udomsakdi C, *et al.* TEL/PDGFbetaR induces hematologic malignancies in mice that respond to a specific tyrosine kinase inhibitor. *Blood* 1999; **93**: 1707–14.

☐ SELF ASSESSMENT QUESTIONS

1   Chronic myeloid leukaemia is defined by:
(a) The presence of the Philadelphia (Ph) chromosome
(b) Clinical and haematological features
(c) The presence of the BCR-ABL fusion gene plus clinical and haematological features
(d) The presence of the Ph chromosome and the BCR-ABL fusion gene
(e) The presence of the Ph chromosome plus clinical and haematological features

2   STI571 has inhibitory activity against:
(a) The ABL, platelet-derived growth factor receptor (PDGFR) β and KIT tyrosine kinases
(b) A broad spectrum of tyrosine kinases
(c) The ABL tyrosine kinase
(d) BCR-ABL
(e) The ABL, PDGFRβ and fibroblast growth factor receptor 1 tyrosine kinases

3   STI571 acts by:
(a) Blocking RAS activity
(b) Blocking the adenosine triphosphate (ATP) binding site within the BCR moiety of BCR-ABL

(c) Blocking the enzymatic active site within the BCR moiety of BCR-ABL
(d) Blocking the enzymatic active site within the ABL moiety of BCR-ABL
(e) Blocking the ATP binding site within the ABL moiety of BCR-ABL

4   Farnesyl transferases block the action of:
(a) RAS only
(b) RAS and many other proteins
(c) RAS and PI3 kinase
(d) RAS, PI3 kinase and many other proteins
(e) RAS and STATs

5   STAT stands for:
(a) Serine/threonine activator of transcription
(b) Signal transducer and activation of transcription
(c) STI571 ABL target
(d) Serine/threonine ABL target
(e) Signal to apoptotic targets

ANSWERS

1a False	2a True	3a False	4a False	5a False
b False	b False	b False	b True	b True
c True	c True	c False	c False	c False
d False	d True	d False	d False	d False
e True	e False	e True	e False	e False

The use of population-based research approaches in haematological malignancy: a generic medical research tool

Stephen Proctor

☐ INTRODUCTION

In a well managed healthcare system such as the NHS the aim is to give a population of patients with cancer a pathway of care which results in all patients receiving prompt investigation, optimal treatment with uniform and consistent evaluation, thus ensuring uniformity of care.

The general perception is that, in order to do this and make progress with new treatments, ever increasing numbers of patients should be entered into randomised control trials (RCTs) which would lead not only to progress but to routine evaluation and optimised care. However, the reality is substantially different in that only a small minority of patients with cancer are entered into trials in the UK (ca 5%) and an even smaller percentage in the USA. Whilst attempts are consistently made via cancer registries to collect information on incidence and time of death, there is a huge gap in knowledge about the detailed investigation, treatment and outcome of the 95% of patients not on trials. As a result of this 'information gap', there are ever increasing numbers of initiatives aimed at individual doctors and NHS trusts, with directives about audit and clinical governance and an explosion of guidelines.

These responses from the Department of Health to try to improve the situation are understandable, but palpably lacking has been the existence of an easily applicable generic process of implementation of routine evaluation and uniformity of care. This chapter will describe the medical population-adjusted clinical epidemiology (PACE) process [1] as it has developed in haematological malignancy, and indicate that this package or process could be applied to other areas of medicine to enable routine and automatic evaluation of 100% of patients, at the same time enhancing entry into classical trials.

☐ DEVELOPMENT OF THE PACE PROGRAMME IN HAEMATOLOGICAL ONCOLOGY IN THE NORTHERN REGION OF THE UK

The process to be described began with the simple idea of collecting an unselected total population-based incidence of treatment and outcome for acute leukaemia for the defined population (3 million) within the Northern Region of England, starting in 1982 [1,2]. Concurrently, a similar process was introduced for the collection of malignant lymphoma information, not only within the Northern Region but also in Scotland (combined population just over 8 million) [3].

Medical PACE has several components, of which the most important relates to the active participation of all the individual doctors interested in the given disease throughout the defined geographical region. The central feature is the development and maintenance of a comprehensive regional register of all patients with a given malignant problem, including demographic details, together with supplemented data on clinical presentation, treatment and outcome of the census population, with annual follow-up information on all patients [1,3,4].

The register is at the heart of the process, but in addition regular group meetings to which all interested parties are invited prevent stagnation. Because all interested physicians are involved, co-operative regional structure and involvement result. The group produces a 'menu book' of agreed treatment strategies based on best practice from regional research and published literature. There is a regular (annual) update of this document, so service frameworks or guideline data can be incorporated. This means that the optimal treatment is available across both regions and, since all cases are collected in a recurring total population study, allows regional audit to be conducted without difficulty (Fig. 1).

The PACE process has been found to lead to improved treatment strategies in patients for whom there are no reliable clinical trials, especially the elderly [5,6]. At the same time, the menu book has maximised recruitment into trials and for other observational studies throughout the two regions. As will be demonstrated, the evaluation and study of Hodgkin's disease have both been enhanced enormously in

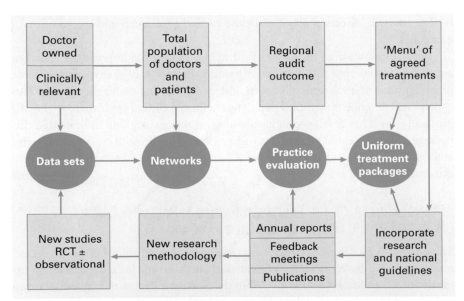

Fig. 1 Diagrammatic representation of how the population-adjusted clinical epidemiology (PACE) programme leads to improved care packages and study approaches in medicine (RCT = randomised clinical trial).

a situation in which 80% of patients within a target study group were offered a randomised trial, 73% of whom accepted [3].

□ SCOTLAND AND NEWCASTLE LYMPHOMA GROUP

A collaboration between the east coast Scottish cities and the Northern Region of England to collect broad-based data on lymphoma patients was started in 1979. Over the ensuing years it has been possible to extend the programme to the whole of Scotland, and to register in great detail over 95% of lymphoma patients in Scotland and Northern England (Fig. 2). Between 1,100 and 1,200 new patients are registered each year. This database now consists of over 14,000 population-representative patients, and has proved to be a major resource for the production of prognostic indices for use in various types of lymphoma, on which RCTs are subsequently superimposed [7–9]. Since 1994, with the co-operation of all concerned in clinical and pathological specialties covered by the Scotland and Newcastle Lymphoma Group (SNLG), it has been possible to demonstrate that such a process can become part of practice, not simply a project.

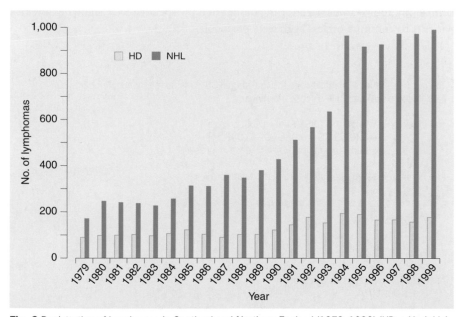

Fig. 2 Registration of lymphomas in Scotland and Northern England (1979–1999) (HD = Hodgkin's disease; NHL = non-Hodgkin's disease).

□ A PROGNOSTIC INDEX FOR HODGKIN'S DISEASE

To give an indication of the possibilities of this approach, the progress made by the SNLG, particularly in Hodgkin's disease, will now be described in more detail. The data sets were used, first, to understand more accurately the risk groups and, secondly, to introduce appropriate study and trial to enhance outcome further.

In 1980, with the chemotherapies then available, it was clear that individuals with advanced stage III and IV Hodgkin's disease would have a 50% chance of survival at five years. In comparison with other malignancies, this was optimistic, but if it were possible to separate more accurately those individuals destined not to respond to the current four drug regimens, new treatment could be introduced for that group of patients. At the same time, it would hopefully be possible to exclude from new treatment those already curable by existing treatments. This was the dawn of the idea of risk-related treatment.

The existence of the register on a broad-based level meant that large numbers of patients had data collected prospectively, with details of treatment received and outcome. There were a large number of suggested prognostic factors in the literature which could be tested with a view to producing a numerical model to help identify poor risk patients. Following an initial assessment on 100 patients, a prognostic index was devised (Fig. 3). This was then validated on a separate cohort of 455 patients [9]. It was found that a cohort of Hodgkin's patients could be divided with 80% accuracy into two groups of patients whose survival at four years would be about 40% and 80%, respectively. This objective numerical prognostic index would pick out only 20% of patients as being true poor risk, but the data were considered sufficiently robust to be used for the design of a prospective RCT, allowing low risk patients to continue on less aggressive protocols.

To calculate the index patient's age, clinical stage (CS), absolute lymphocyte count (LC), haemoglobin (Hb) and bulk disease are required

The index $(I) = 1.5858 - 0.0363$ Age $+ 0.0005$ (Age^2)
$+ 0.0683$ CS $- 0.086$ LC $- 0.0587$ Hb
$+$ additional factor if bulk disease is present*

Age is entered as an absolute figure in the equation

CS is entered according to the key (Ann Arbor Classification):
IA, IIA, IIIA = 1
IB, IIB   = 2
IIIB   = 3
IV   = 4

Absolute LC is entered as a score:
<1.0 x 10^9/l   = 1
1.0–1.5 x 10^9/l = 2
1.5–2.0 x 10^9/l = 3
>2.0 x 10^9/l   = 4

Hb in g/dl is entered as an absolute figure in the equation

* bulk disease (>10 cm) – add 0.3 to index score

Patients with index 0.5 have risk of death from progressive HD of 60–70% in 4 years. Such patients are being entered on a trial protocol in first remission

Fig. 3 Calculation of the prognostic index for Hodgkin's disease (HD) with bulk disease.

Pilot study

It was necessary first to pilot and validate a new chemotherapy schedule for the patients who failed the standard schedule. This was the PVACE-BOP schedule (defined in Fig. 4), a multi-agent schedule given on a continuous 28-day cycle for three consecutive months, with the patient re-commencing chemotherapy immediately having completed the previous month's cycle. A comparator was necessary in this trial of a new generation of chemotherapy as part of primary treatment in a poor risk group. The comparator chosen was high-dose therapy with autologous marrow or stem cell rescue which had demonstrated some capacity to rescue multiply relapsed patients.

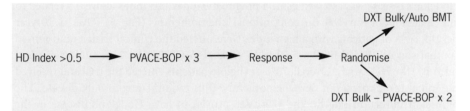

PVACE-BOP SCHEDULE
Continuous schedule for aggressive Hodgkin's disease and relapsed progressive Hodgkin's disease

Day 1	Vinblastine 6 mg/m^2	**Day 8**	Adriamycin 25 mg/m^2
Day 1–3	Etoposide iv 100 mg/m^2 x 1 oral 200 mg/m^2 x 2	**Day 8**	Vincristine 2 mg
Day 1–14	Procarbazine 100 mg/m^2	**Day 15**	Bleomycin 6 mg/m^2
		Day 22	Bleomycin 6 mg/m^2
Day 1–14	Chlorambucil 6 mg/m^2	**Day 14–28**	Prednisolone 40 mg daily
Day 29	= Day 1 of next course		

NB:
(i)   It often happens that in later courses Day 8 injections cannot be given. It is suggested that, rather than interrupt therapy, Day 14–28 sequence is brought forward and Day 8 injections are given on Day 22 instead.
(ii) Omit bleomycin from cycles 4 and 5 if patients have had mantle/mediastinal radiotherapy.
(iii) Give 100 mg hydrocortisone iv with bleomycin.
(iv) Septrin tablets, 2 twice daily, should be given throughout treatment on **Mondays, Wednesdays and Fridays.**

Fig. 4 PVACE-BOP schedule: continuous schedule for aggressive Hodgkin's disease (HD) and relapsed progressive HD (auto BMT = autologous bone marrow transplant; DXT = radiotherapy; iv = intravenous).

The pilot study was conducted on a cohort of patients with a poor prognosis, utilising the following transplant protocol:

☐ high-dose melphalan and etoposide as preconditioning

☐ non-cryopreserved marrow rescue which demonstrated acceptable toxicity with no procedural mortality

☐ good anti-Hodgkin's disease activity.

This became the additional arm of the trial [10].

Trial design

A trial started in 1988 within the geographical area of the SNLG in which every case of Hodgkin's disease was assessed using a prognostic index. An index above 0.5 related to anticipated poor survival on conventional chemotherapy (Fig. 3). Over a 10-year period, 80% of patients with a high index were offered the clinical trial, a randomised comparison of PVACE-BOP × 5 (arm A) versus PVACE-BOP × 3 plus autotransplant (arm B) (the HD3 trial). Overall, 73% of eligible patients entered the trial and received the initial three courses of new chemotherapy plus radiotherapy to bulk disease. The remission induction rate for the 120 cases proven to have Hodgkin's disease in the appropriate category was excellent (93%), much better than previously observed.

☐ INTERNATIONAL PROGNOSTIC INDEX FOR HODGKIN'S DISEASE

While this work was being conducted, an international approach to risk factors in Hodgkin's disease was introduced, led by the German Hodgkin's study group. An international prognostic index for patients with stage IIIB and IV was produced [11], in which the risk factors chosen were similar to those in the SNLG index. It was possible to utilise this index to assess whether the new treatment included in the HD3 trial had demonstrated improvement according to the international scale. In all the risk categories there had been a 10–30% improvement with both arms of the trial. Preliminary analysis of this trial, which closed recently, found that the overall survival at five years for this group of patients had improved from less than 50% to 78%, with no apparent difference between the two arms.

A key strength of this study approach was that it has been possible also to review and analyse all patients not entered in the trial, but who presented with Hodgkin's disease in the geographical area over the same time period. The menu book process ensured that all those patients received an accepted and appropriate form of treatment, as designated by the overall group, and the PACE audit approach ensured uniformity of care.

☐ CONCLUSIONS

Most people would agree that total evaluation of unselected populations and delivery of uniform care are both highly desirable. We suggest that the medical PACE programme [1] is a practical and relatively inexpensive methodology to achieve these goals. Starting with basic data collection, the flow chart in Fig. 1 demonstrates the way in which all the requirements of both healthcare and quality improvement linked to research can be met. Whilst RCTs are key investigative tools when appropriate phase III questions need to be addressed, the majority of patients are not put into clinical trials. As an alternative, the PACE process would provide data accrual for all patients in a given disease area, and undoubtedly enable other trial methodologies to flourish.

Acknowledgements

I should like to thank Dr Penny Taylor, Ms Jo White and the SNLG secretariat for their support, all the members of the Northern Regional Haematology Group and the data management team, and particularly Linda Smith for secretarial help.

REFERENCES

1   Proctor SJ, Taylor PR. A practical guide to continuous population-based data collection (PACE): a process facilitating uniformity of care and research into practice. Review. *QJM* 2000; **93**: 67–73.

2   Charlton B, Taylor PRA, Proctor SJ. The PACE (population-adjusted clinical epidemiology) strategy: a new approach to multi-centred clinical research. *QJM* 1997; **90**: 147–51.

3   Taylor PRA, Angus B, Owen JP, Proctor SJ. Hodgkin's disease: a population-adjusted clinical epidemiology study (PACE) of management at presentation. Northern Region Lymphoma Group. *QJM* 1998; **91**: 131–9.

4   Proctor SJ, Taylor PR, Stark A, Carey PJ, *et al.* Evaluation of the impact of allogeneic transplant in first remission on an unselected population of patients with acute myeloid leukaemia aged 15–55 years. The Northern Regional Haematology Group. *Leukemia* 1995; **9**: 1246–51.

5   Taylor PR, Reid MM, Bown N, Hamilton PJ, Proctor SJ. Acute lymphoblastic leukaemia in patients aged 60 years and over: a population-based study of incidence and outcome. *Blood* 1992; **80**: 1813–7.

6   Taylor PR, Reid MM, Stark AN, Bown N, *et al.* De novo acute myeloid leukaemia in patients over 55-years-old: a population-based study of incidence, treatment and outcome. Northern Region Haematology Group. *Leukemia* 1995; **9**: 231–7.

7   Hayward RL, Leonard RC, Prescott RJ. A critical analysis of prognostic factors for survival in intermediate and high grade non-Hodgkin's lymphoma. Scotland and Newcastle Lymphoma Group Therapy Working Party. *Br J Cancer* 1991; **63**: 945–52.

8   Leonard RC, Hayward RL, Prescott RJ, Wang JX. The identification of discrete prognostic groups in low grade non-Hodgkin's lymphoma. The Scotland and Newcastle Lymphoma Group Therapy Working Party. *Ann Oncol* 1991; **2**: 655–62.

9   Proctor SJ, Taylor P, Donnan P, Boys R, *et al.* A numerical prognostic index for clinical use in identification of poor-risk patients with Hodgkin's disease at diagnosis. Scotland and Newcastle Lymphoma Group (SNLG) Therapy Working Party. *Eur J Cancer* 1991; **27**: 624–9.

10 Taylor PR, Jackson GH, Lennard AL, Lucraft H, Proctor SJ. Autologous transplantation in poor risk Hodgkin's disease using high dose melphalan/etoposide conditioning with non-cryopreserved marrow rescue. *Br J Cancer* 1993; **67**: 383–7.

11 Hasenclever D, Diehl V. A prognostic score for advanced Hodgkin's disease. International Prognostic Factors Project on Advanced Hodgkin's Disease. *N Engl J Med* 1998; **339**: 1506–14.

☐ SELF ASSESSMENT QUESTIONS

1 Randomised controlled trials (RCTs) in cancer are:
   (a) Conducted on 25% of all cancer patients
   (b) Rarely include elderly patients
   (c) Considered as the only form of valid evidence
   (d) Followed by rapid assimilation into routine practice
   (e) Currently rapidly expanding accrual rates

2 In Hodgkin's disease:
   (a) 50% of patients with advanced disease were curable in 1980
   (b) The level of anaemia is a key prognostic factor
   (c) The bulk of disease does not relate to outcome
   (d) Has an incidence double that of non-Hodgkin's lymphoma
   (e) Is now curable in over 80% of cases

3 Population-based studies of a medical condition:
   (a) Provide a more clinically relevant pattern of disease
   (b) Can replace the use of the RCT
   (c) Could be combined with an RCT to the benefit of both methodologies
   (d) Do not work in studying elderly populations

4 In the treatment of advanced Hodgkin's disease:
   (a) The majority of patients need aggressive eight-drug schedules for cure
   (b) Autotransplant after chemotherapy is superior to chemotherapy alone
   (c) Hodgkin's disease in the elderly has a worse prognosis
   (d) Male infertility is a major problem post-chemotherapy

5 The medical PACE programme:
   (a) Could be utilised across most medical specialties
   (b) Is a vehicle for conducting audit and clinical governance
   (c) Is organised by individuals other than doctors
   (d) Is a very expensive option
   (e) Provides denominator population data

ANSWERS

1a False	2a True	3a True	4a False	5a True
b True	b True	b False	b False	b True
c True	c False	c True	c True	c False
d False	d False	d False	d True	d False
e False	e True			e True

Psychiatry and
psychology

The Gulf War and its aftermath

Simon Wessely

□ INTRODUCTION

We have just passed the tenth anniversary of operation Desert Storm, the start of the Persian Gulf War. The facts are clear: Iraq occupied Kuwait on 2 August 1990. Shortly after, coalition forces led by the US began a military deployment known as operation Desert Shield. On 17 January 1991, an active air campaign began against Iraq, operation Desert Storm, and on 24 February a ground war began, lasting only four days. It was a resounding military success: Iraqi forces were beaten in the field and expelled from Kuwait.

The campaign was also a medical success. Traditionally, fighting in hostile environments such as the desert has been associated with morbidity and mortality, often substantial, from causes not related to enemy action such as heat stroke, dehydration and infectious disease. There is no evidence for any deaths from those sources among American or British personnel during the Gulf campaign [1].

□ GULF WAR SYNDROME

Now, ten years later, few will remember the genuine medical achievements of the campaign. Instead, when asked about the Gulf War and health, most people will say that is where Gulf War syndrome began. Shortly after the cessation of hostilities reports started to emerge from the US of clusters of unusual illnesses occurring amongst Gulf War veterans. Claims were made that previously fit veterans had developed unusual diseases, illnesses and symptoms. Reports emerged also of children with birth defects being born to Gulf War veterans. Meanwhile, formal epidemiological research was at last commissioned (see below), but Gulf War syndrome had captured the public imagination by the time these studies had started to report.

This chapter will review the published evidence on the nature and extent of illnesses associated with service in the Gulf War, and offer a tentative explanation for Gulf War syndromes.

□ THE EVIDENCE SO FAR

Case series

The first co-ordinated response to the problem of Gulf War syndrome was to invite any veteran with health problems to come forward for detailed medical evaluation.

This began in the US, and was then repeated in the UK with the establishment of the Medical Assessment Programme. Over 200,000 US and 2,000 UK veterans have now attended these programmes. Studies of these groups have not suggested any unusual pattern of illness. The largest diagnostic category has symptoms and syndromes such as chronic fatigue, pain and others without an adequate medical explanation [2–4]. No new diseases have come to light, nor has any dramatic increase in other known but unusual conditions been documented.

Epidemiological studies

The most comprehensive analyses have been made of the mortality in both the US and UK Gulf cohorts. Contrary to media reports, these show no increase [5,6] other than an increase in accidental death (US and UK) and suicide (US only) – as observed in the aftermath of other conflicts. Likewise, hospitalisations have not increased [7].

US study

The first epidemiological study of Gulf-related illness, a questionnaire-based study of a random sample of Gulf veterans and appropriate military controls from the state of Iowa [8], showed increased rates of symptom reporting in the Gulf cohort. There was an increase in symptom-defined conditions such as chronic fatigue syndrome, depression, post-traumatic stress disorder (PTSD) and others.

UK study

The UK study compared a random sample of 4,246 UK Gulf War veterans, drawn from all three armed services (including both serving and non-serving members), with non-deployed personnel and also with an active duty control group – members of the UK armed forces who had served in Bosnia from the start of the UN Peacekeeping Mission (1992–97) [9].

UK Gulf veterans were 2–3 times more likely to report every one of the 50 symptoms inquired about. Whatever the symptom, the rate was at least twice as high in the Gulf cohort as in either the non-deployed or Bosnia cohorts. The Gulf veterans experienced more symptoms, endorsed more conditions and felt worse than either of the two other cohorts, but were still physically functioning well as a group [9].

Other epidemiological studies

Other epidemiologically based samples from Hawaii, Pennsylvania [10], Boston [11], active service USAAF personnel [12], the SeaBees [13] and the large Veterans Administration study [14] all show similar findings.

Significantly, all these studies are limited by the use of self-report measures. Self-reported symptoms are not of course a good guide to findings on clinical examination [15]. Somatic symptoms in the community are exceedingly common and often persistent, yet fewer than one in five are found to have a discrete physical explanation [16].

Is there a Gulf War syndrome?

The term 'Gulf War syndrome' has acquired remarkable media and popular salience, but is there any such thing? A syndrome implies a unique constellation of signs and/or symptoms. For there to be a Gulf War syndrome, there should be evidence of such a unique constellation found only in the context of the Gulf conflict [17].

Using factor analysis, Haley and colleagues [18] were the first to argue in favour of a unique Gulf War syndrome. However, their data came from a single naval reserve construction battalion, sample size 249, with a 41% response rate and no control group. Of those who responded, 70% reported serious health problems since the Gulf War. This makes it difficult to establish whether or not the proposed new syndrome is linked to Gulf service [19]. A further problem is that any population in which there is a normal distribution of symptoms will yield factors when these are entered into a factor analysis. Hypothesis-driven studies are needed.

Later studies that used epidemiologically defined subjects and appropriate controls have generally not found evidence of a Gulf War syndrome. For example, our study found evidence to support a particular factor structure to symptoms in the Gulf cohort, but this was not significantly different from the factor structure in the Bosnia or Era controls (who went to neither conflict). The Gulf group had experienced more symptoms at greater intensity, but there was no difference in the way these symptoms could be organised [20]. Three controlled US studies drew similar conclusions [12,21,22].

Irrespective of the emerging professional consensus, Gulf War syndrome is established as a popular, media and social reality. Investigating how and why this concept developed is important but the answers will come from social sciences not from statistics.

The position elsewhere

The first country other than the US to publish a detailed examination of its Gulf veterans was Canada [23]. The results were remarkably consistent with those already reported from the US and those to be reported from the UK.

Each country's experience shows examples of natural variations and experiments which will prove informative. For example, Canada sent three vessels to the Gulf, in only two of which those on board were given pyridostigmine bromide (PB) prophylaxis – yet rates of illness were identical [23]. Likewise, Danish Gulf veterans also have elevated rates of symptomatic ill health [24], yet nearly all of them were involved only in peace-keeping duties after the end of hostilities and received neither PB prophylaxis nor vaccinations against biological agents.

The largest enigma remains the French. The pattern of forces' protection used by the French differed from that of the Americans and the British. The French authorities have consistently denied that any health problems have emerged in their

Gulf forces, and there have been few media reports in France – although this has been changing recently [25]. No systematic study has been undertaken. Furthermore, the cultural pattern of illnesses in the Francophone world differs from that in the English-speaking and Scandinavian worlds. Illness entities such as chronic fatigue syndrome or multiple chemical sensitivity are hardly acknowledged or recognised.

The evidence: summary

Gulf service has affected the symptomatic health of large numbers of those who took part in the campaign. At the same time, no evidence has emerged to date of either distinct biomedical abnormalities or premature mortality. It is not that some veterans have been significantly affected whilst the rest have not. There are certainly small numbers of veterans, often with a high media profile, who have developed substantial disability, but on a population basis larger numbers of veterans have experienced small changes in their health.

☐ THE EXPLANATIONS

Hypothesis 1: Gulf War illness is the result of biological hazards in the Gulf

The most popular explanation among the media and, we suspect, the general public is that the cause of Gulf War syndrome lies in the particular hazards of that conflict. Most attention has been given to the measures taken to protect the combatants from the threat of chemical and biological warfare. These included immunisations against biological weapons such as plague and anthrax, and PB tablets to protect against exposure to anticholinesterase-based nerve agents such as sarin. Other hazards included exposure to depleted uranium or to the smoke from the oil fires ignited by the retreating Iraqi forces.

The evidence

Evidence is conflicting for all the hazards.

Vaccination. Some of the most suggestive evidence comes from studies of the possible effects of the vaccination programme used to protect the armed forces against the threat from biological weapons.

The US programme involved immunisation against anthrax and botulism, whilst the UK protected against plague and anthrax, with the use of pertussis vaccine as adjuvant to speed up the response to anthrax vaccine [26]. We found a relationship between receiving both multiple vaccinations in general, and those against chemical and biological warfare agents in particular, and the persistence of symptoms despite controlling for obvious confounders. The finding that multiple vaccinations in other contexts, including deployment to Bosnia, was not associated with any increased experience of symptoms suggests some interaction between multiple vaccination and active service deployment to the Gulf [9,27]. These data are compatible with the hypothesis that Gulf War related illness may be associated with a T helper 2 shift in immune responsiveness [28]. The final test of the hypothesis will come with the results of direct measures of immunological function currently being analysed at King's.

Pyridostigmine bromide. PB, a reversible inhibitor of acetylcholinesterase, was used as a pretreatment for possible exposure to nerve gas. Side effects were frequently reported but they were short lived, and no acute toxicity was observed [29]. This is important because long-term organophosphorus toxicity, which is certainly a hazard, has been clearly documented only in the aftermath of acute toxicity [30]. The Canadian experience (see above) also argues against a prominent role for PB.

PB has been used in civilian practice for the diagnosis of growth hormone disorders and the treatment of myasthenia gravis for many years, and in higher doses than those used by the armed forces, without apparent adverse effect. It has even been used as a treatment for the fatigue associated with post-polio syndrome [31]. Although later studies questioned its efficacy, it was safe and well tolerated [32]. The extensive cumulative experience with PB in civilian neurological practice therefore argues against it having an important role *per se* in Gulf-related illnesses [33,34]. However, there are two caveats:

1   An elegant mouse experiment has suggested that PB may penetrate the blood-brain barrier under stressful conditions [35], but this was not confirmed in guinea pigs [36].

2   Hazard may have resulted from interactions with other agents [37,38]. On the other hand, vaccines and PB given together did not prove toxic to guinea pigs [39].

Organophosphates. It is plausible that polymorphisms in the enzyme detoxification pathways for organophosphate compounds are related to symptoms [40]. One study reports such an association [41], while another does not [42] but instead finds low levels of the detoxification enzyme itself. Such pathways are also probably not involved in PB metabolism [30]. Studies of the King's cohort should clarify this issue.

Large quantities of pesticides in various forms were used by all the combatants to reduce the risk of infectious disease. Certainly, organophosphates have *acute* toxic effects on the human nervous system, but there remains considerable uncertainty and controversy about the effects of low level *chronic* exposure [30,33,43–45].

Sarin. In the US, much attention was given to the possibility that troops had been exposed to low levels of the nerve agent sarin following the probable accidental destruction of an Iraqi arms dump at Khamisiyah. Little evidence has been found that those possibly exposed to the plume had any difference in post-war illness [46]. A recent animal study failed to show any adverse effects from low dose sarin [47].

Depleted uranium. A small group of US Gulf veterans definitely exposed to depleted uranium in the form of shrapnel fragments are being intensively monitored. Some subtle changes have been seen in neuropsychological and neuroendocrine function [48]. No evidence relevant to the vast majority of those deployed has been presented to date.

Smoke from burning oil wells. This was closely monitored. Environmental monitoring studies concluded that, in general, most toxins were below accepted lower limits, but there was an increase in the level of fine particulate, not unusual for a desert region [49]. Levels of polycyclic aromatic hydrocarbon biomarkers were lower in Gulf veterans exposed to the oil fires than in controls who had remained in Germany [50].

Objections to Hypothesis 1

There are two general objections to Hypothesis 1 [33]:

1   Some studies [51,52], but not others [9,8,13,53], have found that certain symptom patterns are related to certain self-reported exposures.

2   The time latency between the war and onset of symptoms is also unusual if symptoms are related to war exposure [53].

Conclusion

There is evidence to suggest that some of the new hazards to which the armed forces were exposed during the Gulf War may be associated with unexpected side effects and perhaps later ill health. On the other hand, some of the evidence needs replication, and other evidence remains implausible. Hypothesis 1 therefore is supported, but not for every claim and instance.

Hypothesis 2: Gulf War illness is a modern manifestation of post-conflict ill health

The first hypothesis would be substantially weakened if it could be shown that similar clinical syndromes have arisen after other conflicts which did not involve the particular hazards of the Gulf War. The second hypothesis is that sending young men to war invariably results in casualties that cannot be explained on a solely physical injury basis, with symptoms similar to those experienced by Gulf War veterans.

This has been most clearly argued by Hyams and colleagues [54]. Interpretable medical records and accounts really started only in the middle of the 19th century, but thereafter the literature contains clinical descriptions of ex-servicemen with conditions that show considerable similarities to the Gulf narratives. These conditions have received many different labels:

□   *Soldier's heart* (later termed effort syndrome) owes its provenance to the Crimean and American Civil War.

□   *Shell shock* and *neurasthenia* dominate the writings of the First World War.

□   *Agent Orange syndrome* and *PTSD* emerge after Vietnam.

Hyams's argument rests entirely on a reading of secondary sources, but the task of assembling primary sources has started. Clinical case histories have already been located from the Crimean War and Indian Mutiny [55] which begin the theme of chronic, unexplained symptoms. More detailed analyses of medical records are being assembled from the Boer War and the First and Second World Wars.

The Gulf War was not a particularly 'stressful' conflict in the traditional sense. The active ground war lasted only a few days (although the deployment itself lasted much longer), and casualties amongst the coalition forces were exceptionally light. It would be historically wrong to extrapolate from the prolonged privation, fear and danger of, for example, the Western Front or the Italian Campaign of the Second World War, to the Gulf War.

The fear of chemical and biological weapons

It would be equally wrong to claim that Gulf veterans were not exposed to stress or fear, and the real threat posed by chemical and biological weapons should not be underestimated [56,57]. Such weapons 'engender fear out of all proportion to their threat' [58] – they are as much, if not more, weapons of psychological as of physical warfare [59]. Even in training, up to 20% of those who took part in exercises using simulated exposure to irritant gases showed moderate to severe psychological anxiety [60]. Iraq had used such weapons during the Iran-Iraq war and against Kurdish civilians. Effective measures, such as wearing the full nuclear-biological-chemical suits, were exceptionally uncomfortable and induced a state of partial sensory deprivation. The threat of chemical and biological warfare was the most commonly expressed fear among the US forces in the coming conflict. During Desert Storm there were several thousand documented chemical alarm alerts. Although subsequently the consensus is that none was truly positive, at the time each alert had to be assumed to be genuine. Believing oneself to have been subject to chemical attack has frequently been found to be associated with the development of symptoms [9,61], sometimes strongly [11,18], even though evidence is against such an attack actually having taken place.

Conclusion

Hypothesis 2, like Hypothesis 1, can be supported. Similar syndromes have occurred previously. There were genuine sources of anxiety during Desert Shield and Desert Storm, chiefly around the threat of chemical and biological warfare, and believing that one was exposed to such weapons is associated with later ill health.

Hypothesis 3: Gulf War syndrome can be found in people who have never been to the Gulf or served in the armed forces

May the features of Gulf War illness have nothing to do with warfare at all? Patients with multiple unexplained symptoms, such as those reported in the narratives of Gulf veterans, are also encountered in civilian medical practice and literature. Such material is found in patient-oriented literature under diverse headings such as myalgic encephalomyelitis (ME), total allergy syndrome, electrical hypersensitivity, dental amalgam disease, silicon breast implant disease, hypoglycaemia, chronic Lyme disease, sick building syndrome and many more. In the professional literature, studies are now reporting that the rates of various symptom-defined conditions originally described in the civilian population are also elevated in the Gulf cohorts. Chief amongst these are chronic fatigue syndrome [62], multiple chemical sensitivity [63,64], fibromyalgia and irritable bowel syndrome. They overlap not only with each other [65] but also with Gulf War illness.

It is not surprising that symptom-based conditions overlap with Gulf War illness, given that Gulf veterans show increased reporting of each of the symptoms that make up the case definitions of the syndromes found in civilian practice. This does not mean, however, that all the syndromes – or indeed Gulf War illnesses – are the same. It means both that they all overlap, with no known discrete boundaries between them, and also that any explanation of Gulf War illness must explain how similar conditions can be found in non-deployed military personnel and civilians.

Conclusion

Hypothesis 3 therefore can also be supported. Illnesses identical to the complaints reported by Gulf veterans are found in civilians who have never served in the armed forces, let alone taken part in the Gulf War.

☐ ATTRIBUTIONS AND EXPLANATIONS

The social and cultural aspects of Gulf War illness

For whatever reason, Gulf War veterans began to experience unusual symptoms on their return from the conflict. Several questions can be asked:

☐   How did these disparate symptoms come together as a new syndrome?

☐   Why did it take the shape it did?

☐   What labels and explanations for these symptoms were advanced by the veterans, the media and many others?

We now suggest that these can be understood not only in terms of human biology, toxicology and psychology, but also in terms of the sociology of illness and the particular position of the veteran in modern society.

The military: from effort syndrome to Gulf War syndrome

Everyone in distress needs some way of explaining it. Research confirms that in the clinical setting patients prefer a firm, albeit inaccurate, label for their symptoms to an honest expression of uncertainty [66]. The ways in which people explain their symptoms can come from many sources, sometimes from doctors but often not [16].

Some of the labels applied to unexplained illnesses in the armed services are related to the particular nature of the recent conflict. Hence:

1   *Soldier's heart* arose because of the contemporary concern that the straps securing the heavy backpacks worn by the Unionist soldiers in the American Civil War were compressing the muscles, arteries and nerves in the region of the heart.

2   The epidemic of *rheumatic conditions* documented after the Boer War was a response to the presumed health dangers of sleeping out in wet conditions on the High Veldt.

3   *Shell shock* took its name from the presumed effects of concussion caused by the passage of the shell, let alone its actual detonation.

4   *Neurasthenia,* another popular term, originally described in civilian life, was a condition affecting successful people as a response to the stresses and strains of contemporary life. When army captains on the Western Front developed similar unexplained conditions associated with extreme exhaustion, it was not difficult to translate the civilian neurasthenia concept into the military context.

5   After Vietnam came two new syndromes, *PTSD* and *Agent Orange syndrome* [67], one ostensibly psychological, the other somatic – a forerunner of Gulf War syndrome.

The civilian perspective

How do the main health concerns of the Gulf campaign discussed above map on to wider civilian health concerns?

The range and scope of symptoms, illnesses and conditions blamed on the environment have increased over about the last decade. This reflects increasing global concern about the effects of chemicals, radiation and infectious diseases, and the collective memories of recent health disasters. The generation that fought the Gulf War was born in a world already sensitised by 'Silent Spring' and thalidomide, and came to maturity to a background of the AIDS epidemic, mad cow disease and numerous well-publicised environmental tragedies such as Chernobyl, Seveso and Bhopal. It is a moot point whether our environment is really more threatening than it was; the food, water and air of any postindustrial revolution city of the 19th century do not bear comparison with its modern counterparts [68,69], but we are more aware of these dangers than were our predecessors.

Environmental attribution provides a link between the otherwise varied new illnesses and health hazards that figure so prominently in the media (eg dental amalgam disease, electromagnetic radiation, ME, organophosphate toxicity, candida, sick building syndrome, multiple chemical sensitivity). The postulated pathophysiological mechanisms are many and varied, but all are associated with the presence of multiple unexplained symptoms, and are in one way or another blamed on some unwelcome external environmental hazard or on a substance introduced into our bodies from outside. The idea that attempts to reduce the hazards of, for example, infections, can also cause unexpected side effects (Hypothesis 1) has echoes in the frequently bitter antivaccination movement [70]. Likewise, the frequently advanced argument that the Gulf War was the 'most high tech war ever', replacing the hazards of previous 'low tech' conflicts with a new set of risks, is directly echoed in the civilian literature on 'techno stress', and thought by many to lie behind the epidemic of syndromes such as repetitive strain injury, VDU complaints that often follow the introduction of new technologies into the workplace [71–73].

One result has been a gradual transformation of popular models of illness and disease. In place of the demons and spirits of yesteryear comes the belief that we as a society are oppressed by mystery gases, viruses and toxins, all invisible and some as elusive as the demons of old. This can be seen in the changing pattern of attributions given by patients with unexplained symptoms [74]. Guy's Poisons Unit, for example, has reported seeing patients with multiple symptoms attributed to environmental poisoning only in the last two decades [75]. Public anxieties over the possible adverse effects of new technologies begin to make sense.

There is a complex relationship between environmental concerns and symptoms. There is no doubt that exposure, whether real or perceived, to environmental hazard such as chemicals leads to increased fears and concerns [76], in turn leading to increased symptom reporting perhaps via activation of the stress response. The strength of a subject's opinions on environmental matters was associated with symptom reporting in those exposed to a hazardous waste site but also in those who were not [77,78]. Those describing themselves as 'very worried' about local environmental conditions were ten times more likely to complain of headaches than those not so concerned [79]. Finally, people who experience more symptoms, for whatever reason, may have an increased level of concern about their environment as they look for explanations for their ill health. The consequence is a vicious circle linking exposure (whether real or perceived), beliefs and symptoms.

Reproductive fears

At the same time as fears over health surfaced, so did fears about reproductive health. It was impossible neither to be moved by individual tragedies described in the media of veterans fathering children with severe birth defects nor to fail to understand and sympathise with the search for explanation by parents of children so afflicted, generally finding these in the father's military service. These fears remain. A common response amongst veterans who have completed our qualitative survey is their intention to delay having children until these issues are resolved. Fortunately, there is no evidence of any increased risk at present [80] – but the longer families delay fertility, the greater the chance that such a risk will develop.

Reproductive fears are largely absent from the records and narratives of the First World War. There is a single Second World War report of Australian veterans returning from the Pacific War expressing these fears, blamed on their malaria prophylaxis. These fears first surface as a major issue in veterans' health during the Vietnam era. The suspicion is that this change was triggered by the cumulative and widespread knowledge of the medical effects of radiation post-Hiroshima and the thalidomide tragedy. Such fears now frequently accompany many environmental accidents and exposures.

The soldier becomes a civilian again

The situation of the soldier returning from war, especially if accompanied by rapid separation from service, is complex. There is readjustment to routine soldiering, and the process of assimilation and accommodation of the experience of war continues. Some may experience guilt or shame at acts of commission or omission. Pride and a feeling of achievement may be felt whilst others may become angry and accusatory at those who they see as letting them down in time of threat. The search for meaning may continue for years.

Apart from the ending of their engagement, leaving the service may be desired for many reasons, including being unable to equal the combat experience or desiring never to have to repeat it. Once 'separated', modern servicemen and women will return to a risk aversive society where individual rights, not duties or obligations, count – the obverse of military society. A realistic knowledge of military experience by civilian society has become less with the end of national conflicts or national service – a decreasing number of civilians will have any contact with the military. Contemporary understanding of military service is more likely to be driven by Hollywood's depictions than personal experience. Films which portray the veteran as victim are common, a situation abhorrent to most servicemen and women. A few will, however, construe their experience in this way, encouraged by the media.

Military and veteran culture also reflects the general changing relationship between the individual and society. One sign of this is the loss of Crown Indemnity by the Ministry of Defence, and the subsequent avalanche of litigation against the military authorities. However, it is simplistic, and probably erroneous, to assume that the rise in symptoms amongst Gulf veterans is related to the rise in litigation. It is more likely that litigation arises as a consequence, rather than a cause, of these concerns. Furthermore, there is little difference in the health complaints and concerns of US and UK veterans [14], but whereas UK veterans can, and are, litigating against the military, their American counterparts are statute barred from any similar activity.

Without subscribing to simplistic notions of war, stress and post-traumatic stress, war cannot be seen as of no psychological or social significance. Nearly everyone is changed by exposure to combat, for better or worse.

Distrust, conspiracy and confidence

The importance of public confidence and political (mis)judgement in shaping health concerns may be illustrated by one US/UK comparison. In the US there has been concern and controversy over the role of the probable accidental discharge of sarin gas at the Khamisiyah arms dump, while a major issue in the UK has been the role of exposure to organophosphate pesticides. Both issues were accompanied by misinformation and mismanagement.

First, in Great Britain, records that now would give crucial information, such as vaccination records, were destroyed. Secondly, when concerns first began to surface in the UK, an attitude was expressed in Parliament that this was a 'storm in a teacup', and hints that those complaining should be able to 'pull themselves together', and that this would not happen to troops properly led and trained. Thirdly, there was a delay in commissioning research that might allay fears.

The result of all these events was a serious lack of trust in governmental and military authorities. Given that risk communication and management are critically dependent upon trust between the community that feels exposed and those responsible for managing that risk [81], misjudgements were probably integral to the further development and shaping of 'Gulf War syndrome' after the conflict.

Another major participant in the story of Gulf War syndrome has been the media, which have both reflected and shaped public concern. Public concern and media coverage go hand in hand – Gulf War syndrome was a 'good story' because it touched on so many contemporary issues of general public concern. They are also consistent with each other, even if neither necessarily reflects an objective appraisal or reality [82]. It is, however, true that the news media are more likely to report negative, trust destroying stories than ones that enhance trust [81].

☐ CONCLUSIONS

What can be said, and what will never be known?

Ten years on, there are some established findings:

- ☐ There is a Gulf health effect, which is neither trivial nor due to selection bias.

- ☐ It is not PTSD in its classic sense.

- ☐ There is no evidence of an increase in well-defined disease categories.

- ☐ There is no evidence to suggest that mortality has increased other than from accidental death or suicide.

More information will be available in the coming months. Key epidemiological studies, such as those conducted by the Veterans Administration in the US and by Manchester University in the UK, will report. The experience of other countries will become clearer. Numerous clinical and animal studies will report, and a flood of reports on neuropsychological, neurological, immunological and other investigations of Gulf veterans is anticipated. If these are based on well-defined, preferably epidemiologically-based, samples, their interpretation will be far easier.

Some informed speculations can also be made. Given that the health effect is not restricted to a small number of individuals but is seen across the population, the exposure or exposures must likewise be distributed across the population. For this reason, exposures that seem only to have affected small numbers of veterans are unlikely candidates. More plausible are exposures that affected the majority of those in theatre: that is, medical countermeasures used to reduce the risk from chemical and biological weapons are more plausible candidates than depleted uranium fragments which affected only a small number.

Likewise, psychosocial factors that might be of relevance are more likely to be general rather than specific. Combat stress disorders leading to post-traumatic stress are unlikely to have affected more than a small proportion of veterans, but the anxiety engendered by the threat of chemical warfare could potentially have influenced virtually everyone. Similarly, few veterans will not have been exposed to the media interest and speculation that began soon after their return.

Reality must be faced. Much will never be known for certain. Ten years after the Gulf conflict the chances of finding new evidence on exposures during the conflict become increasingly unlikely. The possibilities of further direct aetiological research diminish with each year.

The future

It might be argued correctly that each military deployment is unique in its historical and military context, but the story of Gulf War syndrome may not be a 'one off'. Newspaper reports have already appeared about, for example, the 'horrendous range of symptoms' now experienced by Canadian UN peacekeepers in Croatia [83] and Dutch peacekeepers in Cambodia [85,86]. Similar reports have emerged in the German and Belgian press concerning their soldiers in Kosovo.

The current uncertainty over the chronic health effects of low level exposure to chemical and nuclear materials will continue, as will public anxiety. The potential effects of low level chemical and radiation exposure are a long-standing controversy. It is unlikely that these complex scientific and political issues will be resolved in the near term, or that research studies conducted after well-publicised disasters will convincingly answer basic scientific questions because of the difficulties eliminating research biases in highly charged circumstances [81,86,87]. Distrust of medical experts and government officials will continue because blanket assurances that such exposures are associated with no, as opposed to low, risk cannot be provided. As a result, numerous unconfirmed and controversial hypotheses about the effects of low level exposures will continue to flourish.

Gulf War syndrome: the post-modern illness

In a provocative article Gray [88] describes the features of what he calls 'post-modern medicine':

☐   a distrust of science

☐   a readiness to resort to litigation

☐   a greater attention to risk, and

☐   better access to information (of whatever quality).

Like many commentators, he also points out that consumer and patient values have already replaced paternalistic and professional values, and where doctors used to lead they now follow. The monolithic role of the doctor has been challenged by 'lay experts', whose ability to influence public debate and policy increases just as that of the doctor or scientist diminishes. The 'lay expert' may be the survivor of a disaster or the sufferer from a disease [89]. The Gulf War veteran has fulfilled both roles.

The shape of the Gulf War syndrome had been determined in the popular and political imaginations long before scientists or doctors had anything to say on the matter. In the twentieth century popular syndromes often resulted from the combination of charismatic doctors and a receptive public. Gulf War syndrome, we suggest, developed without the assistance of science or medicine. Certainly, populist and occasionally maverick scientists have emerged into the limelight of Gulf War syndrome and have played roles in subsequent events, but Gulf War syndrome may be the first truly post-modern illness, in that it developed from the congruence of veterans' experiences and narratives, their disquiet and distrust, and a powerful media agenda. Medical professionals and scientists generally have reacted to events, not shaped them.

We speculate that the story of Gulf War ill health began with the experiences of veterans reporting symptoms. These may have been triggered as an unexpected reaction to measures taken to protect the armed forces against modern warfare, reinforced by the social and psychological pressures and changes that war brings to all whom it touches. These narratives were taken up by a powerful media, and shaped into a particular syndrome under the influence of popular views of health, disease and illness. Further impetus came from the actions, or inactions, of government, and only recently by the activities of doctors and scientists. How the story will end remains to be seen.

Acknowledgements

The work of the King's College Gulf War Illness Research Unit has been supported by the US Department of Defence, the US Navy, the UK Medical Research Council and the UK Ministry of Defence. None of these organisations has had any input into the conduct, analysis or reporting of any of the research conducted by the unit. The views in this article are entirely our own.

The King's College Gulf War Illness Research Unit

Trudie Chalder, Anthony David, Kate Davies, Lydia Farrin, Matthew Hotopf, Lisa Hull, Khalida Ismail, Edgar Jones, Ian Palmer, Mark Peakman, Steven Reid, Michael Rose, Mohamed Sharief, Catherine Unwin, Simon Wessely.

REFERENCES

1   Hyams KC, Hanson K, Wignall FS, Escamilla J, Oldfield EC. The impact of infectious diseases on the health of U.S. troops deployed to the Persian Gulf during operations Desert Shield and Desert Storm. Review. *Clin Infect Dis* 1995; **20**: 1497–504.

2   Joseph SC. A comprehensive clinical evaluation of 20,000 Persian Gulf War veterans. *Mil Med* 1997; **162**: 149–55.

3   Roy MJ, Koslowe PA, Kroenke K, Magruder C. Signs, symptoms and ill-defined conditions in Persian Gulf war veterans: findings from the Comprehensive Clinical Evaluation Program. *Psychosom Med* 1998; **60**: 663–8.

4   Coker WJ, Bhatt BM, Blatchley NF, Graham JT. Clinical findings for the first 1000 Gulf war veterans in the Ministry of Defence's medical assessment programme. *Br Med J* 1999; **318**: 290–4.

5   Kang HK, Bullman TA. Mortality among U.S. Veterans of the Persian Gulf War. *N Engl J Med* 1996; 335: 1498–504.

6   MacFarlane GJ, Thomas E, Cherry N. Mortality among UK Gulf War veterans. *Lancet* 2000; 356: 17–21.

7   Gray GC, Coate BD, Anderson CM, Kang HK, *et al.* The postwar hospitalization experience of U.S. veterans of the Persian Gulf War. *N Engl J Med* 1996; 335: 1505–13.

8   Self-reported illness and health status among Gulf War veterans. A population-based study. The Iowa Persian Gulf Study Group. *JAMA* 1997; 277: 238–45.

9   Unwin C, Blatchley N, Coker W, Ferry S, *et al.* Health of UK servicemen who served in Persian Gulf War. *Lancet* 1999; 353: 169–78.

10   Stretch RH, Bliese PD, Marlowe DH, Wright KM, *et al.* Physical health symptomatology of Gulf War-era service personnel from the states of Pennsylvania and Hawaii. *Mil Med* 1995; 160: 131–6.

11   Proctor SP, Heeren T, White RF, Wolfe J, *et al.* Health status of Persian Gulf War veterans: self-reported symptoms, environmental exposures and the effect of stress. *Int J Epidemiol* 1998; 27: 1000–10.

12   Fukuda K, Nisenbaum R, Stewart G, Thompson WW, *et al.* Chronic multisymptom illness affecting Air Force veterans of the Gulf War. *JAMA* 1998; 280: 981–8.

13   Gray GC, Kaiser KS, Hawksworth AW, Hall FW, Barrett-Connor E. Increased postwar symptoms and psychological morbidity among U.S. Navy Gulf War veterans. *Am J Trop Med Hyg* 1999; 60: 758–66.

14   Kang HK, Mahan CM, Lee KY, Magee CA, Murphy FM. Illnesses among United States veterans of the Gulf War: a population-based survey of 30,000 veterans. *J Occup Environ Med* 2000; 42: 491–501.

15   McCauley LA, Joos SK, Lasarev MR, Storzbach D, Bourdette DN. Gulf War unexplained illnesses: persistence and unexplained nature of self-reported symptoms. *Environ Res* 1999; 81: 215–23.

16   Kroenke K, Mangelsdorff AD. Common symptoms in ambulatory care: incidence, evaluation, therapy and outcome. *Am J Med* 1989; 86: 262–6.

17   Wegman DH, Woods NF, Bailar JC. Invited commentary: how would we know a Gulf War syndrome if we saw one? *Am J Epidemiol* 1998; 146: 704–11; discussion 712.

18   Haley RW, Kurt TL, Hom J. Is there a Gulf War Syndrome? Searching for syndromes by factor analysis of symptoms. *JAMA* 1997; 277: 215–22.

19   Landrigan PJ. Illness in Gulf War veterans. Causes and consequences. *JAMA* 1997; 277: 259–61.

20   Ismail K, Everitt B, Blatchley N, Hull L, *et al.* Is there a Gulf War syndrome? *Lancet* 1999; 353: 179–82.

21   Knoke JD, Smith TC, Gray GC, Kaiser KS, Hawksworth AW. Factor analysis of self-reported symptoms: does it identify a Gulf War Syndrome? *Am J Epidemiol* 2000; 152: 379–88.

22   Doebbeling BN, Clarke WR, Watson D, Torner JC, *et al.* Is there a Persian Gulf War syndrome? Evidence from a large population-based survey of veterans and nondeployed controls. *Am J Med* 2000; 108: 695–704.

23   *Health study of Canadian Forces Personnel involved in the 1991 conflict in the Persian Gulf.* Ottawa: Goss Gilroy Inc, 1998.

24   Ishoy T, Suadicani P, Guldager B, Appleyard M, *et al.* State of health after deployment in the Persian Gulf: the Danish Gulf War Study. *Dan Med Bull* 1999; 46: 416–9.

25   French army wary of first Gulf War syndrome charge. Reuters 29 May 2000.

26   Ministry of Defence. British chemical warfare defence during the Gulf conflict (1990–1991). London: www.mod.uk/policy/gulfwar/index.htm

27   Hotopf M, David A, Hull L, Ismail K, *et al.* The role of vaccinations as risk factors for ill health in veterans of the Gulf war: cross-sectional study. *Br Med J* 2000; 320: 1363–7.

28   Rook GA, Zumla A. Gulf War syndrome: is it due to a systemic shift in cytokine balance towards a Th2 profile? *Lancet* 1997; 349: 1831–3.

29 Keeler JR, Hurst CG, Dunn MA. Pyridostigmine used as a nerve agent pretreatment under wartime conditions. *JAMA* 1991; **266**: 693–5.

30 Fulco C, Liverman C, Sox H (eds). *Gulf War and health: Vol. 1. Depleted uranium, sarin, pyridostigmine bromide, vaccines.* Washington DC: Institute of Medicine, 2000.

31 Trojan DA, Cashman NR. An open trial of pyridostigmine in post-poliomyelitis syndrome. *Can J Neurol Sci* 1995; **22**: 223–7.

32 Trojan DA, Collet JP, Shapiro S, Jubelt B, *et al.* A multicenter, randomized, double-blinded trial of pyridostigmine in postpolio syndrome. *Neurology* 1999; **53**: 1225–33.

33 *Presidential Advisory Committee on Gulf War Veterans' Illnesses: Final Report.* Washington DC: US Government Printing Office, 1997.

34 Ablers JW, Berent S. Controversies in neurotoxicology: current status. Review. *Neurol Clin* 2000; **18**: 741–64.

35 Friedman A, Kaufer D, Shemer J, Hendler I, *et al.* Pyridostigmine brain penetration under stress enhances neuronal excitability and induces early immediate transcriptional response. *Nat Med* 1996; **2**: 1382–5.

36 Grauer E, Alkalai D, Kapon J, Cohen G, Raveh L. Stress does not enable pyridostigmine to inhibit brain cholinesterase after parenteral administration. *Toxicol Appl Pharmacol* 2000; **164**: 301–4.

37 Abou-Donia MB, Wilmarth KR, Jensen KF, Oehme FW, Kurt TL. Neurotoxicity resulting from coexposure to pyridostigmine bromide, DEET, and permethrin: implications of Gulf War chemical exposures. *J Toxicol Environ Health* 1996; **48**: 35–56.

38 Hoy JB, Cornell JL, Karlix JA, Tebbett IR, van Haaren F. Repeated coadministrations of pyridostigmine bromide, DEET, and permethrin alter locomotor behavior of rats. *Vet Hum Toxicol* 2000; **42**: 72–6.

39 Griffiths GD, Hornby RJ, Stevens DJ, Scott LA, Upshall DG. Biological consequences of multiple vaccine and pyridostigmine pretreatment in the guinea pig. *J Appl Toxicol* 2001; **21**: 59–68.

40 Furlong CE. PON1 status and neurologic symptom complexes in Gulf War veterans. *Genome Res* 2000; **10**: 153–5.

41 Haley RW, Billecke S, La Du BW. Association of low PON1 type Q (type A) arylesterase activity with neurologic symptom complexes in Gulf War veterans. *Toxicol Appl Pharmacol* 1999; **157**: 227–33.

42 Mackness B, Durrington PN, Mackness MI. Low paraoxonase in Persian Gulf War Veterans self-reporting Gulf War Syndrome. *Biochem Biophys Res Comm* 2000; **276**: 729–33.

43 Committee on Toxicity of Chemicals in Food CPatE. *Organophosphates.* London: Department of Health, 1999.

44 United States General Accounting Office. *Gulf War illnesses: improved monitoring of clinical progress and reexamination of research emphasis are needed.* Washington DC: United States General Accounting Office, 1997.

45 Joint Working Group of the Royal College of Physicians and the Royal College of Psychiatrists. *Organophosphate sheep dip: clinical aspects of long-term low-dose exposure.* Salisbury, Wiltshire: Royal College of Physicians, 1998.

46 Gray GC, Smith TC, Knoke JD, Heller JM. The postwar hospitalization experience of Gulf War Veterans possibly exposed to chemical munitions destruction at Khamisiyah, Iraq. *Am J Epidemiol* 1999; **150**: 532–40.

47 Pearce PC, Crofts HS, Muggleton NG, Ridout D, Scott EA. The effects of acutely administered low dose sarin on cognitive behaviour and the electroencephalogram in the common marmoset. *J Psychopharmacol* 1999; **13**: 128–35.

48 McDiarmid MA, Keogh JP, Hooper FJ, McPhaul K, *et al.* Health effects of depleted uranium on exposed Gulf War veterans. *Environ Res* 2000; **82**: 168–80.

49 United States Army Environmental Hygiene Agency. *Biological Surveillance Initiative. Appendix F of Final Report Kuwait Oil Fire Health Risk Assessment, 5 May-3 December 1991.* Aberdeen Proving Ground, MD: US Army Environmental Hygiene Agency, 1994.

50   Poirier M, Weston A, Schoket B, *et al*. Polycyclic aromatic hydrocarbon biomarkers of internal exposure in US Army soldiers serving in Kuwait in 1991. *Polycyclic Aromatic Compounds* 1999; 17: 197–208.

51   Haley RW, Kurt TL. Self-reported exposure to neurotoxic chemical combinations in the Gulf War. A cross-sectional epidemiologic survey. *JAMA* 1997; 277: 231–7.

52   Wolfe J, Proctor SP, Davis JD, Borgos MS, Friedman MJ. Health symptoms reported by Persian Gulf War veterans two years after return. *Am J Ind Med* 1998; 33: 104–13.

53   Kroenke K, Koslowe P, Roy M. Symptoms in 18,495 Persian Gulf War veterans. Latency of onset and lack of association with self-reported exposures. *J Occup Environ Med* 1998; 40: 520–8.

54   Hyams KC, Wignall FS, Roswell R. War syndromes and their evaluation: from the U.S. Civil War to the Persian Gulf War. Review. *Ann Intern Med* 1996; 125: 398–405.

55   Jones E, Wessely S. Case of chronic fatigue syndrome after Crimean War and Indian Mutiny. *Br Med J* 1999; 319: 1645–7.

56   Stokes J, Banderet L. Psychological aspects of chemical defense and warfare. *Mil Psychol* 1997; 9: 395–415.

57   Betts R. The new threat of mass destruction. *Foreign Affairs* 1998; 77: 26–41.

58   O'Brien LS, Payne RG. Prevention and management of panic in personnel facing a chemical threat – lessons from the Gulf War. *J R Army Med Corps* 1993; 139: 41–5.

59   Holloway HC, Norwood AE, Fullerton CS, Engel CC Jr, Ursano RJ. The threat of biological weapons. Prophylaxis and mitigation of psychological and social consequences. *JAMA* 1997; 278: 425–7.

60   Fullerton CS, Ursano RJ. Behavioral and psychological responses to chemical and biological warfare. *Mil Med* 1990; 155: 54–9.

61   Nisenbaum R, Barrett DH, Reyes M, Reeves WC. Deployment stressors and a chronic multisymptom illness among Gulf War veterans. *J Nerv Ment Dis* 2000; 188: 259–66.

62   Kipen HM, Hallman W, Kang H, Fiedler N, Natelson BH. Prevalence of chronic fatigue and chemical sensitivities in Gulf Registry Veterans. *Arch Environ Health* 1999; 54: 313–8.

63   Black DW, Doebbeling BN, Voelker MD, Clarke WR, *et al*. Multiple chemical sensitivity syndrome: symptom prevalence and risk factors in a military population. *Arch Intern Med* 2000; 160: 1169–76.

64   Reid S, Hotopf M, Hull L, Ismail K, *et al*. Multiple chemical sensitivity and chronic fatigue syndrome in British Gulf War veterans. *Am J Epidemiol* 2001; 153: 604–9.

65   Wessely S, Nimnuan C, Sharpe M. Functional somatic syndromes: one or many? Review. *Lancet* 1999; 354: 936–9.

66   Thomas KB. The consultation and the therapeutic illusion. *Br Med J* 1978; 1: 1327–8.

67   Hall W. The logic of a controversy: the case of Agent Orange in Australia. *Soc Sci Med* 1989; 29: 537–44.

68   Shorter E. Multiple chemical sensitivity: pseudodisease in historical perspective. *Scand J Work Environ Health* 1997; 23(Suppl 3): 35–42.

69   Dalrymple T. *Mass listeria: the meaning of health scares*. London: Andre Deutsch, 1998.

70   Jefferson T. Real or perceived adverse effects of vaccines and the media – a tale of our times. *J Epidemiol Community Health* 2000; 54: 402–3.

71   Berg M, Arnetz BB, Liden S, Eneroth P, Kallner A. Techno-stress. A psychophysiological study of employees with VDU-associated skin complaints. *J Occup Med* 1992; 34: 698–701.

72   Smith M, Carayon P. Work organization, stress and cumulative trauma disorders. In: Moon S, Sauter S (eds). *Beyond biomechanics: psychosocial aspects of musculoskeletal disorders in office work*. London: Taylor & Francis, 1996: 23–44.

73   Arnetz BB, Wiholm C. Technological stress: psychophysiological symptoms in modern offices. *J Psychosom Res* 1997; 43: 35–42.

74   Stewart DE. The changing faces of somatization. *Psychosomatics* 1990; 31: 153–8.

75   Hutchesson EE, Volans GN. Unsubstantiated complaints of being poisoned. Psychopathology of patients referred to the national poisons unit. *Br J Psychiatry* 1989; 154: 34–40.

76   Bowler RM, Mergler D, Huel G, Cone JE. Psychological, psychosocial, and psychophysiological sequelae in a community affected by a railroad chemical disaster. *J Trauma Stress* 1994; 7: 601–24.

77   Roht LH, Vernon SW, Weir FW, Pier SM, *et al.* Community exposure to hazardous waste disposal sites: assessing reporting bias. *Am J Epidemiol* 1985; **122**: 418–33.

78   Lipscomb JA, Satin KP, Neutra RR. Reported symptom prevalence rates from comparison populations in community-based environmental studies. *Arch Environ Health* 1992; **47**: 263–9.

79   Shusterman D, Lipscomb J, Neutra R, Satin K. Symptom prevalence and odor-worry interaction near hazardous waste sites. *Environ Health Perspect* 1991; **94**: 25–30.

80   Cowan DN, DeFraites RF, Gray GC, Goldenbaum MB, Wishik SM. The risk of birth defects among children of Persian Gulf War veterans. *N Engl J Med* 1997; **336**: 1650–6.

81   Slovic P. Trust, emotion, sex, politics, and science: surveying the risk-assessment battlefield. *Risk Anal* 1999; **19**: 689–701.

82   Funkhouser G. The issues of the sixties: an exploratory study in the dynamics of public opinion. *Public Opin Q* 1973; **37**: 62–75.

83   Gilmour B. Hazardous duty. *Edmonton J* 9 September 1999.

84   Soetekouw PM, De Vries M, Preijers FW, Van Crevel R, *et al.* Persistent symptoms in former UNTAC soldiers are not associated with shifted cytokine balance. *Eur J Clin Invest* 1999; **29**: 960–3.

85   De Vries M, Soetekouw PM, Van Der Meer JW, Bleijenberg G. Fatigue in Cambodia veterans. *QJM* 2000; **93**: 283–9.

86   Neutra RR. Epidemiology for and with a distrustful community. *Environ Health Perspect* 1985; **62**: 393–7.

87   David AS, Wessely SC. The legend of Camelford: medical consequences of a water pollution accident. Review. *J Psychosom Res* 1995; **39**: 1–9.

88   Gray JA. Postmodern medicine. *Lancet* 1999; **354**: 1550–3.

89   Bury M. Postmodernity and health. In: Scambler G, Higgs P (eds). *Modernity and health*. London: Routledge, 1998: 1–28.

Alzheimer's disease: from palliation to modification

Simon Lovestone

☐ INTRODUCTION

Alzheimer's disease (AD) wreaks havoc in the brain, havoc in the family and, because of the costs of caring for sufferers, havoc to health service budgets. Described by Alzheimer in 1907 in a woman called Auguste D who died in her fifties, this early onset dementia is now known to be essentially the same condition as that which so commonly causes dementia in older people. Perhaps two of the most important developments over the past 20 years has been the consigning to the history books of senile dementia or 'just ageing', and the recognition that AD is one of the most important causes of morbidity and mortality in the elderly. Approximately 600,000 people are affected in the UK and the costs have been estimated at over £1 billion per year.

In the late 1960s the first steps were taken towards finding interventions. These resulted in a licensed drug being released in 1997, with the class of compounds approved for use in the UK by the National Institute for Clinical Excellence (NICE) in 2001. These drugs are symptomatic or palliative only, and are complementary to existing and – in most parts of the UK – comprehensive services for people with dementia and their families. Current research is rapidly heading towards a more complete understanding of the molecular pathogenesis of AD and has the more ambitious aim of moving to beyond mere palliation towards disease modification.

☐ CHOLINERGIC HYPOTHESIS OF ALZHEIMER'S DISEASE

The first wave of research with therapy in mind resulted in the understanding that AD was a predominantly cholinergic disorder [1]. Broadly speaking, three pieces of evidence attest to this:

1   Neuropathology demonstrated marked neuronal loss within the cholinergic tracts, in particular the nucleus basalis Meynert, the origin of cholinergic forebrain projection fibres.

2   Post-mortem indices of cholinergic function show attrition; in particular, markers such as cholinesteryltransferase are lower in AD brain.

3   Studies in animals show that lesioning of cholinergic tracts either surgically or with cholinergic inhibitors such as scopolamine decreases cognitive ability in rodents and other animals. The first two lines of evidence are consistent with this finding.

Although cholinergic deficiencies are clearly present in AD brain, the cholinergic receptors, in particular muscarinic receptors, are either unaltered or upregulated. It follows that there is residual capacity in the brain for using cholinergic replacement therapy.

The cholinergic hypothesis resulting from this work has limitations, in that careful examination of AD brain demonstrates other neurochemical deficits and the evidence for cholinergic loss early in the process (as opposed to end-stage disease) is necessarily limited.

□ THERAPEUTIC APPROACHES TO RESTORE CHOLINERGIC FUNCTION

On the basis of the cholinergic hypothesis, compounds were developed with the aim of rectifying the cholinergic loss using three distinct approaches (Fig. 1):

1   Precursors of acetylcholine, notably lecithin: trials of these were largely negative.

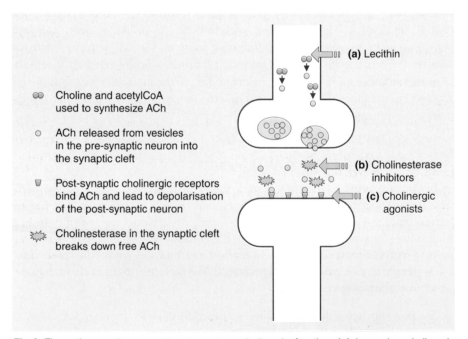

Fig.1 Three therapeutic approaches to restore cholinergic function: **(a)** increasing cholinergic function in Alzheimer's disease, driving synthesis of acetylcholine (ACh) using lecithin; **(b)** decreasing ACh breakdown by inhibiting cholinesterases; **(c)** direct stimulation of the post-synaptic receptors. Only cholinesterase inhibition has so far been successful (acetylCoA = acetyl co-enzyme A).

2   Cholinesterase inhibitors: this class of compounds, which prevent or attenuate acetylcholine breakdown in the synaptic cleft, have proved successful.

3   Direct muscarinic agonists: recent trials with these compounds have been disappointing.

□ CHOLINESTERASE INHIBITORS

The first cholinesterase inhibitor shown to be useful in randomised control trials (RCTs) was tacrine, but this drug had adverse effects on the liver. Subsequently, three compounds have proved efficacious and safe in RCTs and have therefore been licensed for use in AD:

□   rivastigmine

□   donepezil

□   galanthamine.

In general, effects are consistent with a significant placebo treatment group difference on cognitive tests at six months, with the treatment group showing modest improvement or no change relative to a decrease in cognitive ability in the placebo group. A number-needed-to-treat analysis suggests 3–7 treatments result in significant benefits for at least one recipient [2]. Effects on function and behaviour, as well as on global change, have also been reported.

Some aspects of the pharmacological profiles of the three compounds are different, but few data are currently available to allow rational decisions regarding which one to use. There are as yet no published head-to-head studies.

Long-term effects

The long-term effects of cholinesterase inhibitors are less well established and have not been assessed in RCTs. Open label extension studies suggest a possible continuing effect beyond six months because the decline observed is perhaps less than would have been predicted from previous untreated serially assessed groups [3]. However, these data are weak.

In practical terms, relatively few people meet the strict criteria for prescription of these drugs (mild to moderate AD with assured compliance). The monitoring of therapy using repeated measures of function, behaviour and cognition has implications for services. It is possible that the availability of specific treatments will increase recognition of dementia in the community, and hence provision of services to a wider group of needy patients. Perhaps this will be one of the more important consequences of these novel therapeutics.

□ MOLECULAR PATHOGENESIS OF ALZHEIMER'S DISEASE

Amyloid precursor protein

Molecular research in AD can be dated to 1984 with the discovery by Glenner and Wong [4] that the amyloid core of plaques (Fig. 2) was a peptide derived from a

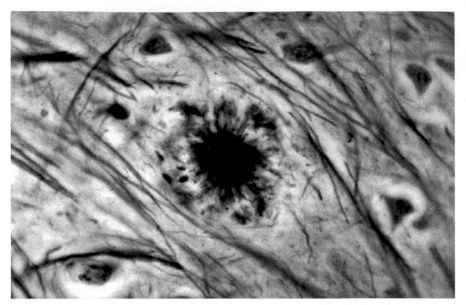

Fig. 2 Neuritic plaque: an extracellular plaque consisting of a core of amyloid peptide surrounded by neuritic change, revealed by silver staining in Alzheimer disease brain.

protein, amyloid precursor protein (APP), the gene for which is carried on chromosome 21 (Fig. 3). This work led to the amyloid cascade hypothesis in which it was stated that genetic and/or environmental factors alter the metabolism of APP such that more Aβ peptide is generated and deposited in plaques [5]. Neurofibrillary

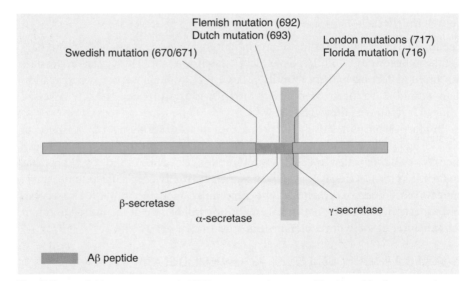

Fig. 3 The amyloid precursor protein (APP) spans membranes and is cleaved by three secretases (β, α and γ). Mutations in the gene at chromosome 21 are a cause of early onset autosomal dominant Alzheimer's disease. The Aβ peptide forms the core of plaques and is produced from APP. (Numbers in brackets represent amino acid positions of the mutations.)

tangles, the other lesion described by Alzheimer, were thought to be a downstream consequence of amyloid deposition (Fig. 4). All subsequent work has tended to confirm this core hypothesis. Most dramatically, it has been demonstrated in early onset autosomal dominant familial AD (FAD), a rare cause of AD, that altered metabolism of APP can be a primary aetiopathogenetic event. The evidence for this is convincing (reviewed in detail in [6]). It may be briefly summarised:

☐   Mutations in APP associated with FAD increase the production of Aβ or the more fibrillinogenic and pathogenic Aβ42.

☐   The presenilin gene, mutations in which also cause FAD (more frequently than APP mutations), is either γ-secretase or closely associated with it [7].

☐   Late onset AD has been linked to chromosome 10 and the same region of the chromosome that is linked to variability in serum amyloid [8,9].

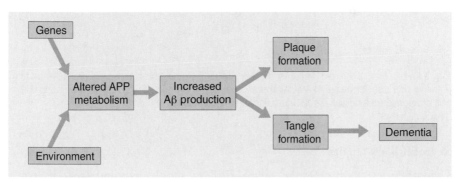

Fig. 4 The amyloid cascade hypothesis. Both genetic and environmental influences can alter the metabolism of amyloid precursor protein (APP) leading to more Aβ production. The Aβ peptide aggregates, forms the core of plaques and stimulates tau phosphorylation, one of the processes involved in neurofibrillary tangle formation. Tangles result in neuronal loss and hence dementia, but whether plaques do is a matter of dispute.

Apolipoprotein E

The other gene associated with late onset AD as a quantitative trait locus (as opposed to an autosomal dominant single gene of major effect) is apolipoprotein E (apoE). Polymorphic variation in apoE is associated with AD, with apoEε4 increasing risk and/or decreasing age of onset, and apoEε2 decreasing risk.

It is not known how apoE affects pathogenesis, but some evidence suggests that it too alters APP metabolism or deposition. It is clear that the APP protein is metabolised either by β- and then γ-secretase enzymes to yield Aβ, or by α-secretase to yield non-amyloidogenic fragments (Fig. 5). Furthermore, this metabolism is altered by mutations in genes in early onset FAD and by normal variation in genes in late onset AD. Environmental effects on APP processing are less easy to determine, but it would appear that head injury also increases Aβ deposition [10].

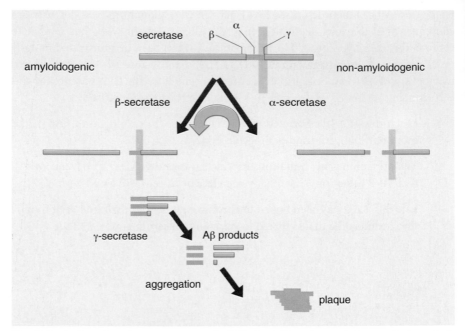

Fig. 5 Metabolism of amyloid precursor protein (APP). Amyloidogenic metabolism results from, first, β- then γ-secretase cleavage of APP. Aggregation of the Aβ products leads to plaque formation. Non-amyloidogenic metabolism results from α-secretase cleavage.

Neurofibrillary tangles

The other lesion of AD, the neurofibrillary tangle, is composed of highly phosphorylated aggregates of tau (Fig. 6). Tau is a microtubule-associated protein, normally expressed only in axons where it functions to stabilise microtubules, and hence participates in structural stability and fast axonal transport. Tau phosphorylation regulates this function, and highly phosphorylated tau does not bind to microtubules [11]. In the fetus, high levels of tau phosphorylation contribute to the necessary neuronal plasticity. Although tau phosphorylation is regulated by a number of kinases, glycogen synthase (GSK)-3 appears to be the predominant kinase in normal brain as its inhibition by either lithium or insulin reduces tau phosphorylation in neurons. In AD brain, highly phosphorylated tau is aggregated into paired helical filaments (in tangles), but it is not yet known whether phosphorylation precedes or follows tangle formation (Fig. 7). Mutations in tau are a primary aetiological cause in some familial frontal lobe dementias, resulting in disruption of the normal isoform expression of tau, reduced ability to bind microtubules, and increased propensity to aggregate [12].

The predominant hypothesis integrating these observations is probably that decreased binding of tau to microtubules, caused by increased phosphorylation, mutations or auto-isoform expression, results in increased cytoplasmic tau and hence abnormal self-aggregation and subsequent neuronal death. How Aβ and tau aggregation connect in pathological terms is not known. In cells in culture,

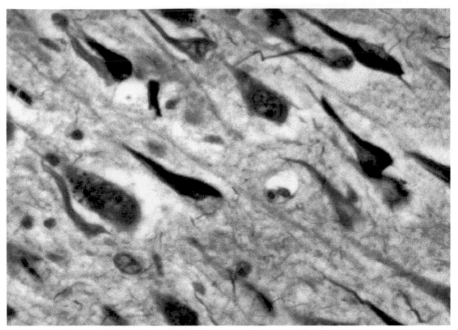

Fig. 6 Intraneuronal neurofibrillary tangles in Alzheimer disease brain.

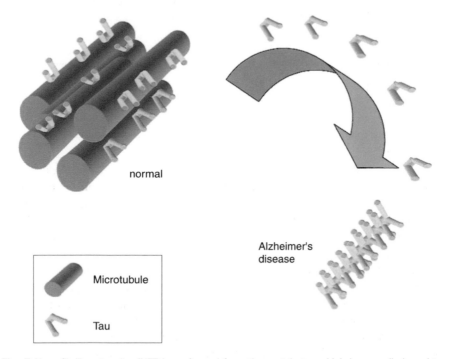

Fig. 7 Neurofibrillary tangles (NFTs) are formed from the protein tau which is normally bound to microtubules. Both increased phosphorylation (found in Alzheimer's disease) and mutations in tau (found in some forms of frontotemporal dementia) result in decreased binding of tau to microtubules. However, it remains to be proven that tau phosphorylation precedes NFT formation.

however, Aβ results in neurotoxicity and increased tau phosphorylation. This neurotoxicity is prevented by GSK-3 inhibitors. It is therefore possible – but far from proven – that tau phosphorylation by GSK-3 is the missing link between amyloid and tau pathology.

☐ THERAPEUTIC APPROACHES

The molecular cascade of events established to date suggests a number of therapeutic strategies of possible use over the forthcoming years. One of those showing most promise at present is the 'amyloid vaccine'. Both passive and active immunisation in transgenic mice overexpressing the human APP gene carrying the FAD mutations has arrested, and even reduced, plaque formation and reversed acquired cognitive deficits [13]. Clinical studies in man are currently underway. It remains to be seen whether this or any of the other potential disease modifications prove to be useful in the near future. None the less, 100 years after Alzheimer's case description of Auguste D we are probably on the threshold of a true Alzheimer treatment.

REFERENCES

1 Francis PT, Palmer AM, Snape M, Wilcock GK. The cholinergic hypothesis of Alzheimer's disease: a review of progress. *J Neurol Neurosurg Psychiatry* 1999; **66**: 137–47.

2 Livingston G, Katona C. How useful are cholinesterase inhibitors in the treatment of Alzheimer's disease? A number needed to treat analysis. Review. *Int J Geriatr Psychiatry* 2000; **15**: 203–7.

3 Rogers SL, Doody RS, Pratt RD, Ieni JR. Long-term efficacy and safety of donepezil in the treatment of Alzheimer's disease: final analysis of a US multicentre open-label study. *Eur Neuropsychopharmacol* 2000; **10**: 195–203.

4 Glenner GG, Wong CW. Alzheimer's disease: initial report of the purification and characterization of a novel cerebrovascular amyloid protein. *Biochem Biophys Res Commun* 1984; **120**: 885–90.

5 Hardy JA, Higgins GA. Alzheimer's disease: the amyloid cascade hypothesis. Review. *Science* 1992; **256**: 184–5.

6 Storey E, Cappai R. The amyloid precursor protein of Alzheimer's disease and the Aβ peptide. Review. *Neuropathol Appl Neurobiol* 1999; **25**: 81–97.

7 Da Silva HAR, Patel AJ. Presenilins and early-onset familial Alzheimer's disease. *Neuroreport* 1997; **8**: I–XII.

8 Ertekin-Taner N, Graff-Radford N, Younkin LH, Eckman C, *et al.* Linkage of plasma Abeta42 to a quantitative locus on chromosome 10 in late-onset Alzheimer's disease pedigrees. *Science* 2000; **290**: 2303–4.

9 Myers A, Holmans P, Marshall H, Kwon J, *et al.* Susceptibility locus for Alzheimer's disease on chromosome 10. *Science* 2000; **290**: 2304–5.

10 Horsburgh K, Cole GM, Yang F, Savage MJ, *et al.* β-amyloid (Aβ)42(43), Aβ42, Aβ40 and apoE immunostaining of plaques in fatal head injury. *Neuropathol Appl Neurobiol* 2000; **26**: 124–32.

11 Lovestone S, Reynolds CH. The phosphorylation of tau: a critical stage in neurodevelopment and neurodegenerative processes. Review. *Neuroscience* 1997; **78**: 309–24.

12 Heutink P. Untangling tau-related dementia. Review. *Hum Mol Genet* 2000; **9**: 979–86.

13 Janus C, Pearson J, McLaurin J, Mathews PM, *et al.* A beta peptide immunization reduces behavioural impairment and plaques in a model of Alzheimer's disease. *Nature* 2000; **408**: 979–82.

☐ SELF ASSESSMENT QUESTIONS

1 The amyloid precursor protein (APP):
  (a) Gene carries mutations in late onset Alzheimer's disease (AD)
  (b) Is expressed only in neurons
  (c) Is metabolised to produce the amyloid peptide by α- and γ-secretases
  (d) Produces the peptide that aggregates into extracellular plaques in AD
  (e) Is a potential target for new therapies in AD

2 Approved disease-specific treatments for AD:
  (a) Include ginkgo biloba and vitamin E
  (b) Have been shown to have effects on behaviour and function in AD
  (c) Are most suitable for severe dementia
  (d) Increase neurotransmitter function through direct agonist action
  (e) Increase cholinergic activity

3 Tau:
  (a) Is a microtubule-associated protein
  (b) Is abnormally expressed in neurons in AD
  (c) Is less phosphorylated in AD than in normal tissue
  (d) Carries mutations in frontal lobe dementia when familial
  (e) Is present in the core of the neuritic plaque

4 AD:
  (a) Affects approximately 200,000 people in the UK
  (b) Was described by Alzheimer first in an old man
  (c) Is accompanied by loss of cholinergic neurons
  (d) The origin of cholinergic neurons is the locus caeruleus
  (e) Scopolamine was an early experimental treatment

5 The molecular genetics of the dementia has shown:
  (a) A genetic effect on the production of Aβ peptide in life
  (b) That polymorphic variation in apolipoprotein E is a risk factor for AD
  (c) That mutations in APP are the main cause of familial early onset AD
  (d) That mutations in tau are the main cause of familial early onset frontal lobe dementia
  (e) That polymorphic variation in APP is associated with late onset AD

ANSWERS

1a False	2a False	3a True	4a False	5a True
b False	b True	b False	b False	b True
c False	c False	c False	c True	c False
d True	d False	d True	d False	d True
e True	e True	e False	e False	e False

Serotonin and the pathophysiology of depression

Philip Cowen

☐ MAJOR DEPRESSION

Significance and burden

Major or 'clinical' depression is a common disorder with a lifetime risk in the general population of 10–15%. In about 50% of cases, depression is recurrent and associated with a substantial morbidity and significant mortality. In the developed world, recurrent depression measured in disability-adjusted life-years (DALYs) is second only to cardiovascular disease in terms of illness burden. Worldwide there are about one million suicides each year, about 70% of which are probably due to clinical depression [1].

Symptomatology

Major depression, the name given to clinical depression in the Diagnostic and Statistical Manual of Mental (DSM) Disorders (Table 1), is a term covering much,

Table 1 Abridged Diagnostic and Statistical Manual of Mental (DSM)-IV criteria for major depressive episode.

Over the last two weeks, five of the following features should be present most of the day, or nearly every day (must include one or two):

- Depressed mood
- Loss of interest or pleasure in almost all activities
- Significant weight loss or gain (more than 5% change in one month) or an increase or decrease in appetite nearly every day
- Insomnia or hypersomnia
- Psychomotor agitation or retardation (observable by others)
- Fatigue or loss of energy
- Feelings of worthlessness or excessive or inappropriate guilt (not merely self-reproach about being sick)
- Diminished ability to think or concentrate, or indecisiveness (either by subjective account or observation of others)
- Recurrent thoughts of death (not just fear of dying), or suicidal ideation, or a suicide attempt, or a specific plan for committing suicide

---

rather disparate, symptomatology. For example, as well as depressed mood, patients can suffer crippling anxiety, and changes in psychomotor function, sleep and appetite. Loss of the normal capacity for pleasure is a common feature of severe depression, as is some degree of suicidal ideation. Cognitive impairment is also common.

Risk factors and pathophysiology

The range of neuropsychological abnormalities seen in clinical depression suggests a complex underlying neurobiology. Knowledge of the relevant pathophysiology is still rudimentary. The main neurochemical theory of depression (the 'monoamine' theory) is based on knowledge of the actions of drugs that were discovered by chance to be effective antidepressant agents about 40 years ago. Thus, tricyclic antidepressants such as imipramine block the pre-synaptic reuptake of noradrenaline and serotonin (5-HT), while monoamine oxidase inhibitors inhibit the breakdown of monoamines by preventing metabolism by monoamine oxidase. Many antidepressant compounds have been introduced since then, but it is still true to say that all marketed antidepressant drugs potentiate the synaptic actions of noradrenaline and/or 5-HT by one mechanism or another [1].

It has been much harder to establish whether or not brain monoamine function is lowered in patients with depression. However, recent investigations, particularly those using positron emission tomography (PET) and single-photon emission tomography, have provided reliable evidence that brain 5-HT function is abnormal in unmedicated depressed patients (Table 2). It is not clear, though, whether these abnormalities are important in pathophysiology or epiphenomena simply associated with the state of being depressed.

Rather more is known about personal and psychosocial risk factors for depression. These include genetic predisposition (often referred to as family history

Table 2 Serotonin (5-HT) abnormalities in major depression.

- Low plasma tryptophan
- Diminished 5-HT neuroendocrine responses
- Decreased platelet 5-HT uptake
- Decreased brain binding potential of 5-HT1A and 5-HT2A receptors (PET)
- Decreased brain binding potential of 5-HT transporters (SPET)

PET = positron emission tomography; SPET = single-photon emission tomography.

Table 3 Risk factors for depression.

• Family history of depression	• Neuroticism
• Female gender	• Low social support
• Childhood adversities	• Recent stressful life events
• Personal history of depression	

of mood disorder), adverse childhood experiences and recent stressful life events [2] (Table 3). A past history of depression is a high risk factor for future episodes, and it is possible that depression itself might produce neurobiological effects that predispose to future episodes.

☐ TRYPTOPHAN AND SEROTONIN

The synthesis of brain 5-HT is dependent on the availability of tryptophan (TRP), the amino acid precursor of 5-HT, from plasma. This is because TRP hydroxylase, the enzyme which converts TRP to 5-hydroxy TRP in the brain, is normally unsaturated with its substrate. TRP is an essential amino acid, therefore dietary manipulations can alter plasma levels of TRP and thereby brain 5-HT levels.

One such dietary manipulation, called 'TRP depletion', involves administering an oral mixture of amino acids which lacks TRP. This mixture produces an acute reduction in brain 5-HT levels by lowering the amount of TRP available for brain 5-HT synthesis. Two mechanisms probably account for this reduction in TRP availability:

1   The TRP-free amino acid mixture decreases plasma TRP via stimulation of protein synthesis in the liver and utilisation of endogenous TRP stores.

2   The neutral amino acids present in the mixture compete with endogenous plasma TRP for transport across the blood-brain barrier [3].

Tryptophan depletion and mood

TRP depletion causes little change in mood in healthy volunteers, suggesting that diminished brain 5-HT function by itself is insufficient to produce clinical depressive symptomatology. Our hypothesis was that lowering brain 5-HT function in subjects vulnerable to depression might produce clinical depressive symptomatology. To test this, 15 women were studied who had suffered recurrent episodes of major depression who were clinically recovered and free of drug treatment for at least three months [4]. Such subjects are known to be at high risk of episodes of depression in the future [2].

The subjects received two amino acid mixtures in a double-blind, balanced-order, cross-over design. One of the mixtures was nutritionally balanced and contained TRP (balanced mixture), while the other was identical except for the omission of TRP (TRP-free mixture). Subjects were rated on the Hamilton Rating Scale for Depression before and seven hours following ingestion of each mixture. The TRP-free mixture produced a 75% reduction in plasma TRP concentration; following its administration, 10 of the women (67%) experienced temporary, but clinically significant, depressive symptoms. No changes in mood were seen following the balanced mixture (Fig. 1). Interestingly, the full range of depressive symptoms was seen when subjects relapsed, suggesting that deficient 5-HT function could produce the return of all the complex symptomatology of major depression.

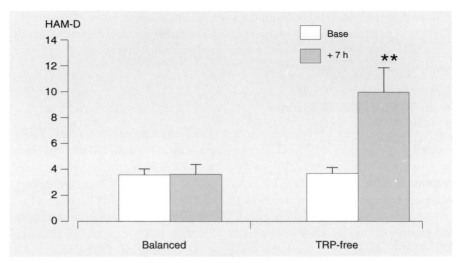

Fig. 1 Mean (± SEM) scores on the Hamilton Rating Scale for Depression (HAM-D) in 15 recovered depressed patients before and seven hours following ingestion of two amino acid mixtures. One mixture was nutritionally balanced (Balanced); the other mixture was identical except for the omission of tryptophan (TRP-free) (** significantly greater than Balanced treatment ($p < 0.01$)).

These findings suggest that acute lowering of brain 5-HT function can precipitate clinical depressive symptoms in well, untreated individuals at risk of depression. There seem to be two possible explanations for this occurring in those vulnerable to depression but not in healthy subjects. In those at risk of depression:

1   5-HT pathways may modulate brain regions critical for mood regulation that are potentially dysfunctional. Lowering brain 5-HT function may enable this dysfunction to become clinically manifest.

2   Brain 5-HT itself may be regulated abnormally so that a situation of precursor deficit produces a particularly large impairment in brain 5-HT neurotransmission.

Brain regions involved in depressive relapse induced by tryptophan depletion

It is important to determine the brain regions involved in depressive relapse because this might give further information about pathophysiology and possible means of prevention. The use of TRP depletion in a PET imaging paradigm allows changes in regional cerebral blood flow to be measured during the process of relapse. Eight recovered depressed men were studied with $^{15}H_2O$ PET after both TRP depletion and a control (balanced) amino acid mixture.

Increasing levels of depression after TRP depletion were found to be associated with diminished neural activity in the ventral anterior cingulate, orbitofrontal cortex and caudate nucleus. These areas have been implicated in previous brain imaging studies of depression, and they all receive a heavy 5-HT innervation. TRP depletion may therefore induce depression by impairing activity in these brain regions [5].

☐ IMPLICATIONS OF LOW BRAIN SEROTONIN FUNCTION

These findings suggest that people at risk of depression are psychologically vulnerable to low brain 5-HT function. 5-HT synthesis depends on TRP availability, so it is possible that situations that result in lowered plasma TRP levels might lead to depression in vulnerable individuals. Such situations might occur during dieting or under life stresses which can lower plasma TRP, probably via increasing cortisol secretion [6]. In contrast, manipulations that help maintain plasma TRP at optimal levels could prevent depression in those at risk.

Acknowledgements

The work of the author was supported by the Medical Research Council.

REFERENCES

1   Gelder MG, Mayou RA, Cowen PJ. *Shorter Oxford Textbook of Psychiatry*. Oxford: Oxford University Press, 2001.

2   Kendler KS, Kessler RC, Neale MC, Heath AC, Eaves LJ. The prediction of major depression in women: toward an integrated etiologic model. *Am J Psychiatry* 1993; 150: 1139–48.

3   Young SN, Smith SE, Pihl RO, Ervin FR. Tryptophan depletion causes a rapid lowering of mood in normal males. *Psychopharmacology (Berl)* 1985; 87: 173–7.

4   Smith KA, Fairburn CG, Cowen PJ. Relapse of depression after rapid depletion of tryptophan. *Lancet* 1997; 349: 915–9.

5   Smith KA, Morris JS, Friston KJ, Cowen PJ, Dolan RJ. Brain mechanisms associated with depressive relapse and associated cognitive impairment following acute tryptophan depletion. *Br J Psychiatry* 1999; 174: 525–9.

6   Maes M, Schotte C, Scharpe S, Martin M, Blockx P. The effects of glucocorticoids on the availability of L-tryptophan and tyrosine in the plasma of depressed patients. *J Affect Disord* 1990; 18: 121–7.

☐ SELF ASSESSMENT QUESTIONS

1   Clinical depression:
   (a) Has a lifetime risk of about 5%
   (b) Is rarely recurrent
   (c) Is known as 'major depression' in DSM-IV
   (d) Is responsible for about 70% of suicides
   (e) Is equally common in men and women

2   Risk factors for major depression include:
   (a) Past history of depression
   (b) Low levels of social support
   (c) Lack of religious belief
   (d) Recent use of antibiotics
   (e) Childhood adversity

3   Common symptoms of major depression include:
   (a) Loss of pleasure

(b) Early morning waking
(c) Visual hallucinations
(d) Cognitive impairments
(e) Stereotypies

4   Abnormalities in serotonin (5-HT) function found in depression include:
(a) Low plasma tryptophan
(b) Low plasma 5-HT
(c) Decreased brain 5-HT1A receptor binding
(d) Diminished 5-HT neuroendocrine responses
(e) Lowered urine 5-hydroxyindoleacetic acid

5   Depressive relapse is associated with changes in regional blood flow in the following brain areas:
(a) Orbitofrontal cortex
(b) Locus ceruleus
(c) Caudate nucleus
(d) Cingulate cortex
(e) Brain stem

ANSWERS

1a False	2a True	3a True	4a True	5a True
b False	b True	b True	b False	b False
c True	c False	c False	c True	c True
d True	d False	d True	d True	d True
e False	e True	e False	e False	e False

Rheumatology

Amyloidosis

Philip Hawkins

□ INTRODUCTION

Amyloidosis is a disorder of protein folding in which normally soluble proteins are deposited as abnormal, insoluble fibrils that disrupt tissue structure and cause disease. Some 20 different unrelated proteins can form amyloid *in vivo* and amyloidosis is classified clinically according to the fibril protein type (Table 1) [1]. In systemic amyloidosis, deposition may occur in all tissues except the brain, and amyloid fibrils are present in the walls of blood vessels throughout the body. Systemic amyloidosis is often fatal, although its prognosis has been improved by haemodialysis, kidney, liver and heart transplantation, and by increasingly effective treatment of the various conditions that underlie amyloid deposition [2]. There are also various local forms of amyloidosis in which deposits are confined to specific foci or to a particular organ or tissue. These may be clinically silent or trivial or may be associated with serious disease, such as heart failure in senile cardiac amyloidosis, or haemorrhage in local respiratory or urogenital tract amyloid. In addition, there are important diseases associated with local amyloid deposition in which the pathogenetic role of the amyloid is still unclear, for example, Alzheimer's disease, the prion disorders and type 2 diabetes mellitus. Although these conditions will not be discussed in this chapter, therapeutic strategies aimed at inhibiting amyloid fibrillogenesis and/or promoting regression of amyloid deposits in systemic amyloidosis may also be applicable to localised amyloidosis and vice versa.

In addition to the fibrils, amyloid deposits always contain the plasma protein serum amyloid P (SAP) component which undergoes specific calcium-dependent binding to amyloid fibrils. SAP contributes to amyloidogenesis, and radiolabelled SAP is a specific, quantitative and highly informative tracer for scintigraphic imaging of systemic amyloid deposits [3,4].

The treatment of amyloidosis comprises measures to support impaired organ function, including dialysis and transplantation, together with vigorous efforts to control underlying conditions responsible for production of fibril precursors. Serial SAP scintigraphy has demonstrated that reduction of the supply of amyloid fibril precursor proteins leads to regression of amyloid deposits and clinical benefit in many cases.

□ ACQUIRED SYSTEMIC AMYLOIDOSIS

Reactive systemic (AA) amyloidosis (Table 2) is a complication of chronic infections and inflammatory diseases in which there is sustained overproduction of the

Table 1 Classification of amyloidosis.

Type	Fibril precursor protein	Clinical syndrome
AA	Serum amyloid A protein	Reactive systemic amyloidosis associated with acquired or hereditary chronic inflammatory diseases Formerly known as secondary amyloidosis
AL	Monoclonal immunoglobulin light chains	Systemic amyloidosis associated with myeloma, monoclonal gammopathy, occult B cell dyscrasia Formerly known as primary amyloidosis
ATTR	Normal plasma transthyretin Genetically variant transthyretin	Senile systemic amyloidosis with prominent cardiac involvement Familial amyloid polyneuropathy, usually with systemic amyloidosis Sometimes prominent amyloid cardiomyopathy or nephropathy
Aβ₂M	β₂-microglobulin	Peri-articular and occasionally systemic amyloidosis associated with renal failure and long-term dialysis
Aβ	β-protein precursor (and rare genetic variants)	Cerebrovascular and intracerebral plaque amyloid in Alzheimer's disease Occasional familial cases
AapoAI	Apolipoprotein AI	Autosomal dominant systemic amyloidosis Predominantly non-neuropathic with prominent visceral involvement
AFib	Fibrinogen α-chain	Autosomal dominant systemic amyloidosis Non-neuropathic with prominent visceral involvement
ALys	Lysozyme	Autosomal dominant systemic amyloidosis Non-neuropathic with prominent visceral involvement
ACys	Cystatin C	Hereditary cerebral haemorrhage with cerebral and systemic amyloidosis
AGel	Gelsolin	Autosomal dominant systemic amyloidosis Predominant cranial nerve involvement with lattice corneal dystrophy
AIAPP	Islet amyloid polypeptide	Amyloid in islets of Langerhans in type 2 diabetes mellitus and insulinoma

Amyloid composed of peptide hormones, prion protein and unknown proteins not included.

acute-phase protein, serum amyloid A (SAA) protein. The amyloid fibrils are composed of AA protein, an N-terminal fragment of SAA. AA amyloidosis occurs in up to 10% of patients with rheumatoid arthritis, juvenile inflammatory arthritis and Crohn's disease. Most patients present with nephropathy, there may be liver and gastrointestinal involvement at a late stage, but the heart and nerves are rarely affected.

Table 2 Conditions associated with AA amyloidosis.

Chronic inflammatory disorders
- Rheumatoid arthritis
- Juvenile chronic arthritis
- Ankylosing spondylitis
- Psoriasis and psoriatic arthropathy
- Reiter's syndrome
- Adult Still's disease
- Behçet's syndrome
- Crohn's disease

Chronic microbial infections
- Leprosy
- Tuberculosis
- Bronchiectasis
- Decubitus ulcers
- Chronic pyelonephritis in paraplegics
- Osteomyelitis
- Whipple's disease

Neoplastic disorders
- Castleman's disease tumours
- Hodgkin's disease
- Renal carcinoma
- Carcinoma of gut, lung, urogenital tract

Monoclonal immunoglobulin light chain (AL) amyloidosis is a complication of monoclonal gammopathies, which in most patients are subtle. AL fibrils are derived from monoclonal light chains which have a unique structure in each patient. Any organ other than the brain may be affected, commonly including the heart, and the prognosis is usually poor. About one in 1,500 deaths in the UK is due to AL amyloidosis.

Dialysis-associated (Aβ₂M) amyloidosis is a complication of long-term haemodialysis for renal failure. β_2-microglobulin (β_2M), the light chain of cell surface HLA class I molecules, is normally catabolised in the proximal renal tubule. The plasma concentration of β_2M rises with renal failure and remains very high on both peritoneal dialysis and haemodialysis. Aβ_2M amyloid starts to accumulate in bones and joints after about five years of dialysis. Arthralgia and carpal tunnel syndrome are typical symptoms but minor visceral and vascular deposits can occur.

Senile systemic (ATTR) amyloidosis is a disease of the elderly that occurs with increasing frequency after the age of 70 years, predominantly affecting the heart and often asymptomatic. The fibrils are composed of normal wild type transthyretin (TTR).

☐ HEREDITARY SYSTEMIC AMYLOIDOSIS

The different forms of hereditary systemic amyloidosis are caused by deposition of genetically variant proteins as amyloid fibrils associated with mutations in the genes for transthyretin, cystatin C, gelsolin, apolipoprotein (apo) AI, lysozyme and fibrinogen A α-chain. These diseases are all inherited in an autosomal dominant pattern with variable penetrance and present clinically at various times from the teens to old age, though usually in adult life:

☐ By far the commonest hereditary amyloidosis is caused by *transthyretin variants*, usually presenting as familial amyloid polyneuropathy (FAP) with peripheral and autonomic neuropathy.

☐ *Cystatin C amyloidosis* presents as cerebral amyloid angiopathy with recurrent cerebral haemorrhage and clinically silent systemic deposits. It has been reported only in Icelandic families.

☐ *Gelsolin amyloidosis* presents with cranial neuropathy but is also extremely rare.

☐ *Apo AI, lysozyme* and *fibrinogen α-chain amyloidosis* present as non-neuropathic systemic amyloidosis that can affect any or all the major viscera, with renal involvement usually prominent. These conditions are readily misdiagnosed as acquired AL amyloidosis, and are less rare than previously thought.

☐ PATHOGENESIS

Despite the structural diversity of amyloid forming proteins, the ultrastructural morphology of all amyloid fibrils is remarkably similar. They all share a common core structure of twisted anti-parallel β-pleated sheets. Amyloid fibril formation evidently involves substantial refolding of the native structures of the various fibril precursor proteins to generate structures rich in β-sheets that autoaggregate in a highly ordered manner to form the fibrils.

Amyloid deposition occurs *in vivo* under several conditions:

1   When a normal protein is present for a sufficient time at an abnormally high concentration (eg SAA or β_2M).

2   In the presence of an ordinary concentration of a normal, but inherently amyloidogenic, protein over a prolonged period (eg transthyretin in senile systemic amyloidosis).

3   When there is an acquired or inherited variant protein with abnormal structure (eg monoclonal immunoglobulin light chains or amyloidogenic variants of transthyretin, lysozyme, apo AI, fibrinogen A α-chain, etc).

Most known amyloidogenic proteins are capable of partly unfolding and then refolding and aggregating to form typical amyloid fibrils *in vitro* [5]. The amyloidogenic variant proteins associated with hereditary amyloidosis are less stable than their normal wild type counterparts. As a result, under physiological conditions, the amyloidogenic proteins exist as partly unfolded intermediate states much more readily than normal, and then proceed to assemble spontaneously as amyloid fibrils [6].

The mechanisms by which amyloid deposits damage tissues and compromise organ function are poorly understood. Massive deposits, which may amount to kilograms, are structurally disruptive and incompatible with normal function, as are strategically located small deposits, for example in the glomeruli or nerves. However, the relationship between quantity of amyloid and organ dysfunction differs greatly between individuals. There is a strong impression that the *rate* of new amyloid deposition is at least as important a determinant of progressive organ failure as the amyloid load itself. *In vitro* studies have suggested that isolated amyloid fibrils, in particular newly formed fibrils, are toxic and may induce death of cultured cells by both necrosis and apoptosis. Organ function in amyloidosis is extremely brittle. Renal or cardiac failure is easily precipitated, even in individuals with apparently normal organ function, as a result of salt and water imbalance, intravascular volume depletion, intercurrent infection, etc.

Major unanswered questions concern the tissue distribution and time of appearance of amyloid deposits as well as their variable clinical consequences. Many features of the various forms of amyloidosis overlap, but the clinical phenotype associated with a particular fibril type can also be enormously variable, even between families with identical amyloidogenic mutations and within single kindreds. Clearly, there are major genetic and environmental influences on *in vivo* amyloidogenesis other than simply the presence of an amyloidogenic variant protein, but there are few clues as to the nature of these factors.

□ DIAGNOSIS

The diagnosis of amyloidosis usually requires histological confirmation. The pathognomonic tinctorial property of amyloidotic tissue is apple green/red birefringence when stained with Congo red dye and viewed under intense cross-polarised light. However, histology can neither provide information about the overall whole-body load or the distribution of amyloid deposits nor permit monitoring of the natural history of either amyloidosis or its response to treatment.

To overcome these problems, we developed radiolabelled human SAP as a specific, non-invasive, quantitative *in vivo* tracer for amyloid deposits. It has now been used as a routine tool in our clinical practice for 10 years and over 2,000 studies have been performed. Scintigraphy and metabolic turnover studies with labelled SAP have contributed greatly to the knowledge of amyloidosis, especially its diagnosis, monitoring and response to treatment (Fig.1) [1,2].

□ NATURAL HISTORY OF AMYLOID DEPOSITS

The impression that amyloid deposition is irreversible and inexorably progressive is misleading and largely reflects the persistent nature of the acquired or hereditary

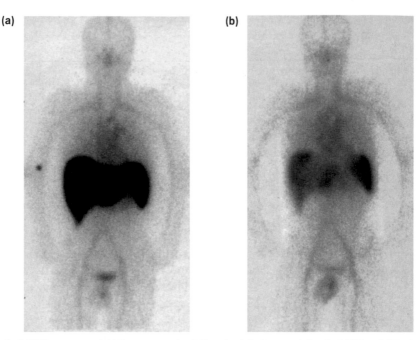

Fig. 1 Serial ^{123}I-serum amyloid P component scintigraphy **(a)** at presentation in 1998 and **(b)** at follow-up two years later, demonstrating regression of hepatic and splenic AA amyloid deposits in a patient with rheumatoid arthritis. The inflammatory disease activity was completely suppressed by treatment with oral chlorambucil.

conditions that are complicated by amyloidosis. Many case reports have described improvement in organ function when underlying conditions have been controlled, and serial SAP scintigraphy has systematically shown regression of amyloid in these circumstances. This has been observed in the following situations:

☐ when supply of amyloid fibril precursor proteins has been reduced in AA amyloidosis by vigorous control of rheumatic inflammation [7]

☐ in AL amyloidosis with clonal suppression by cytotoxic drugs [1]

☐ in haemodialysis-associated amyloidosis after renal transplantation, and

☐ in hereditary transthyretin and fibrinogen α-chain amyloidosis following liver transplantation [8,9].

It is now clear that amyloid deposits are in a state of dynamic turnover, the rate varying greatly between patients and with different types of amyloidosis. The existence of such turnover has encouraging implications for patient management.

☐ TREATMENT OF SYSTEMIC AMYLOIDOSIS (Table 3)

There has been much recent progress in the management of patients with systemic amyloidosis involving:

Table 3 Principles of treatment in systemic amyloidosis.

Disease	Aim of treatment	Example of treatment
AA amyloidosis	Suppress acute-phase response, thereby reducing SAA production	Immunosuppression in rheumatoid arthritis, colchicine in FMF
AL amyloidosis	Suppress production of monoclonal light chains	Chemotherapy for myeloma and monoclonal gammopathy
Hereditary amyloidosis	Reduce/eliminate production of genetically variant amyloidogenic protein	Orthoptic liver transplantation for variant transthyretin-associated FAP, and selected cases of fibrinogen A α-chain amyloidosis
Dialysis-related amyloidosis	Reduce plasma concentration of β_2M	Renal transplantation

AA = reactive systemic; AL = monoclonal immunoglobulin light chain; β_2M = β_2-microglobulin; FAP = familial amyloid polyneuropathy; FMF = familial Mediterranean fever; SAA = serum amyloid A.

☐ careful preservation of the function of organs damaged by amyloid

☐ replacement of end-stage organ failure by dialysis and transplantation, and

☐ innovative and aggressive measures to reduce the supply of amyloid fibril precursor proteins.

Reactive systemic (AA) amyloidosis

The aim of treatment in AA amyloidosis is to suppress as completely as possible the inflammatory process responsible for sustained overproduction of SAA. Extremely good results have been obtained in patients with rheumatoid arthritis using oral chlorambucil, an approach justified by the otherwise poor prognosis of AA amyloidosis. Follow-up studies have demonstrated that amyloid deposition is halted in all patients when SAA values are restored to normal, with partial or complete regression in about half the cases. Frequent monitoring of the circulating SAA concentration is therefore an essential guide to treatment.

Monoclonal immunoglobulin light chain (AL) amyloidosis

In AL amyloidosis the goal of treatment is to suppress the B cell clone producing the amyloidogenic monoclonal immunoglobulin light chain, using chemotherapy regimens based on those used in multiple myeloma, including:

☐ prolonged low-dose oral therapy

☐ cyclical infusions, and

☐ autologous stem cell transplantation.

All these treatments are hazardous and stem cell transplantation carries a substantial procedural mortality. However, the median survival of untreated patients with newly diagnosed systemic AL amyloidosis is less than two years, whereas that of selected patients receiving aggressive cytotoxic regimes in our practice now exceeds five years. Life saving heart or liver transplantation may be appropriate in certain cases, but only in conjunction with chemotherapy.

Dialysis-associated amyloidosis

Renal transplantation is the only therapy in dialysis-associated amyloidosis that removes β_2M and is of major clinical benefit. Following successful renal allografting, the circulating β_2M concentration immediately falls to normal. Although there is rapid relief of amyloid-related symptoms, regression of amyloid deposits occurs only very gradually in the long term.

Familial amyloid polyneuropathy

In FAP associated with transthyretin mutations, orthoptic liver transplantation can halt amyloid deposition because the variant amyloidogenic protein is produced mainly in the liver. Successful liver transplantation has been reported in hundreds of cases. Although the peripheral neuropathy usually only stabilises, autonomic function may improve and the associated visceral amyloid deposits regress in many cases.

Fibrinogen A α-chain amyloidosis

Fibrinogen is synthesised solely by the liver and hepatic transplantation is therefore potentially curative in fibrinogen A α-chain amyloidosis.

Future therapeutic possibilities

Both improved understanding of the protein folding mechanisms underlying amyloid fibrillogenesis and the recognition that relative instability of the precursor molecules is a key factor in amyloidogenesis have identified novel therapeutic possibilities. These include investigation of small molecules, peptides and glycosaminoglycan analogues that:

- □ bind to and stabilise fibril precursors [10]

- □ interfere with refolding and/or aggregation into the cross-β core structure common to amyloid fibrils, or

- □ bind to mature amyloid fibrils and promote their refolding back towards the native conformation.

Some of these agents have already been shown to be effective in experimental murine AA amyloidosis. Our efforts to develop specific therapy are focused on the avid binding of SAP to amyloid fibrils, which significantly contributes to the pathogenesis of amyloidosis [11]. The removal of SAP from amyloid deposits may facilitate their clearance, and we have identified a compound that inhibits the SAP-fibril interaction which is now being tested in patients.

REFERENCES

1 Hawkins PN. The diagnosis, natural history and treatment of amyloidosis. The Goulstonian Lecture 1995. Review. *J R Coll Physicians Lond* 1997; **31**: 552–60.

2 Gillmore JD, Hawkins PN, Pepys MB. Amyloidosis: a review of recent diagnostic and therapeutic developments. Review. *Br J Haematol* 1997; **99**: 245–56.

3 Hawkins PN, Lavender JP, Pepys MB. Evaluation of systemic amyloidosis by scintigraphy with 123I-labeled serum amyloid P component. *N Engl J Med* 1990; **323**: 508–13.

4 Hawkins PN, Wootton R, Pepys MB. Metabolic studies of radioiodinated serum amyloid P component in normal subjects and patients with systemic amyloidosis. *J Clin Invest* 1990; **86**: 1862–9.

5 Kelly JW. Alternative conformations of amyloidogenic proteins govern their behaviour. Review. *Curr Opin Struct Biol* 1996; **6**: 11–7.

6 Booth DR, Sunde M, Bellotti V, Robinson CV, *et al.* Instability, unfolding and aggregation of human lysozyme variants underlying amyloid fibrillogenesis. *Nature* 1997; **385**: 787–93.

7 Hawkins PN, Richardson S, Vigushin DM, David J, *et al.* Serum amyloid P component scintigraphy and turnover studies for diagnosis and quantitative monitoring of AA amyloidosis in juvenile rheumatoid arthritis. *Arthritis Rheum* 1993; **36**: 842–51.

8 Holmgren G, Ericzon BG, Groth CG, Steen L, *et al.* Clinical improvement and amyloid regression after liver transplantation in hereditary transthyretin amyloidosis. *Lancet* 1993; **341**: 1113–6.

9 Rydh A, Suhr O, Hietala SO, Åhlström KR, *et al.* Serum amyloid P component scintigraphy in familial amyloid polyneuropathy: regression of visceral amyloid following liver transplantation. *Eur J Nucl Med* 1998; **25**: 709–13.

10 Kisilevsky R, Lemieux LJ, Fraser PE, Kong X, *et al.* Arresting amyloidosis *in vivo* using small-molecule anionic sulphonates or sulphates: implications for Alzheimer's disease. *Nat Med* 1995; **1**: 143–8.

11 Botto M, Hawkins PN, Bickerstaff MC, Herbert J, *et al.* Amyloid deposition is delayed in mice with targeted deletion of the serum amyloid P component gene. *Nat Med* 1997; **3**: 855–9.

☐ SELF ASSESSMENT QUESTIONS

1 Immunoglobulin light chain (AL) amyloidosis:
   (a) May be localised to one particular anatomical site
   (b) Always occurs in association with a monoclonal proliferation of B cells
   (c) May regress following stem cell transplantation
   (d) Can occur in patients with rheumatoid arthritis
   (e) Is occasionally hereditary

2 Reactive systemic amyloidosis:
   (a) Usually presents with nephropathy
   (b) Frequently gives rise to cardiomyopathy
   (c) Often regresses when the underlying inflammatory disease is suppressed
   (d) Can complicate any disorder that gives rise to a sustained acute-phase inflammatory response
   (e) Has a prognosis that is strongly influenced by the circulating concentration of serum amyloid A protein

3   Hereditary systemic amyloidosis:
(a) Is caused by deposition of genetically variant proteins
(b) Is inherited in an autosomal recessive manner
(c) In its common form presents with neuropathy
(d) Can be indistinguishable clinically from AL amyloidosis
(e) Gives rise to clinical phenotypes that vary substantially in association with particular gene mutations

4   Amyloid deposition:
(a) Involves abnormal folding of various proteins
(b) Occurs only when the abundance of the respective amyloid precursor protein is substantially increased
(c) Is associated with Alzheimer's disease
(d) Is associated with maturity-onset diabetes mellitus
(e) Is associated with the prion diseases, for example Creutzfeldt-Jakob disease

ANSWERS

1a True	2a True	3a True	4a True
b True	b False	b False	b False
c True	c True	c True	c True
d True	d True	d True	d True
e False	e True	e True	e True

Infectious diseases

Methicillin-resistant *Staphylococcus aureus*: infection out of control

Mark Farrington

☐ INTRODUCTION

Within the past decade there has been an explosion in the prevalence of methicillin-resistant *Staphylococcus aureus* (MRSA) infection in hospitals in many countries worldwide. Although knowledge of the microbiology and molecular biology of MRSA is increasing, and the ability to type strains affecting different hospitals is expanding in ingenious ways, there is still only limited scientific knowledge about the best ways to prevent transmission of the organism within hospitals. In the UK, this leads to the incongruous position of being able to describe in considerable scientific detail the loss of control of MRSA in hospitals, while being apparently powerless to slow it down.

Although the techniques needed to control MRSA efficiently in an individual hospital probably differ depending on whether the organism is endemic or uncommon, there is none the less much to learn from studying the recent loss of control of MRSA in the UK. This knowledge may be applied to reducing the prevalence of MRSA in the future and to problems which may yet be faced with other *S. aureus* strains. The events of the past decade need to be a stimulus to high quality epidemiological research in the future.

☐ THE ORGANISM

MRSA strains were first described by Jevons in 1961 shortly after the introduction into routine clinical practice of the new antibiotic, methicillin [1]. Possession of the methicillin resistance (*mec*) genes is common within many staphylococcal species and had been found within culture collections of *S. aureus* before Jevons's work. Methicillin-resistant populations express an altered penicillin-binding protein (PBP-2') in a small number of cells which confers clinical resistance against all clinically useful beta-lactam antibiotics. The proportion of cells expressing this protein within a methicillin-resistant population is affected by culture conditions, including temperature and salt concentrations, and is also increased by growing the organisms in the presence of beta-lactam antibiotics. MRSA populations appear to be genetically closely related, and methicillin resistance genes have possibly been introduced to *S. aureus* only a few times in recent history. A few clones appear to be widespread across many countries. It follows that MRSA is much more commonly acquired by cross-infection than selected from an initially susceptible population by antibiotic exposure in an individual patient. Treatment of patients with antibiotics renders them more susceptible to acquiring MRSA when exposed because it eliminates the commensal flora normally occupying their mucosal binding sites.

Treatment of methicillin-resistant staphylococcal infections

Most strains of MRSA prevalent in developed countries are also resistant to a range of other antibiotics useful for routine treatment of staphylococcal infection, including the macrolides, tetracycline, 4-quinolones, and occasionally rifampicin and fusidic acid. Currently, treatment of clinically serious MRSA infections requires the use of the injectable glycopeptide agents, vancomycin or teicoplanin. These agents are expensive, associated with an increased risk of side effects and, at least in seriously infected patients, require monitoring by serum assay. A recent worrying trend is the emergence of MRSA strains with intermediate resistance to the glycopeptides – the so-called vancomycin intermediate-resistant *S. aureus* (VISA) strains – which appear to be associated with extensive use of glycopeptide agents. They were described first in Japan [2]) and are sometimes known as glycopeptide intermediate-resistant (GISA), vancomycin-resistant *S. aureus* (VRSA) or glycopeptide-resistant *S. Aureus* (GRSA) strains. A number of new antibiotics that may have useful activity against MRSA have recently been released or are under development, but clinical experience with these is limited and they will undoubtedly be very expensive.

☐ EPIDEMIC METHICILLIN-RESISTANT *STAPHYLOCOCCUS AUREUS* STRAINS

The Staphylococcus Reference Laboratory of the Division of Hospital Infection, Central Public Health Laboratory, Colindale, has documented a startling rise in the number of hospitals in England and Wales reporting problems with two so-called 'epidemic' MRSA strains, EMRSA-15 and EMRSA-16 (Fig. 1) [3]. These strains were first described in the early 1990s and have demonstrated remarkable abilities to colonise and infect patients throughout the UK healthcare system. Earlier EMRSAs (eg EMRSA-3) have not increased in prevalence. Surprisingly little is known about the microbiological factors that fit EMRSA strains for such successful exploitation of the healthcare environment.

Whether the average MRSA strain is more or less virulent than the average methicillin-sensitive strain of *S. aureus* (MSSA) has been made largely irrelevant by the massive rise in EMRSA prevalence in the UK, which has been accompanied by increased reports of *S. aureus* bacteraemia in England and Wales [4]. MRSA bacteraemia has been added to a broadly unchanged prevalence of MSSA bacteraemia. This presumably results from the propensity of MRSA strains to colonise and infect a different population from that affected by MSSA: patients with MRSA have been in hospital for longer, received more antibiotics, undergone more medical procedures, and are more likely to be in intensive care units. Hence, EMRSA has expanded into a new ecological niche within hospitals.

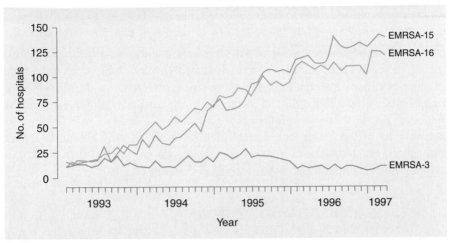

Fig.1 Hospitals in the UK affected by epidemic methicillin-resistant *Staphylococcus aureus* (EMRSAs) 1993–97 (first quarter) (reproduced, with permission, from [3]).

Many UK hospitals have described rapid loss of control of MRSA and the establishment of endemicity soon after detection of an EMRSA-15 or -16 outbreak [5]. In MRSA epidemiology, a hospital is said to have endemic MRSA when local transmission between patients on the wards is continuously occurring. In the early 1990s, the UK standard of practice [6] advocated a strict 'search-and-destroy' policy to seek out, isolate and attempt to eradicate MRSA within hospitals. The reasons for the failure of this policy are unproven, but published experience and informal discussions point to the importance of late detection of outbreaks and incomplete reaction to MRSA introduction to certain hospital services. In many UK hospitals, including Addenbrooke's [7], the critical outbreaks leading to loss of control began in departments of medicine for the elderly and other chronic care environments where little prospective screening was performed and highly aggressive control policies were felt to be inappropriate. Low MRSA infection/colonisation ratios were usually reported in patients on such units, but with their transfer to acute hospital services MRSA was repeatedly introduced to high risk areas, resulting in outbreaks of serious infection. Continuing new introductions rendered stringent control measures impossible to maintain at a time when budgetary restrictions were severe, waiting list initiatives pressing, and maintenance of 'spare capacity' for isolation and other infection control purposes was unpopular [7].

During the early and mid-1990s a number of other changes were detected within Addenbrooke's Hospital (which were probably common throughout the NHS) which were subjectively associated with the rise in MRSA prevalence [7]. These included:

☐ loss of flexibility of accommodation of affected patients within the hospital

☐ rising nursing workload, and

☐ less free exchange of information between hospital trusts.

☐ NATIONAL GUIDELINES FOR METHICILLIN-RESISTANT *STAPHYLOCOCCUS AUREUS* CONTROL

In the face of the advancing tide of MRSA infection, and after a difficult gestation period, new national guidelines were produced in 1998 which recognised the impracticability of maintaining attempts at stringent control in the face of rising numbers of introductions [8]. Unfortunately, in this author's opinion, support can be found within these new guidelines for virtually any level of infection control response to MRSA. It is noteworthy that stringent control measures applied throughout the Netherlands are still apparently effective within their healthcare system, which is undoubtedly better resourced than our own [9].

☐ METHICILLIN-RESISTANT *STAPHYLOCOCCUS AUREUS* AT ADDENBROOKE'S NHS TRUST

Over the long term, the experience of MRSA at Addenbrooke's is different from that in a number of other UK centres. Addenbrooke's NHS Trust is a 1,300-bed teaching tertiary referral and district general hospital. There are 150 single rooms available for isolation within the wards, 19 with exhaust ventilation. Twelve of these are on a specialist infectious diseases unit.

MRSA was first detected in the hospital in 1985. This introduction resulted in an outbreak on the transplant unit, with high rates of clinical infection and bacteraemia among the unit's vulnerable patients [7]. This experience convinced the infection control team that a particularly stringent and comprehensive MRSA control policy was required (summarised in Table 1). Over a 10-year period the infectious diseases ward was used to house all known MRSA-positive patients. The successful eradication from the hospital of multiple MRSA introductions was demonstrated by means of prospective information gathering, typing of most first MRSA patient-isolates, together with the use of standard definitions of outbreaks, clearance and strain origin. In other centres, MRSA became endemic shortly after it was first detected [5].

Figure 2 shows the number of patient isolates with MRSA detected at Addenbrooke's during six-month periods between 1985 and 1996. Until the first half

Table 1 Stringent methicillin-resistant *Staphylococcus aureus* control policy, Addenbrooke's Hospital 1985–95 (for details see [7]).

Epidemiological definitions	Standard definitions of 'outbreak', 'clearance', 'source of outbreak'
Prospective and reactive screening	High risk patients and units Interhospital transfers
Action on first isolate	Screening regimen Movement restrictions on patients and staff
Action on confirmation of local outbreak (ie 2 linked isolates on same ward)	Closure to new admissions Screening regimen Transfer positives to infectious diseases ward Attempt clearance

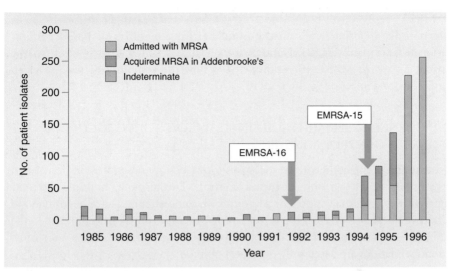

Fig. 2 Methicillin-resistant *Staphylococcus aureus* (MRSA) at Addenbrooke's Hospital 1985-96 (orange bars = patients admitted to Addenbrooke's with MRSA acquired elsewhere; purple bars = patients who acquired MRSA *de novo* in Addenbrooke's NHS Trust). The source of the MRSA was not determined in 1996 (green bars) (EMRSA = epidemic MRSA).

of 1994 more than half the cases of MRSA in the hospital had been acquired outside Addenbrooke's rather than while the patients were inpatients. From 1993, there was a progressive rise in the number of patients admitted with MRSA and a corresponding rise in local acquisitions. During this period, Addenbrooke's isolation facilities were overwhelmed by the number of patients carrying MRSA within the hospital. From 1995 it became no longer possible to survey MRSA cases within the hospital prospectively. Hence, for 1996 only the total number of isolates are shown, this information being based on less active screening.

The influence of epidemic strains of MRSA on the situation in Addenbrooke's is not simple. EMRSA-16 was first seen in late 1991, and in the next four years was introduced eight times with only six secondary associated cases. Our stringent control measures (with the resources available at the time) prevented establishment of endemicity of this strain. However, when EMRSA-15 was first introduced in 1994 there was a marked increase in cases of both epidemic strains. This was interpreted as showing that the stringent policy adopted could cope with about 15 introductions per six months, even of epidemic strains. The hospital's capacity to cope with MRSA introductions was exceeded in mid-1994 and was rapidly followed by the establishment of frequent local transmission.

In common with the national guidelines adopted in 1998 [8], the hospital was forced to relax the stringent policy of the previous 10 years. The new policy allows much more flexibility in ward closures (only in response to clusters of infection rather than mere colonisation) and promotes 'cohorting' of patients and staff on individual bays of affected wards rather than single room isolation on a specialist ward.

MRSA cases have been added to MSSA bacteraemias since 1995 in Addenbrooke's Hospital on a background of rising numbers of blood cultures performed per year (Fig. 3). National surveillance schemes further attest to the current impact of MRSA: for example, it is now the commonest cause of clean surgical wound infection in the UK [10].

☐ EVIDENCE-BASED METHICILLIN-RESISTANT *STAPHYLOCOCCUS AUREUS* CONTROL MEASURES

Most studies of infection control measures for MRSA are descriptive in design and have usually employed only historical controls. Furthermore, multiple different interventions are usually applied. Although welcome attempts have been made to adduce evidence-based measures for control of nosocomial infection [11], the difficulty of performing truly comparative trials in this area means that most recommendations are based only on expert opinion.

Two commonly advocated measures, hand hygiene, and cohorting of staff and patients, will be discussed to illustrate different problems within this area.

Hand hygiene

The importance of hand hygiene in MRSA control has been highlighted in several recent publications. Many studies have demonstrated poor compliance with hand hygiene standards in most hospitals, and even intensive intervention measures have produced only limited and transient improvements. A recently published innovative study by Pittet *et al* [12] employed a multidisciplinary approach to improving hand hygiene in a large Swiss hospital, and studied a wide variety of direct and surrogate end-points to establish the effectiveness of the intervention. Repeated detailed

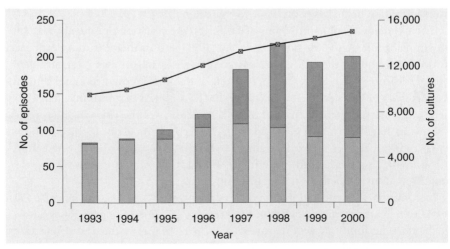

Fig. 3 *Staphylococcus aureus* bacteraemia in Addenbrooke's Hospital 1993–2000 (⊠ = number of blood cultures performed; orange bars = methicillin-susceptible *S. aureus* bacteraemia; purple bars = rising number of additional methicillin-resistant *S. aureus*-positive cultures).

prevalence studies of hospital infections, including MRSA, were performed throughout a six-year period. A multidisciplinary project team designed and monitored the interventions and, crucially, there was active senior managerial participation. Use of alcoholic hand-rub was promoted on all wards, and small bottles of this were carried by individuals. Adequate funding was provided for the whole programme, and advertising of the project's methods, aims and continuing outcomes was widespread in all areas of the hospital.

Figure 4 demonstrates the beneficial and sustained effects on MRSA infection of the programme. There was only a modest increase in performance of hand hygiene (48–66% of the recommended occasions), but the result was an impressive five-fold increase in alcoholic hand-rub use and total hospital-acquired infections fell from 17% to 10%. Although the programme cost £155,000, it was estimated to have prevented 900 infections and saved over £1.2 million.

Even though historical controls were used, the sustained improvement in all variables strongly suggests a causal relationship.

Shortcomings of the study

Before expectations are raised too highly, however, it is important to note that this study was performed in a very large hospital with extensive financial and isolation

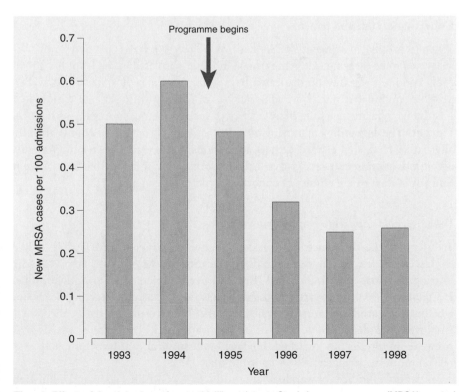

Fig. 4 Effect of hand hygiene for methicillin-resistant *Staphylococcus aureus* (MRSA) control (reproduced, with permission, from [12]).

resources, with a relatively low MRSA background prevalence and an enormous hospital infection control team – certainly far larger than any to be found in UK hospitals of comparable size. Few details are given in the report of other MRSA control measures that were applied, for example:

☐   Which patients were screened?

☐   Were high risk carriers isolated before their screening results were known?

☐   Were attempts made to clear carriage from patients or staff?

☐   Were all known carriers nursed in single rooms?

Furthermore, performance of hand hygiene is known to fall as staff workload increases. This study should be repeated in other units with facilities and procedures more in line with the UK average before hand hygiene advocacy can be seen as the ultimate and sole solution.

It has been the subject of discussion for many years among UK microbiologists whether general measures such as hand washing alone are capable of bringing MRSA prevalence within reasonable levels, or whether active 'search-and-destroy' procedures are necessary. It is hoped that it will soon be possible to perform studies to answer the question scientifically.

Cohorting of staff and patients

When a hospital's stringent MRSA control policy is relaxed, patients known or suspected to be carrying MRSA are usually no longer isolated in single rooms but are often cohorted together on dedicated bays within ordinary hospital wards. Where possible, nominated nurses are allocated to work only with patients within such positive bays on any one shift. Maintenance of such cohorting arrangements has been thought to be demanding of nursing time, but is generally felt less disruptive than the alternative of closing a ward to new admissions, particularly when no alternative accommodation or extra staff is available. Unfortunately, it has proved impossible to find any studies of the efficacy of cohorting as an independent variable.

Grace Reynolds Application of the Study of Peto

To quantify the differences in workload between stringent and flexible MRSA control strategies, the Grace Reynolds Application of the Study of Peto (GRASP) nursing workload system was used (this had been implemented at Addenbrooke's Hospital in 1993). At the ward and shift levels GRASP assesses nursing needs and whether they are being met by available staff [13]. Prospective data collection is employed and data quality assessed at the ward level. The system was used to compare outbreaks on matched medical and surgical wards before and after relaxation of the stringent MRSA control policy [13].

A variety of indices of workload are produced by GRASP. Figs. 5 and 6 illustrate how two of these indices vary on the matched wards according to whether they were closed (in the stringent control period) or left open with cohorting in bays (after

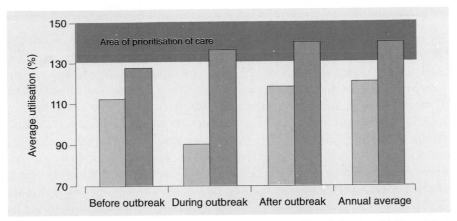

Fig. 5 The different effects of stringent (orange bars) and relaxed (purple bars) methicillin-resistant *Staphylococcus aureus* control procedures on nursing workload, defined as average utilisation expressed as per cent of the optimal workload for a quality care environment.

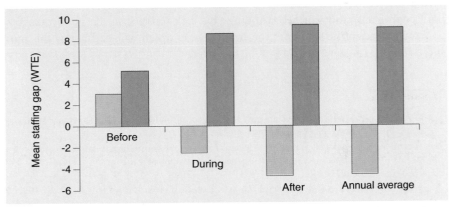

Fig. 6 The different effects of stringent (orange bars) and relaxed (purple bars) methicillin-resistant *Staphylococcus aureus* control procedures on quality of nursing services in affected areas, expressed as the mean staffing gap between the number of whole time equivalents (WTEs) needed to bring the average utilisation into the range of quality care and the number of WTEs available.

relaxation of the policy in mid-1995). During outbreaks in the stringent policy period, workload on affected wards dropped sharply, returning to baseline at the end of the outbreak (Fig. 5). In contrast, on the introduction of cohorting, workload rose into the area of 'necessary prioritisation of care' in which nurses have to limit the necessary tasks they are able to perform for those patients judged to be of low priority. The marked increase in the number of nurses required to ensure a quality care environment with cohorting (ie the period of relaxed control measures) is shown in Fig. 6.

These results have obvious implications for the design of future studies comparing different interventions. It has not been possible to find any study showing whether or not increasing nurse staffing resources during an outbreak is an effective control measure.

☐ CONCLUSIONS

We are beginning to learn more about the details of controlling MRSA during and between outbreaks in modern hospitals. Unfortunately, most of the interventions used are not based on high quality evidence. They are interdependent, and focusing on one or another at the expense of others may be counterproductive. There is a need to know, for example, in what circumstances drives to improve hand hygiene are sufficient and, in particular, what baseline staffing and isolation resources are necessary to ensure a reasonable level of control. Setting norms within the NHS for staffing and workload is currently unfashionable. The approach favoured by the NHS Executive will probably be limited to placing hospitals' MRSA prevalence rates in the public domain and promoting application of the current highly flexible national MRSA guidelines [8]. It is of concern that the issues and variables involved in MRSA control are so complex and intertwined that leaving all the important decisions to local hospitals is unlikely to lead to efficient and uniform control.

On the positive side, there is now wide recognition in the NHS that MRSA is both controllable and worth controlling. We look forward to the performance of good quality scientific studies in the coming years which will clarify how this most successful of pathogens should best be managed.

REFERENCES

1   Chambers HF. Methicillin resistance in staphylococci: molecular and biochemical basis and clinical implications. Review. *Clin Microbiol Rev* 1997; **10**: 781–91.

2   Hiramatsu K, Aritaka N, Hanaki H, Kawasaki S, *et al.* Dissemination in Japanese hospitals of strains of *Staphylococcus aureus* heterogeneously resistant to vancomycin. *Lancet* 1997; **350**: 1670–3; comment 1644–5.

3   Epidemic methicillin resistant *Staphylococcus aureus. Commun Dis Rep CDR Wkly* 1997; **7**: 191.

4   Methicillin resistance in *Staphylococcus aureus* isolated from blood in England and Wales: 1994 to 1998. *Commun Dis Rep CDR Weekly* 1999; **9**: 65, 68.

5   Cox RA, Conquest C, Mallaghan C, Marples RR. A major outbreak of methicillin-resistant *Staphylococcus aureus* caused by a new phage-type (EMRSA-16). *J Hosp Infect* 1995; **29**: 87–106.

6   Revised guidelines for the control of epidemic methicillin-resistant *Staphylococcus aureus.* Report of a working party of the Hospital Infection Society and British Society for Antimicrobial Chemotherapy. *J Hosp Infect* 1990; **16**: 351–77.

7   Farrington M, Redpath C, Trundle C, Coomber S, Brown NM. Winning the battle but losing the war: methicillin-resistant *Staphylococcus aureus* (MRSA) infection at a teaching hospital. *QJM* 1998; **91**: 519–21.

8   Revised guidelines for the control of methicillin-resistant *Staphylococcus aureus* infection in hospitals. British Society for Antimicrobial Chemotherapy, Hospital Infection Society and the Infection Control Nurses Association. *J Hosp Infect* 1998; **39**: 253–90.

9   Vandenbrouke-Grauls CMJE. Management of methicillin-resistant *Staphylococcus aureus* in the Netherlands. *Rev Med Microbiol* 1998; **9**: 109–16.

10   Nosocomial Infections National Surveillance Scheme: Surveillance of Surgical Site Infection in English Hospitals 1997–1999. http://www.phls.co.uk/publications/index.htm.

11   Pratt RJ, Pellowe C, Loveday HP, Robinson N, *et al.* The epic project: developing national evidence-based guidelines for preventing healthcare associated infections. Phase I: Guidelines

for preventing hospital-acquired infections. Department of Health, England. *J Hosp Infect* 2001; 47(Suppl): S3–82.

12   Pittet D, Hugonnet S, Harbarth S, Mourouga P, *et al*. Effectiveness of a hospital-wide programme to improve compliance with hand hygiene. Infection Control Programme. *Lancet* 2000; **356**: 1307–12.

13   Farrington M, Trundle C, Redpath C, Anderson L. Effects on nursing workload of different methicillin-resistant *Staphylococcus aureus* (MRSA) control strategies. *J Hosp Infect* 2000; **46**: 118–22.

□ SELF ASSESSMENT QUESTIONS

1   Methicillin resistance in *Staphylococcus aureus*:
   (a) Is mediated by a modification of penicillin binding protein 3
   (b) Is mediated by enzymic destruction of beta-lactam antibiotics
   (c) Was first described within a year of the introduction of methicillin to clinical practice
   (d) Implies resistance to all clinically useful beta-lactam antibiotics
   (e) Is conferred by possession of the chromosomal *mec* gene complex

2   The rise in prevalence of methicillin-resistant *Staphylococcus aureus* (MRSA) in the UK in the 1990s:
   (a) Has involved dissemination of multiple, highly distinct strains of MRSA
   (b) Has been mainly restricted to a few large specialist hospitals
   (c) Has not been matched with a corresponding rise in serious clinical infections caused by MRSA
   (d) Has been associated with a rise in the reported total prevalence of staphylococcal infection
   (e) Has been associated with transfer of patients carrying MRSA between hospitals

3   Hand hygiene by healthcare workers:
   (a) May be increased by education drives, but only transiently
   (b) May be increased by wide provision of alcoholic hand-rub
   (c) Is the only control measure needed to control MRSA outbreaks
   (d) When increased by education drives, is probably both clinically and cost effective
   (e) Probably requires multidisciplinary support throughout a hospital for sustained improvement

4   Nursing workload:
   (a) When high, leads to reduced performance of hand hygiene
   (b) Rises at the end of outbreaks as new patients are admitted
   (c) If reduced by appointing more nurses to a ward, is known to reduce infection rates
   (d) Has been consistently found to be high at the start of outbreaks
   (e) Rises when cohorting is used to control outbreaks

ANSWERS

1a	False	2a	False	3a	True	4a	True
b	False	b	False	b	True	b	True
c	True	c	False	c	False	c	False
d	True	d	True	d	True	d	False
e	True	e	True	e	True	e	True

Sexual ill health

Michael Adler

☐ INTRODUCTION

There have been success stories in the ways in which new and emerging threats to sexual health have been tackled. For example, the control of HIV in England, which has one of the lowest rates in Western Europe, has been achieved through health promotion, open access to genitourinary medicine (GUM) clinics and needle-exchange schemes. Likewise, the availability of a broad range of contraceptive methods provided free by the NHS has given many the opportunity to plan their families and avoid unwanted pregnancy. However, despite these achievements, there can be little room for complacency. This chapter outlines the considerable and disturbing level of sexual ill health which still exists in England, and ways in which a start can be made to tackling this major social and public health problem. The extent of the problem can be illustrated by looking at five areas:

1 Morbidity/disease impact.

2 Sexual behaviour/knowledge.

3 Social exclusion.

4 Inequity of current service provision.

5 Costs.

Good sexual health is an important contributor to people's general health and well-being, but in all these five areas we are not doing well in achieving this goal.

☐ MORBIDITY/DISEASE IMPACT

Virtually all the sexually transmitted infections (STIs) are increasing in frequency, which must reflect increased risk taking and less than adequate control. The annual number of attendances at departments of GUM/sexually transmitted diseases in England is now over one million which represents a doubling over the last decade (Fig. 1) [1]. The commonest conditions seen in clinics are chlamydial infections, non-specific urethritis and wart virus infections. Most diseases have increased: for example, the numbers of cases of gonorrhoea, chlamydia and genital wart virus infections seen in GUM departments in England have risen by 56%, 74% and 20%, respectively, between 1995 and 1999 (latest figures) (Fig. 2). In addition, surveys of

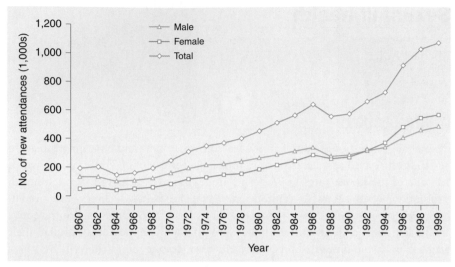

Fig. 1 New attendances at genitourinary medicine clinics, England, 1960–99 [1].

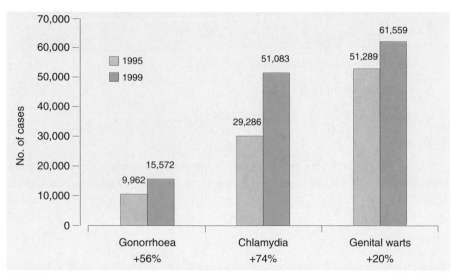

Fig. 2 Changes in cases seen in departments of genitourinary medicine and sexually transmitted diseases, England, 1995–99.

women seeking medical help other than at departments of GUM show that infection rates for chlamydial infections of up to 12% can be found (Table 1) [2]. Part of this increase will be an ascertainment bias due to new diagnostic methods and publicity which mean that more people will be screened or seek care. Chlamydia is of increasing concern because of its long-term complications. For example, 10–40% of cases of untreated chlamydial infection will result in pelvic inflammatory disease with subsequent ectopic pregnancy and infertility [3].

Table 1 Median prevalence rates of chlamydia reported from various clinical settings.

Survey population	Median prevalence (%)	Range (%)
General practice	4.5	1–12
Antenatal or obstetric units	4.6	2–7
Gynaecology clinics	4.8	3–6
Family planning clinics	5.1	3–7
Women seeking terminations	8.0	7–12
Genitourinary medicine clinics	16.4	7–29

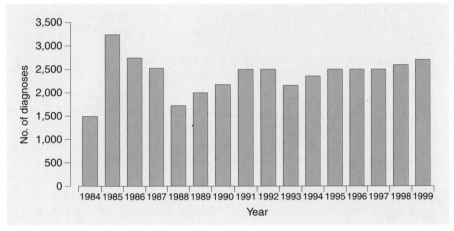

Fig. 3 UK HIV diagnoses by year of diagnosis, 1984–1999 (last three years adjusted for reporting delay) [4].

Although, as indicated earlier, this country has one of the lowest rates of HIV infection in Western Europe, there is a need to be concerned since the number of new HIV infections diagnosed in 1999 (latest figures) was the highest since 1985 (and equal to that in 1986) (Fig. 3) [4]. Also in 1999, for the first time more infections were acquired through heterosexual sexual intercourse than by men having sex with men. Currently, there are estimated to be approximately 30,000 people living with HIV in the UK, of whom it is thought about a third are undiagnosed. The percentage varies between different groups: amongst homosexual men it has been estimated that 28% are undiagnosed but, alarmingly, for heterosexual men and women it is 49%.

Since the advent of highly active antiretroviral therapy (HAART) the long-term survival has improved for people with HIV. In association with steadily increasing new infections, this means that the number of people living with HIV constantly expands. Figure 4 indicates the increase in HIV diagnosis together with the decline in AIDS diagnoses and deaths. This increase in the number of people living with HIV presents challenges for long-term clinical treatment, care and social support, as well as for health promotion and the avoidance of further transmission.

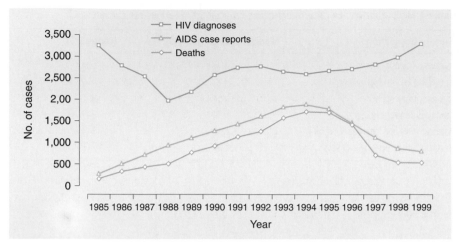

Fig. 4 HIV diagnoses, AIDS case reports and deaths in HIV infected individuals by year of diagnosis/occurrence, 1985–99 (last three years adjusted for reporting delay).

☐ SEXUAL BEHAVIOUR/KNOWLEDGE

Recent information on sexual behaviour suggests that there is increased risk taking behaviour and a lack of knowledge. The average age of first intercourse has now declined to 17 years, whereas 40 years ago it was 21 years for women and 20 for men [5]. Despite this, 57% of women and 24% of men who had sex before 16 years old thought it was 'too soon'. A decrease in the age of first intercourse does not necessarily mean that people are having more sexual partners, although over 13% of men and 9% of women have had more than one partner in the last year. Clearly, partner change is a crucial variable in the acquisition and transmission of STIs. It is worrying that 30% of men and 25% of women aged 16–24 years do not use contraception at first intercourse since failure to do so exposes them to potential infection and pregnancy [5]. It is also alarming that the message of barrier contraception is not understood adequately: 25% of 14–15 year olds think that the pill on its own will protect against STIs [6]. Nearly 60% of young gay men do not always use condoms when having intercourse, and reports suggest inconsistent or non-use of condoms even among HIV infected men [7]. The high level of new HIV infection in England has to be tackled by better health promotion.

Concerns about the level of knowledge around contraception and protection against infections are compounded by surveys indicating that the level of knowledge about common infections such as chlamydia is extremely low. For example, in a survey carried out in 1998, 87% of men and 65% of women reported either not having heard of chlamydia or not knowing what it is [8].

☐ SOCIAL EXCLUSION

Sexual ill health is associated with poverty and social exclusion. The major burden of sexual infection is experienced by women, gay men, teenagers, young adults and black ethnic minorities. The rates of gonorrhoea in some inner city black minority ethnic groups are 10–11 times higher than in whites [9]. Members of the population groups most affected by HIV may already be disadvantaged and experience social exclusion, for example because of race, sexual orientation or drug misuse.

Teenage pregnancy is often both a cause and a consequence of social exclusion. The risk of teenage parenthood is greatest for young people who have grown up in poverty and disadvantage, or for those with poor educational attainment. Overall, teenage parenthood is more common in areas of deprivation and poverty. The poorest areas in England have a teenage conception and birth rate up to six times higher than the most affluent areas [10] – but even in the most prosperous areas in the UK the teenage birth rates are higher than the average rates in some comparable European countries. There is a similar correlation between deprivation and gonorrhoea rates: the higher the deprivation score, the higher the rate of gonorrhoea (Fig. 5).

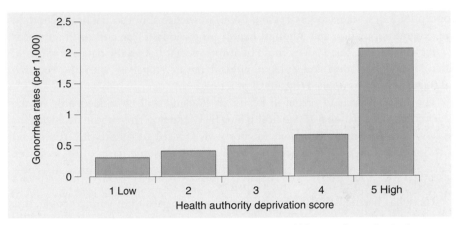

Fig. 5 Gonorrhoea rates per 1,000 men and women (all ages), 1999, according to deprivation score.

☐ INEQUITY OF CURRENT SERVICE PROVISION

There are significant geographical variations in current service provision in terms of access, quality and range of services available. For example, the number of NHS funded abortions varies from 46–96% in different health authorities, with no evidence that this relates to need. Recent surveys in GUM departments have suggested that the pressures on services have led to unacceptable delays. Waiting times for urgent and routine appointments were up to one and four weeks, respectively, in some areas, while only 54% of patients trying to get access for acute STI, or who were a named contact, could do so within 24 hours. The same percentage of patients had to wait more than seven days to obtain a routine appointment [11].

☐ COSTS

Major costs are associated with the burden of sexual ill health. Prevention of sexual health problems offers significant scope not only for improving public health but also for more effective use of NHS funds. For example, the cost of preventable infertility could be dramatically reduced, releasing funds to be spent more effectively. The prevention of unplanned pregnancy through the NHS provision of contraception services has been estimated to save over £2.5 billion a year in NHS costs alone [12]. There are also considerable costs associated with treatment of HIV-positive individuals. Recent data suggest an average lifetime treatment cost ranges between £135,000 and £181,000 for each HIV-positive patient. The number of known HIV-positive individuals is currently just over 20,000, so the lifetime treatment cost for these individuals (apart from those as yet undiagnosed) is extremely high at £2.7–3.6 billion.

☐ WHAT HAS BEEN LEARNT AND POSSIBLE SOLUTIONS

The evidence suggests that there are a number of indicators of sexual ill health in this country, with significant inequalities in terms of infection and unintended conception rates, access to services and poor knowledge about sexual health, both in the general population and amongst health professionals. The current fragmented *ad hoc* approach to these issues could be improved. Although the data are soft, and often of a behavioural and epidemiological nature, together with the research findings they can be applied to clinical practice.

The current levels of sexual ill health in England will be tackled only by the development of a national sexual health and HIV strategy. This should deal with the issues of services being fragmented, too narrowly focused and poorly advertised, and with unacceptable waiting times for access to care in some parts of the country. Work on the strategy for sexual health and HIV, which started 18 months ago, is now complete and the findings are with Ministers.

There has been particular concern over the sexual health of young people. It is acknowledged that young people have specific needs, but the strategy also recognises both that sexual health is important throughout people's lives and that information/health promotion and service needs will vary according to age, life stage and sexual orientation.

☐ SEXUAL HEALTH AND HIV STRATEGY FOR ENGLAND

The strategy has two straightforward objectives:

1   To ensure that all individuals have better access to knowledge to achieve good sexual health.

2   To make services and information more available and accessible to all those who require them at all ages.

The strategy aims to achieve the following outcomes:

1   To reduce transmission of HIV and STIs.

2   To reduce the prevalence of undiagnosed HIV and STIs.

3   To reduce the unintended pregnancy rate.

4   To improve health and social care for people living with HIV.

5   To reduce the stigma associated with HIV and sexuality.

The headline proposals of the strategy recognise the need to increase access to services, HIV/STI prevention and health promotion (Table 2). In addition, the strategy will attempt to reduce the inequalities of access to services and to set standards for all services provided for sexual health. Thus, we hope to provide nurses and practitioners with all the necessary skills to deliver better and more holistic services for sexual health. Currently, for example, a physician working in GUM may be providing an excellent service for the screening of infection and the management of HIV, but not for contraception, while those working effectively in contraception may lack the skills for screening for infection. Certainly, within primary care, the ability to screen for infections is variable. None of this will undermine the specialist – rather, skills will be raised overall so that patients can receive agreed minimum standards of care wherever it is sought. This will require programmes of professional education and training. It is also fair to say that there is a lack of evidence for effective health promotion and HIV prevention. It is therefore important to have a research base to collect evidence of good practice and to set up pilot studies looking at different ways of delivering care.

Table 2 Sexual ill health and HIV strategy: headline proposals.

- To increase access by developing wider professional roles, particularly for those working in primary care and for nurses more generally

- To increase prevention of HIV and sexually transmitted infections and health promotion through improvements in promoting testing, better information, and health promotion delivered through a wider range of services, including primary care

- To reduce inequalities, for example of access to NHS services such as abortion, contraception and genitourinary medicine clinics

- To set standards for services

- To develop an underpinning programme of professional education and training

- To develop a research/agenda/evidence base

☐ CONCLUSIONS

Sexual ill health is a considerable social and public health problem, as illustrated by the data outlined in this chapter. The development and implementation of a national strategy recognise this and will pave the way for tackling this problem.

REFERENCES

1   Trends in sexually transmitted infection in the United Kingdom, 1990–1999. New episodes seen at genitourinary medicine clinics. PHLS (England, Wales & Northern Ireland), DHSS & PS (Northern Ireland) and the Scottish ISD(D)5 Collaborative Group (ISD, SCIEH and MSSVD), December 2000.

2 Chief Medical Officer's Expert Advisory Group. *Chlamydia trachomatis.* London: Department of Health, 1998.

3 Stamm WE, Guinan ME, Johnson C, Starcher T, *et al.* Effect of treatment regimens for *Neisseria gonorrhoeae* on simultaneous infection with *Chlamydia trachomatis. N Engl J Med* 1984; **310**: 545–9.

4 Public Health Laboratory Service. Press Release, 25 January 2001.

5 Wellings K, Field J, Johnson AM, Wadsworth J. *Sexual behaviour in Britain.* The National Study of Sexual Attitudes and Lifestyles. London: Penguin, 1994.

6 Health Education Authority. *Young people and health.* London: HEA, 1999.

7 *Findings from the National Gay Men's Sex Survey 1999.* London: Sigma Research Vital Statistics, July 2000.

8 Rainford L, Meltzer M. *Contraception and sexual health 1998.* A report on research using the ONS Omnibus survey produced on behalf of the Department of Health. London: Office for National Statistics, 2000. ISBN 185774 4136.

9 Low N, Daker-White G, Barlow D, Pozniak AL. Gonorrhoea in inner London: results of a cross sectional study. *Br Med J* 1997; **314**: 1719–23.

10 *Teenage pregnancy.* Social Exclusion Unit, CM4342. London: The Stationery Office, 1999.

11 Djuretic T, *et al.* Genitourinary medicine services in the United Kingdom are failing to meet the current demand (in press).

12 McGuire Hughes D. *The economics of family planning services.* A report prepared for the Contraceptive Alliance Family Planning Association. London: Contraceptive Alliance, 1995.

Invasive meningococcal disease

William Lynn

□ INTRODUCTION

Invasive meningococcal disease is one of the most fulminant and frightening bacterial infections seen in the UK [1]. Other bacterial pathogens such as *Streptococcus pneumoniae* or *Staphylococcus aureus* may be responsible for more deaths, but the ability of *Neisseria meningitidis* to kill previously fit children and young adults within a few hours of the onset of illness merits specific attention. Furthermore, meningococcal infection may occur in small clusters or mini-epidemics, causing much public anxiety and media attention. These factors make it essential that all physicians involved in acute medicine should be aware of the diagnosis and management of meningococcal infection.

□ EPIDEMIOLOGY

N. meningitidis has a worldwide distribution. There are a number of sero-groups (types) of the organism based on the antigenic determinants of the outer membrane of the bacterial cell wall. Most cases of invasive meningococcal disease occur in children and young adults with an overall mortality of 10% [1]. Survivors may suffer from serious sequelae, particularly neurological damage or amputations.

Neisseria meningitidis types B and C

Historically, *N. meningitidis* type B has been the predominant cause of invasive disease in the UK, but there has been an increase in infections due to type C over the past few years [2]. Invasive meningococcal infection is reported in around six per 100,000 people per year in the UK with a peak incidence during the winter months. The incidence fell steadily following the Second World War until there was a rise in cases during the 1990s possibly related to increased outbreaks due to type C strains (Fig 1).

Currently, types B and C are each responsible for approximately 40–45% of cases. Following the introduction of a specific polysaccharide meningococcal type C vaccine in 1998 there has been an approximately 80% fall in infections due to this organism in children. No vaccine is available for *N. meningitidis* type B.

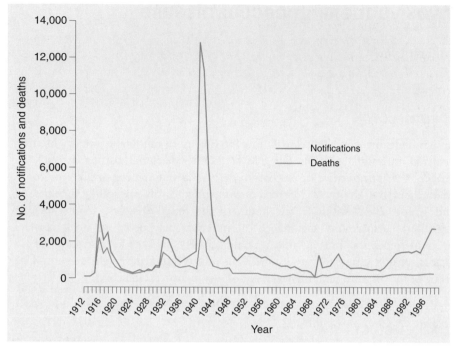

Fig. 1 Meningococcal notifications and deaths in England and Wales, 1912–1996 (reproduced, with permission, from [2]).

Neisseria meningitidis type A

Type A and other serotypes are seen less commonly in the UK but are prevalent in other parts of the world. Type A, for example, is endemic in sub-Saharan Africa and vaccination is recommended for travellers to this area.

□ PATHOGENESIS

N. meningitidis is a common commensal (coloniser) of the upper respiratory tract. About 5–10% of the adult population may carry *N. meningitidis* at any one time, with higher rates of carriage in children, adolescents and during outbreaks [1]. Thus, the vast majority of the time we live in peaceful co-existence with this microorganism. The question is why catastrophic infection may occur in some individuals. For invasive disease, the organism must possess virulence factors allowing penetration of epithelia, and survival and dissemination within the body.

Invasion of respiratory epithelium

N. meningitidis gains entry via the respiratory tract. The first hurdle facing a pathogenic strain of the organism will be attachment to respiratory mucosa, followed by passage through or between epithelial cells (Fig. 2). Contact between *N. meningitidis* and epithelial cells is mediated by surface proteins and polysaccharides presented on small projections (pili) of the bacterial cell [3,4]. The organism has to survive within the mucosal surface layer before penetrating the epithelium, so organisms able to resist mucosal defences have a greater chance of persisting. Meningococcal strains that possess immunoglobulin (Ig) A protease activity in their outer membrane proteins can avoid IgA-mediated mucosal immunity. Most strains of *N. meningitidis* recovered from invasive human disease express IgA protease activity [5]. Furthermore, antigenic variation in the outer membrane protein has been described during the invasion process as effectively presenting a 'moving target' to host immune responses [4].

In addition to intrinsic bacterial factors, any epithelial damage is likely to increase susceptibility to invasion in a host colonised by *N. meningitidis*. This explains increased susceptibility following respiratory virus infections. There is some evidence to suggest that children of parents who smoke are at increased risk of invasive meningococcal disease.

Survival in blood

To cause invasive disease, the organism must survive, multiply and disseminate. Blood is a hostile environment with many factors in both cellular and fluid phases that directly kill or inhibit bacterial growth. For *N. meningitidis*, host factors are essential in the initial (innate) response to bloodstream invasion (Fig. 2). *N. meningitidis* activates complement, which may lead to direct bacterial lysis or enhanced opsonophagocytosis and clearance from the circulation. Pathogenic

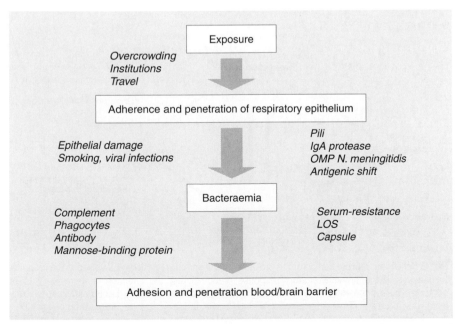

Fig. 2 Schematic representation of the processes involved in the pathogenesis of meningococcal meningitis (Ig = immunoglobulin; OMP = outer membrane protein; LOS = lipooligosaccharide).

neisseria species have mechanisms that help them avoid these host defences, such as sialylation of outer bacterial proteins [6].

Shock and organ failure

The clinical picture of fulminant meningococcal sepsis is one of hypotension, organ failure and severe coagulopathy (purpura fulminans). The key events will be described briefly in this chapter (for full description, see [1,7]).

Whole bacteria, bacterial fragments (eg endotoxin) or bacterial products (eg exotoxins) provoke a vigorous inflammatory reaction [8]. Ideally, inflammation will localise and then eliminate any infection. However, the overwhelming nature of this host response may sometimes lead to tissue damage, organ failure and even death (Fig. 3) [9].

Pro-inflammatory responses do not occur in isolation but are balanced by a variety of counter-regulatory homeostatic mechanisms that reduce inflammation and may lead to relative immunosuppression. This is a complicated situation in which clinical outcome is likely to be determined by the balance between pro-inflammatory and anti-inflammatory pathways (Fig. 3).

Disseminated intravascular coagulation may complicate any cause of severe bacterial sepsis. Meningococcal infection is exceptional in the frequency and severity of coagulopathy complicating invasive disease. Furthermore, damage as a result of

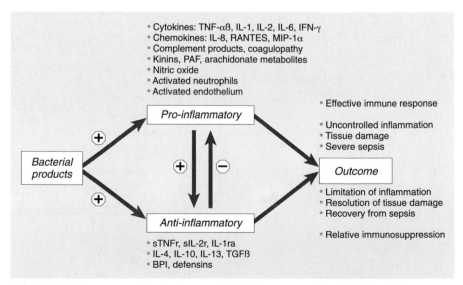

Fig. 3 Schematic representation of the pro- and anti-inflammatory pathways involved in the response to infection. If the pro-inflammatory response predominates, the infection is more likely to be controlled but at the risk of severe sepsis and organ damage (BPI = bactericidal/permeability-increasing protein; IFN = interferon; IL = interleukin; IL-1ra = IL-1 receptor antagonist; MIP = macrophage inhibitory protein; PAF = platelet activating factor; sIL-2r = soluble IL-2 receptor; TGFβ = transforming growth factor β; sTNFr = soluble TNF receptor; TNF = tumour necrosis factor) (reproduced, with permission, from [9]).

micro- and macrovascular thrombosis results in some of the most severe complications including amputation. Meningococcal products activate the endothelium and coagulation cascade by a number of mechanisms (Fig. 4).

Severe bacterial sepsis leads to vasodilatation and lowered systemic vascular resistance mediated by endothelial damage and release of nitric oxide. This is partially compensated by a rise in cardiac output responsible for the bounding peripheral pulse seen in many patients. Myocardial depression may occur in fulminant meningococcal infection, probably due to multiple factors including the effects of cytokines and meningococcal endotoxin and myocardial ischaemia. It may result in circulatory collapse and rapid death.

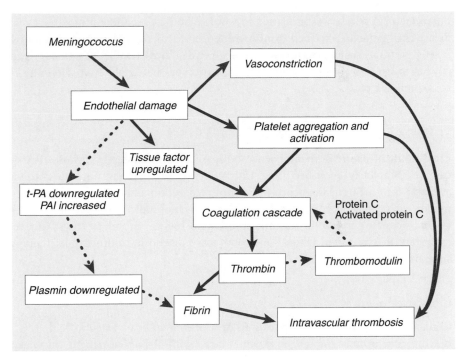

Fig. 4 Pathways leading to disseminated intravascular coagulation in meningococcal sepsis (PAI = plasminogen activator inhibitor; t-PA = tissue-plasminogen activator) (adapted, with permission, from [1]).

Genetic variation in the host response to meningococcal infection

In addition to the bacterial virulence factors important in disease pathogenesis (some of which have been described above) and the host responses implicated in organ failure, it has become apparent in recent years that variation in the host defence is a major determinant of whether infection occurs and of the outcome. It has been known for a long time that deficiency of terminal components of the complement pathway increases susceptibility to meningococcal infection [10]. Complement deficiency may be acquired (as in active systemic lupus erythematosus) or genetically determined, and a number of families with such deficiencies have been described. Interestingly, although the risk of infection is increased, these patients appear to be partially protected from some severe manifestations of systemic meningococcal sepsis. This was demonstrated in a C6-deficient patient who was given fresh frozen plasma for disseminated intravascular coagulation complicating meningococcal bacteraemia, leading to endotoxin release and shock [11].

Genetic polymorphisms in several areas of the immune response to bacterial infection have been linked to outcome from meningococcal disease, including mannose-binding protein [12], cytokine responses [13,14] and genes involved in coagulation [15–17]. The genetic influence on the balance between inflammatory mechanisms was shown in a unique study by Westendorp et al [13]. Interleukin (IL)-10 (anti-inflammatory) and tumour necrosis factor (TNF)α (pro-inflammatory) release was measured in whole blood exposed to endotoxin ex vivo. Relatives of patients who died from meningococcal infection demonstrated a high IL-10:TNFα ratio compared to relatives of survivors. Thus, families of non-survivors appear to express an anti-inflammatory phenotype that could have difficulty in containing infection.

□ MANAGEMENT OF MENINGOCOCCAL INFECTION

The fulminant nature of meningococcal disease means that death in those affected can be completely abolished only with effective vaccination. With no vaccine available for type B meningococcus, prompt recognition and antimicrobial therapy remain of critical importance. In addition, chemoprophylaxis and vaccination (where possible) are useful to limit spread and reduce secondary cases. Current management consists of clinical and laboratory diagnosis, antimicrobial therapy, supportive care and public health aspects.

Clinical features

Clinical presentations and complications of N. meningitidis are listed in Table 1. It is not difficult to make the diagnosis when faced with a shocked patient who has a purpuric rash (Fig. 5) or obvious signs of meningitis. The challenge lies in spotting early disease when symptoms are frequently non-specific. Rash is often not present in the early stages, or may be erythematous rather than purpuric. Breathlessness is not a feature of uncomplicated influenza and suggests more serious disease including bacterial sepsis. Any patient who presents with fever or headache and is a known contact of meningococcal disease should be taken seriously. A petechial or purpuric rash on the peripheries and the conjunctivae should be looked for carefully (Fig. 6).

Triage approach

1   If there is a strong suspicion of meningococcal infection, therapy should be started immediately.

Table 1. Disease manifestations of *Neisseria meningitidis*.

Manifestation	Comments
Meningococcal septicaemia	Meningitis may or may not be present
Purpura fulminans	Rapidly progressive confluent purpura with limb ischaemia and shock
Meningitis	May or may not have features of severe sepsis
Septic arthritis	May complicate severe sepsis or present as localised disease
Chronic meningococcaemia	Rare, mainly occurs in the elderly
	Easily confused with systemic vasculitis
Pneumonia	Uncommon
Conjunctivitis	Uncommon, risk of progressing to meningitis

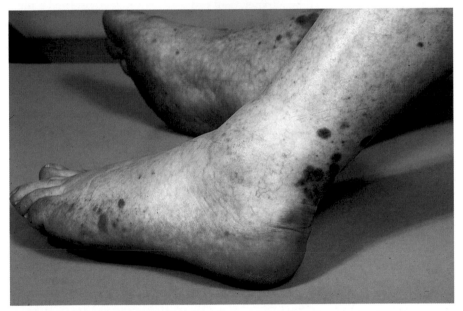

Fig. 5 Typical peripheral purpuric rash of meningococcal septicaemia.

2   If it is absolutely certain that the patient has a simple viral infection, reassurance should be given with a warning to seek medical help immediately if a non-blanching rash develops.

3   In doubtful cases, the patient should be kept under close observation whilst awaiting blood test results as meningococcal sepsis may progress rapidly.

Laboratory tests

At presentation of meningococcal sepsis the white cell and platelet counts are usually low but early in infection may be normal. If meningococcal infection is suspected, a

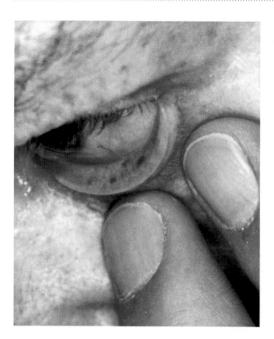

Fig. 6 Subconjunctival petechial haemorrhages.

coagulation screen should always be performed because this is often abnormal [18]. Arterial blood gas measurement should be performed in all breathless patients and may reveal a metabolic acidosis with a compensatory respiratory alkalosis.

Blood cultures must be performed in all cases. *N. meningitidis* may also be cultured by disrupting and swabbing purpuric lesions. The organism can be recovered from a throat swab in many cases.

Lumbar puncture should be considered where there is doubt about either the clinical diagnosis or the infecting organism, but is not necessary where there is a clear-cut clinical diagnosis of meningococcal infection [18]. A lumbar puncture must not be performed if raised intracranial pressure is suspected. If computed tomography scanning is readily available, it is prudent to perform a scan prior to lumbar puncture in any case of suspected intracranial infection.

Meningococcal antigen can be looked for in cerebrospinal fluid using latex agglutination testing. Polymerase chain reaction testing for meningococcal DNA can be obtained via the Public Health Laboratory Service meningococcal reference laboratory [19].

Antimicrobial therapy

In the UK, *N. meningitidis* is fully sensitive to both penicillins and cephalosporins, although there are concerns about emerging penicillin resistance in other parts of the world [20]. There is, however, increasing penicillin resistance in *S. pneumoniae* which influences the choice of antimicrobial therapy in cases of meningitis where the organism is not known. Current guidelines recommend that a third-generation cephalosporin is used in meningitis of unknown aetiology, but penicillin remains acceptable where there is a strong clinical or confirmed laboratory diagnosis of meningococcal infection [18]. Most general practitioners (GPs) do not carry injectable cephalosporins, and penicillin is still recommended for use in the community prior to hospitalisation. Administration of antibiotics before transfer to hospital is associated with a lower mortality and complication rate. A recent US study linked delay in antibiotic administration after arrival in accident and emergency with disease progression and poor outcome for patients with community-acquired meningitis [21]. Despite this, there is still evidence that parenteral penicillin is not being given by all GPs for cases of suspected meningitis [22] and it is likely that delay in antibiotic delivery is common within hospital. Antibiotics should not be delayed to perform or await diagnostic tests.

Adjunctive corticosteroid use

There are no large randomised trials of corticosteroids in meningococcal meningitis. Dexamethasone should be considered in the presence of raised intracranial pressure [1], but there are insufficient data to warrant corticosteroids in all patients.

Supportive care

Patients with meningococcal infection may deteriorate rapidly; this can occur in the few hours after antibiotics have been given. Patients should not be left alone in a darkened side room. Early involvement of the high dependency or intensive care unit facilities is essential where there is evidence of organ failure or significant impairment of consciousness. Supportive care aims to maximise oxygenation, prevent circulatory collapse and minimise neurological damage [1].

☐ PUBLIC HEALTH ASPECTS

Invasive meningococcal disease at any body site is notifiable. This is a statutory obligation for the clinician looking after the patient. Prompt notification is essential to ensure appropriate chemoprophylaxis and for the detection of outbreaks. Meningococcal infection should be notified urgently by telephone to the local consultant in communicable disease control (CCDC), followed by written notification. The CCDC will need to know the age, address, GP, occupation, work address or site of education and whether there has been any recent travel. A list should be made of close contacts. The CCDC will advise on the need for chemoprophylaxis and, when the organism has been typed, whether vaccination is required for contacts.

Chemoprophylaxis is usually given only to household or 'kissing' contacts. The aim is to break the chain of transmission rather than to protect individuals. Staff members rarely need prophylaxis, and treatment should be considered only for staff who have been involved in mouth-to-mouth resuscitation. Wider prophylaxis, for example to a school or other organisation, will be considered by the CCDC where there is evidence for an outbreak related to a specific place. Penicillin is not sufficient to eradicate carriage. Standard prophylaxis has been rifampicin 600 mg every 12 hours for two days (dose adjusted for children). A single 500 mg dose of ciprofloxacin is as effective and is used by many people in the UK, although it is not licensed for this indication. Chemoprophylaxis should be given to the index case as well as to the contacts [23].

☐ IMMUNOTHERAPY

Patients presenting with shock or organ failure have a high mortality even with prompt administration of antibiotics and good supportive care. There is a need for therapies that modify the host response to infection and preserve organ function. A full description of the myriad of possible therapeutic approaches is not possible here (they are summarised in Table 2). Anti-endotoxin agents have shown some activity, but probably need to be given very early for significant benefit and have not shown unequivocal mortality benefit in randomised trials [24]. Anti-cytokine agents have been disappointing in the treatment of bacterial sepsis, with many failed studies.

Agents that modify the coagulation cascade seem to be the most promising of the adjunctive therapies on the immediate horizon. Protein C depletion is associated with poor outcome in meningococcal sepsis, and replacement of protein C improves the coagulopathy and outcome in experimental models of bacterial sepsis. A number of small studies of protein C replacement in fulminant meningococcal sepsis suggest reversal of coagulopathy and reduced mortality [25]. Recently, a phase III placebo-controlled study of recombinant activated protein C in 1,690 patients with severe bacterial sepsis demonstrated an absolute reduction in the risk of death of 6.1% ($p = 0.005$) [26].

☐ CONCLUSIONS

Meningococcal disease remains a significant cause of morbidity and mortality in children and young adults despite the fact that *N. meningitidis* is sensitive to readily available antibiotics. The introduction of a type C polysaccharide vaccine has resulted in a large fall in type C cases in children, but immediate prospects for a vaccine against type B meningococcus remain poor. Meningococcal infection may progress rapidly to organ failure and death, making early recognition and prompt antimicrobial therapy essential. Both community and hospital practitioners need to try to minimise delays in antibiotic administration. Initiation of coagulopathy is central to the pathogenesis of meningococcal disease and agents that modify this process may have a future role in therapy.

REFERENCES

1   Pathan N, Nadel S, Levin M. Pathophysiology and management of meningococcal septicaemia. *J R Coll Physicians Lond* 2000; **34**: 436–44.
2   Ramsay M, Kaczmarski E, Rush M, Mallard R, *et al.* Changing patterns of case ascertainment and trends in meningococcal disease in England and Wales. *Commun Dis Rep CDR Rev* 1997; **7**: R49–54.

Table 2. Immunotherapeutic approaches to severe bacterial sepsis.

Anti-endotoxin	Anti-LPS MAbs	Phase II studies in Gram-negative sepsis and one phase II trial in meningococcal disease No overall mortality benefit
	$rBPI_{21}$	Phase III study in meningococcal disease in children No overall mortality benefit Reduction in amputation rate and improved functional status just reached significance
Anti-inflammatory mediators	Studies of anti-TNF, anti-IL-1, bradykinin and PAF antagonists	Many large phase II and phase III studies No overall mortality benefit detected in any of the studies
Anti-coagulopathy	Activated protein C	Phase III study in severe sepsis discontinued early due to significant reduction in mortality in treated group
	Anti-thrombin III	Promising phase II studies Larger trial awaited
Removal of multiple mediators	Haemofiltration/perfusion	Anecdotal reports of benefit No trial data

IL = interleukin; LPS = lipopolysaccharide; Mab = monoclonal antibody; PAF = platelet activating factor; $rBPI_{21}$ = recombinant bactericidal/permeability-increasing protein; TNF = tumour necrosis factor.

3   Virji M, Kayhty H, Ferguson DJ, Alexandrescu C, *et al.* The role of pili in the interactions of pathogenic Neisseria with cultured human endothelial cells. *Mol Microbiol* 1991; **5**: 1831–41.

4   de Vries FP, van Der Ende A, van Putten JP, Dankert J. Invasion of primary nasopharyngeal epithelial cells by *Neisseria meningitidis* is controlled by phase variation of multiple surface antigens. *Infect Immun* 1996; **64**: 2998–3006.

5   Vitovski S, Read RC, Sayers JR. Invasive isolates of *Neisseria meningitidis* possess enhanced immunoglobulin A1 protease activity compared to colonizing strains. *FASEB J* 1999; **13**: 331–7.

6   Estabrook MM, Griffiss JM, Jarvis GA. Sialylation of *Neisseria meningitidis* lipooligosaccharide inhibits serum bactericidal activity by masking lacto-N-neotetraose. *Infect Immun* 1997; **65**: 4436–44.

7   Brealey D, Singer M. Multi-organ dysfunction in the critically ill: epidemiology, pathophysiology and management. *J R Coll Physicians Lond* 2000; **34**: 424–7.

8   Noursadeghi M, Cohen J. Immunopathogenesis of severe sepsis. *J R Coll Physicians Lond* 2000; **34**: 432–6.

9   Lynn WA. Severe sepsis. In: Pusey C (ed). *Horizons in Medicine*, vol 11. London: Royal College of Physicians of London, 1999: 55–68.

10 Ross SC, Densen P. Complement deficiency states and infection: epidemiology, pathogenesis and consequences of neisserial and other infections in an immune deficiency. Review. *Medicine (Baltimore)* 1984; **63**: 243–73.

11 Lehner PJ, Davies KA, Walport MJ, Cope AP, *et al.* Meningococcal septicaemia in a C6-deficient patient and effects of plasma transfusion on lipopolysaccharide release. *Lancet* 1992; **340**: 1379–81.

12 Hibberd ML, Sumiya M, Summerfield JA, Booy R, Levin M. Association of variants of the gene for mannose-binding lectin with susceptibility to meningococcal disease. Meningococcal Research Group. *Lancet* 1999; **353**: 1049–53.

13 Westendorp RG, Langermans JA, Huizinga TW, Verweij CL, Sturk A. Genetic influence on cytokine production in meningococcal disease. *Lancet* 1997; **349**: 1912–3.

14 Booy R, Nadel S, Hibberd M, Levin M, Newport MJ. Genetic influence on cytokine production in meningococcal disease. *Lancet* 1997; **349**: 1176.

15 Hermans PW, Hibberd ML, Booy R, Daramola O, *et al.* 4G/5G promoter polymorphism in the plasminogen-activator-inhibitor-1 gene and outcome of meningococcal disease. Meningococcal Research Group. *Lancet* 1999; **354**: 556–60.

16 Kondaveeti S, Hibberd ML, Booy R, Nadel S, Levin M. Effect of the Factor V Leiden mutation on the severity of meningococcal disease. *Pediatr Infect Dis J* 1999; **18**: 893–6.

17 Westendorp RG, Hottenga JJ, Slagboom PE. Variation in plasminogen-activator-inhibitor-1 gene and risk of meningococcal septic shock. *Lancet* 1999; **354**: 561–3.

18 Begg N, Cartwright KA, Cohen J, Kaczmarski EB, *et al.* Consensus statement on diagnosis, investigation, treatment and prevention of acute bacterial meningitis in immunocompetent adults. Review. British Infection Society Working Party. *J Infect* 1999; **39**: 1–15.

19 Kaczmarski EB, Ragunathan PL, Marsh J, Gray SJ, Guiver M. Creating a national service for the diagnosis of meningococcal disease by polymerase chain reaction. *Commun Dis Public Health* 1998; **1**: 54–6.

20 Arreaza L, de La Fuente L, Vazquez JA. Antibiotic susceptibility patterns of *Neisseria meningitidis* isolates from patients and asymptomatic carriers. *Antimicrob Agents Chemother* 2000; **44**: 1705–7.

21 Aronin SI, Peduzzi P, Quagliarello VJ. Community-acquired bacterial meningitis: risk stratification for adverse clinical outcome and effect of antibiotic timing. *Ann Intern Med* 1998; **129**: 862–9.

22 Ragunathan L, Ramsay M, Borrow R, Guiver M, *et al.* Clinical features, laboratory findings and management of meningococcal meningitis in England and Wales: report of a 1997 survey. Meningococcal meningitis: 1997 survey report. *J Infect* 2000; **40**: 74–9.

23 Kaczmarski EB, Cartwright KA. Control of meningococcal disease: guidance for microbiologists: CCDC. Consultant in Communicable Disease Control, England. *Commun Dis Rep CDR Rev* 1995; **5**: R196–8.

24 Levin M, Quint PA, Goldstein B, Barton P, *et al.* Recombinant bactericidal/permeability-increasing protein (rBPI21) as adjunctive treatment for children with severe meningococcal sepsis: a randomised trial. rBPI21 Meningococcal Sepsis Study Group. *Lancet* 2000; **356**: 961–7.
25 Betrosian AP, Balla M, Kofinas G, Papanikolaou M, Georgiadis G. Protein C in the treatment of coagulopathy in meningococcal sepsis. *Crit Care Med* 1999; **27**: 2849–50.
26 Bernard GR, Vincent JL, Laterre PF, La Rosa SP, *et al.* Efficacy and safety of recombinant human activated protein C for severe sepsis. *N Engl J Med* 2001; **344**: 699–709.

☐ SELF ASSESSMENT QUESTIONS

1 In meningococcal infection:
   (a) A blanching macular rash is characteristic
   (b) Pneumonia may occur
   (c) Osteomyelitis is a common complication
   (d) Type B is the commonest serotype encountered in the UK
   (e) A neutrophil leucocytosis is characteristic

2 In the laboratory diagnosis of *Neisseria meningitidis*:
   (a) Polymerase chain reaction is available to confirm the diagnosis
   (b) Cerebrospinal fluid examination should be performed in all patients
   (c) *N. meningitidis* can frequently be cultured from a throat swab in patients with meningitis
   (d) Serology is used to confirm the diagnosis
   (e) Abnormal coagulation is a late finding

3 The following are important bacterial virulence factors:
   (a) Sialylation of meningococcal surface proteins
   (b) Immunoglobulin G protease
   (c) Secretion of proteolytic enzymes
   (d) Antigenic variation
   (e) Surface pili

4 Management of meningococcal disease:
   (a) Any staff potentially exposed to the patient should receive chemo-prophylaxis
   (b) Lumbar puncture should be performed before antibiotic administration
   (c) Penicillin effectively eliminates nasopharyngeal carriage
   (d) Ceftriaxone is a suitable choice for empirical therapy
   (e) Dexamethasone has been shown to reduce mortality

5 The following statements about meningococcal disease are true:
   (a) Genetic factors influence susceptibility to meningococcal infection
   (b) There is an increased risk of meningococcal infection when travelling to Africa
   (c) Cell-mediated immunodeficiency increases the risk of invasive meningococcal disease
   (d) Infection may be spread by animals
   (e) Mannose-binding protein enhances plasma clearance of *N. meningitidis*

ANSWERS

1a	False	2a	True	3a	True	4a	False	5a	True
b	True	b	False	b	False	b	False	b	True
c	False	c	True	c	False	c	False	c	False
d	True	d	False	d	True	d	True	d	False
e	False	e	False	e	True	e	False	e	True

Common chronic diseases

Evidence-based management of hypertension?

Gordon McInnes

☐ INTRODUCTION

The evidence base in support of the drug treatment of hypertension is amongst the strongest in medicine. Prospective, randomised clinical trials (RCTs) in 50,000 individuals demonstrated conclusively that pharmacological reduction of blood pressure reduces the risk of cardiovascular events and all-cause mortality [1].

The magnitude of reduction in stroke events in the trials is exactly that predicted from long-term epidemiological studies for the differences in systolic and diastolic blood pressure achieved (Fig. 1) [1]. However, although the reduction in coronary heart disease (CHD) events (the predominant complication of hypertension in Western populations) is significant, it is rather less than expected. The shortfall in CHD prevention might be explained by deleterious metabolic effects of diuretics which formed the basis of therapy in almost all the trials. Other antihypertensive agents should avoid these unwanted actions and could have advantages in cardioprotection.

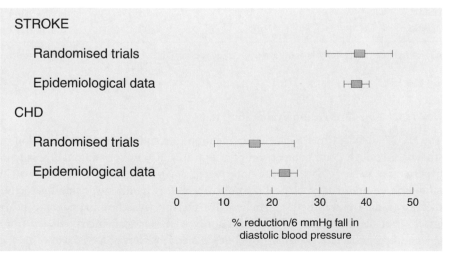

Fig. 1. Results of randomised trials of antihypertensive therapy for stroke and coronary heat disease (CHD) in relation to predictions from epidemiological data. Mean (horizontal bars 95% confidence intervals) risk reduction for 6 mmHg difference in diastolic blood pressure [1].

☐ EVIDENCE FROM TRIALS

The first contenders were the beta-blockers. In the 1980s, there were great expectations that these drugs would be superior to diuretics, particularly since beta-blockers reduce the risk of reinfarction or death in patients with CHD. This hypothesis was tested in a series of large-scale controlled trials. The results were inconclusive.

Large outcome trials with the newer drugs, angiotensin-converting enzyme (ACE) inhibitors and calcium-channel blockers (CCBs), in hypertension were slow to appear. The first results did not appear until 20 years after their introduction. The wait was hardly worthwhile. No trial detected a significant difference in CHD events between therapy based on newer drugs and that based on conventional agents. However, the precision of comparisons in individual trials was weak, with wide 95% confidence intervals for differences (Table 1). Since clinically useful differences in CHD events between therapies could not be excluded in any of the trials, individually the trials were not informative.

Table 1 Relative risk (RR) of myocardial infarction and 95% confidence intervals (CI) in comparisons of newer drugs and conventional drugs (diuretics and beta-blockers).

Trial	Ref.	Drug	RR	95% CI
STOP-2	4	ACEI	0.90	0.72–1.13
		CCB	1.18	0.96–1.47
CAPPP	5	ACEI	0.96	0.77–1.19
INSIGHT	6	CCB	1.09	0.76–1.58
NORDIL	7	CCB	1.16	0.94–1.44
ALLHAT	8	AB	1.03	0.90–1.17

AB = alpha-blocker; ACEI = angiotensin-converting enzyme inhibitor; CCB = calcium-channel blocker.

Heart Outcomes Prevention Evaluation Study

The HOPE study [2] merits particular mention (see end of text for explanation of studies). Although not a comparison of a new drug against conventional therapy in hypertensive patients, it has been interpreted as showing an advantage of ACE inhibition beyond that of blood pressure control. It is hardly surprising that active therapy (ramipril) was better than inactive therapy (placebo) in reducing heart attacks, but the magnitude of the reduction was greater than that predicted from epidemiological data for the small difference in blood pressure observed. However, the reduction in cardiovascular events per mmHg difference in blood pressure was no greater than that seen in other high risk populations (eg patients with diabetes) treated with other forms of antihypertensive therapy [3]. In the absence of a positive control group treated with another agent providing equivalent blood pressure control no definitive conclusions can be reached. A better acronym for HOPE might be 'HYPE'. (The HOPE trial in the context of diabetes is discussed in the chapter by Rudy Bilous.)

Reasons for failure of trials of newer versus older drugs

The recent trials of newer drugs against older drugs have failed because they were too small, the event rate was low, almost 50% of deaths were not cardiovascular and strokes were almost as common as CHD events (Table 2). The pattern of events in recent trials (relatively low proportion of cardiovascular deaths and high rate of stroke events) was not anticipated from epidemiological data or from trials comparing active therapy against placebo in which cardiovascular deaths and CHD predominated [1]. In early trials [1], the ratio of CHD to stroke events was 3:2, while in the recent trials [4–7] the ratio is 1:1. Therefore, the newer drugs appear to have been tested in a very different environment from that in which older drugs were evaluated and the hypothesis of a shortfall in CHD prevention generated. Insufficient power and the large proportion of non-vascular mortality make it difficult to detect differences between treatments for the outcome of interest: CHD. Clinical trials provide short-term answers to long-term problems and are in effect surrogates for real life where treatment is often given for a lifetime.

Table 2 Coronary heart disease (CHD) and stroke events in recent outcome trials.

Trial	Ref.	CHD	Stroke	Ratio
STOP-2	4	614	659	0.93
CAPPP	5	343	337	1.02
INSIGHT	6	191	163	1.17
NORDIL	7	443	355	1.25
Overall		*1,591*	*1,514*	*1.05*

☐ OTHER FORMS OF EVIDENCE

In the face of uncertainty from the trials, it is reasonable to examine other forms of evidence. Observational studies are generally frowned upon since the introduction of chance bias may confound interpretation. However, recently published meta-analyses [9,10] have indicated that well-conducted studies of this type can provide estimates of treatment effects qualitatively and quantitatively similar to those from RCTs.

☐ GLASGOW BLOOD PRESSURE CLINIC

The Glasgow blood pressure clinic, established in 1968, provides a suitable environment to observe the long-term effects of antihypertensive drug therapy. The clinic now has a computerised database of almost 11,000 patients. This provides standardised records of clinical findings, drug treatment and investigations. Patients are record-linked with the Registrar General (Scotland) and the West of Scotland Cancer Registry which provide information on dates and causes of death, and fatal and non-fatal cancer. The database has several attributes:

☐   prolonged follow-up

☐   large number of subjects

☐   structured clinical records

☐   accurate data on outcome

☐   high mortality rate (ie a large number of patients died in a short time).

The potential value of this resource is illustrated by the findings in a recent analysis of over 5,000 patients prescribed antihypertensive medication at the clinic between 1 January 1980 and 31 December 1995. This population was selected to examine the influence on outcome of newer antihypertensive drugs. Both dihydropyridine CCBs and ACE inhibitors were introduced into clinical practice in 1980. The drugs received by these patients included CCBs (2,295 patients), ACE inhibitors (1,599), beta-blockers (3,679) and diuretics (3,297). As would be expected, most patients received more than one drug during the 16-year observation period.

This analysis addressed several objectives:

1   Do CCBs predispose to cancer?

2   Influence of ACE inhibitors.

3   Possible outcome differences between newer antihypertensive agents.

Do calcium-channel blockers predispose to cancer?

No association was found between the use of CCBs and occurrence of cancer. However, an unexpected observation was that incident (fatal and non-fatal) and fatal cancers were reduced in patients who had received ACE inhibitors [11]. Survival curves showed that benefit was apparent only after 3–4 years of therapy (Fig. 2), providing plausibility for this finding.

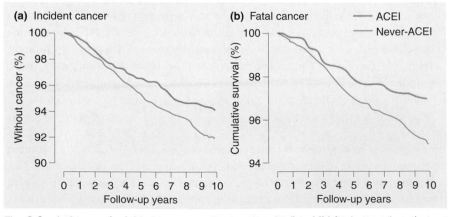

Fig. 2 Survival curves for **(a)** incident cancer (fatal and non-fatal) and **(b)** fatal cancer in patients at the Glasgow blood pressure clinic who received or never received an angiotensin-converting enzyme inhibitor (ACEI) [11].

Influence of angiotensin-converting enzyme inhibitors

By the end of 1995, over 850 patients had died, with all-cause mortality significantly lower in patients who had received ACE inhibitors. In observational studies, a possible explanation for such a finding is bias which might arise if, by chance, ACE inhibitors had been prescribed for low risk patients. No such bias was identified, and an analysis using a Cox proportional hazard model to adjust for confounding factors confirmed the survival advantage in ACE inhibitor-treated subjects (Table 3).

Table 3 Relative hazard ratio and 95% confidence intervals (CI) for patients treated with angiotensin-converting enzyme inhibitors (ACEIs) compared with never-ACEI treated patients.

		Relative hazard		Relative hazard	
Cause of death	No. of deaths	Ratio*	95% CI	Ratio**	95% CI
All causes	857	0.76	0.63–0.91	0.75	0.63–0.91
Vascular:					
all	564	0.81	0.65–1.01	0.78	0.62–0.98
CHD	349	0.76	0.57–1.02	0.75	0.56–0.99
stroke	132	0.81	0.51–1.29	0.79	0.49–1.25
other	83	1.02	0.58–1.81	0.96	0.54–1.74
Other non-cancer	121	0.72	0.45–1.14	0.76	0.48–1.22

* adjusted for age, gender and year of entry.
** adjusted for all patient characteristics (including age, gender, year of entry, smoking, blood pressure, creatinine, urea, anti-diabetic, lipid lowering and anti-platelet medication).
CHD = coronary heart disease.

Possible outcome differences between newer antihypertensive agents

The final question addressed was whether there were any outcome differences between newly introduced antihypertensive agents: ACE inhibitors and CCBs. Over 90% of CCB-treated patients received dihydropyridines (more than 50% long-acting preparations, nifedipine gastrointestinal-transport-system (GITS) or amlodipine). The comparisons were between patients who had received an ACE inhibitor but never a CCB (680 patients), a CCB but never an ACE inhibitor (1,416), an ACE inhibitor and also a CCB (879), and those who had received neither an ACE inhibitor nor a CCB (2,232). After adjustment for the patient characteristics indicated in Table 3, all-cause mortality was found to be significantly reduced in patients who had received an ACE inhibitor but never a CCB, and significantly increased in patients who had taken a CCB but never an ACE inhibitor, compared with those who had received neither. Patients who had received both classes of drugs had intermediate risk of death. Qualitatively similar differences, but of greater magnitude, were seen for all vascular mortality and CHD mortality.

The differences between treatment groups were particularly extreme for CHD mortality for which survival curves separated early – unlike the findings for cancer (Fig. 2) – and continued to separate over 10 years of follow-up (Fig. 3). This suggests

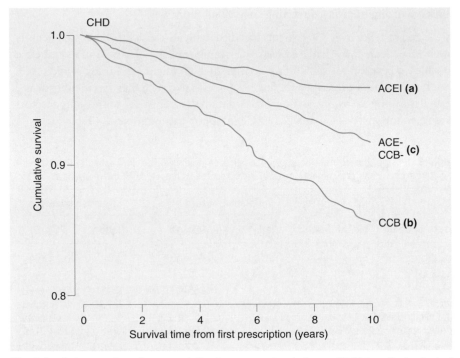

Fig. 3 Survival curves from first prescription for coronary heart disease (CHD) in patients who had received **(a)** angiotensin-converting enzyme inhibitors (ACEI) but never calcium-channel blockers (CCB), **(b)** CCB but never ACEI and **(c)** neither.

that relatively short-term prospective randomised trials may underestimate long-term differences between treatments.

The high CHD mortality in CCB-treated patients might be explained if these drugs were given preferentially to patients with CHD who might be expected to have high CHD mortality. CCBs are used to treat symptomatic CHD, but treatment with the most frequently used anti-anginal drugs, beta-blockers, was not associated with excess CHD mortality, suggesting that the results were not confounded by indication.

Short-acting CCBs (such as nifedipine capsules) have been reported to increase CHD risk, and were widely used during the early period of observation. This could have influenced the results. However, when CHD mortality was examined in four-year periods between 1980 and 1995, the excess risk associated with CCB treatment did not decline with time. Thus, increased CHD mortality seems to have persisted even after the widespread introduction of long-acting dihydropyridines.

☐ HEALTH IMPLICATIONS

These findings may have substantial health implications. Based on 857 deaths over 34,519 patient-years, it can be estimated that use of ACE inhibitors might spare 35 deaths per 1,000 patients treated for five years. In contrast, use of CCBs might lead to the loss of 45 lives which would otherwise be spared (Fig. 4). These

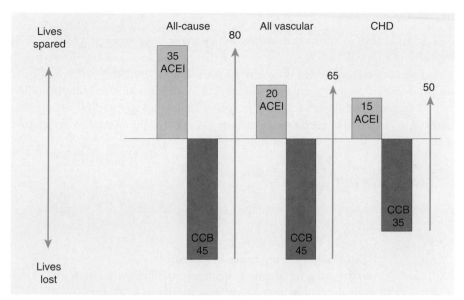

Fig. 4 Outcome differences between angiotensin-converting enzyme inhibitors (ACEI) and calcium-channel blockers (CCB). Lives spared or lives lost per 1,000 patients treated for five years. Data for ACEI-treated patients and CCB-treated patients relative to patients who received neither of these drug classes, based on 857 deaths (564 vascular and 349 coronary heart disease (CHD)) over 34,519 patient-years.

calculations offer no support for the widespread use of CCBs and the relative underuse of ACE inhibitors in hypertension.

A recent meta-analysis [12] of prospective outcome trials found a significantly reduced risk of CHD events in ACE inhibitor-treated hypertensive patients in direct comparison with those receiving CCBs (Table 4). This finding is compatible with the results of the Glasgow blood pressure clinic observational study, despite a low event rate for CHD relative to stroke and a low proportion of cardiovascular deaths. Longer follow-up of patients with high cardiovascular (and CHD) risk, as in the UK, might have produced results even closer to those from the Glasgow study.

Table 4 Meta-analysis of direct comparison between angiotensin-converting enzyme inhibitors (ACEIs) and calcium-channel blockers (CCBs) (4,871 patients) [12].

Outcome	No. of patients	OR	95% CI
Coronary heart disease events	261	0.81	0.68–0.97
Stroke	240	1.02	0.85–1.21
Major cardiovascular events	1,178	0.92	0.83–1.01
Congestive heart failure	353	0.82	0.67–1.00
Mortality	774	1.03	0.91–1.18

CI = confidence interval; OR = odds ratio for ACEIs vs CCBs.

☐ CONCLUSIONS

The evidence base for the drug treatment of hypertension is strong, but trials seeking evidence of outcome differences between active agents have been uninformative. If differences are to be detected, future trials must have more CHD events and be of longer duration. Meanwhile, observational data merit consideration. Large numbers of well documented fatal events and prolonged follow-up in the clinic setting may allow demonstration of mortality differences not apparent in short-term prospective trials.

☐ TRIAL ACRONYMS

ALLHAT   Antihypertensive and Lipid-Lowering Treatment to Prevent Heart Attack
CAPP   Captopril Prevention Project
HOPE   Heart Outcomes Prevention Evaluation
INSIGHT   International Nifedipine gastrointestinal-transport-system (GITS) study: Intervention as a Goal in Hypertension
NORDIL   Nordic Diltiazem
STOP-2   Swedish Trial in Old Patients with Hypertension-2

REFERENCES

1 Collins R, MacMahon S. Blood pressure, antihypertensive drug treatment and the risks of stroke and of coronary heart disease. Review. *Br Med Bull* 1994; **50**: 272–98.

2 Effects of an angiotensin-converting-enzyme inhibitor, ramipril, on cardiovascular events in high-risk patients. The Heart Outcomes Prevention Evaluation Study Investigators. *N Engl J Med* 2000; **342**: 145–53.

3 Hansson L, Zanchetti A, Carruthers SG, Dahlof B, *et al.* Effects of intensive blood-pressure lowering and low-dose aspirin in patients with hypertension: principal results of the Hypertension Optimal Treatment (HOT) randomised trial. HOT Study Group. *Lancet* 1998; **351**: 1755–62.

4 Hansson L, Lindholm LH, Ekbom T, Dahlof B, *et al.* Randomised trial of old and new antihypertensive drugs in elderly patients: cardiovascular mortality and morbidity. The Swedish Trial in Old Patients with Hypertension-2 Study. *Lancet* 1999; **354**: 1751–6.

5 Hansson L, Lindholm LH, Niskanen L, Lanke J, *et al.* Effect of angiotensin-converting-enzyme inhibition compared with conventional therapy on cardiovascular morbidity and mortality in hypertension: the Captopril Prevention Project (CAPPP) randomised trial. *Lancet* 1999; **353**: 611–6.

6 Brown MJ, Palmer CR, Castaigne A, de Leeuw PW, *et al.* Morbidity and mortality in patients randomised to double-blind treatment with a long-acting calcium-channel blocker or diuretic in the International Nifedipine GITS study: Intervention as a Goal in Hypertension Treatment (INSIGHT). *Lancet* 2000; **356**: 366–72.

7 Hansson L, Hedner T, Lund-Johansen P, Kjeldsen SE, *et al.* Randomised trial of effects of calcium antagonists compared with diuretics and beta-blockers on cardiovascular morbidity and mortality in hypertension: the Nordic Diltiazem (NORDIL) study. *Lancet* 2000; **356**: 359–65.

8 Major cardiovascular events in hypertensive patients randomized to doxazosin vs chlorthalidone: the antihypertensive and lipid-lowering treatment to prevent heart attack trial (ALLHAT). ALLHAT Collaborative Research Group. *JAMA* 2000; **283**: 1967–75.

9   Benson K, Hartz AJ. A comparison of observational studies and randomized controlled trials. *N Engl J Med* 2000; **342**: 1878–86.

10   Concato J, Shah N, Horwitz RI. Randomized, controlled trials, observational studies, and the hierarchy of research designs. *N Engl J Med* 2000; **342**: 1887–92.

11   Lever AF, Hole DJ, Gillis CR, McCallum IR, *et al.* Do inhibitors of angiotensin-I-converting enzyme protect against risk of cancer? *Lancet* 1998; **352**: 179–84.

12   Neal B, MacMahon S, Chapman N. Effects of ACE inhibitors, calcium antagonists, and other blood-pressure-lowering drugs: results of prospectively designed overviews of randomised trials. Blood Pressure Lowering Treatment Trialists' Collaboration. *Lancet* 2000; **356**: 1955–64.

☐ SELF ASSESSMENT QUESTIONS

1   Reduction of diastolic blood pressure by 6 mmHg using conventional antihypertensive therapy (based on diuretic or beta-blocker):
   (a) Reduces stroke events by 38%
   (b) Reduces stroke events by the magnitude expected from epidemiological data
   (c) Has no significant effect on coronary heart disease (CHD) events
   (d) Reduces CHD events by significantly less than expected from epidemiological data
   (e) Reduces all-cause mortality by 12%

2   In prevention of CHD events, outcome trials have demonstrated that:
   (a) Beta-blockers are superior to diuretics
   (b) Angiotensin-converting enzyme (ACE) inhibitors are superior to diuretics or beta-blockers
   (c) Calcium-channel blockers (CCBs) are superior to diuretics and beta-blockers
   (d) Alpha-blockers are inferior to diuretics
   (e) ACE inhibitors are superior to CCBs

3   Possible reasons why long-term randomised trials have failed to demonstrate differences between antihypertensive agents for CHD mortality include:
   (a) There are no differences
   (b) Event rates were too low
   (c) There was a high proportion of non-cardiovascular deaths
   (d) Many patients withdrew from randomised therapy
   (e) Confidence intervals were too narrow

4   Possible advantages of observational studies in evaluating treatment effects include:
   (a) Large number of events
   (b) Long duration of follow-up
   (c) Real-life clinical setting
   (d) No need for careful design and analysis
   (e) Eliminate need for prospective trials

5 Properties of observational studies of treatment effects include:
   (a) Produce results qualitatively different from those obtained in randomised controlled trials
   (b) Systematically overestimate the magnitude of the effects of treatment
   (c) Subject to bias
   (d) May be confounded by indication
   (e) Should not be used alone to decide on treatment decisions

ANSWERS

1a True	2a False	3a True	4a True	5a False
b True	b False	b True	b True	b False
c False	c False	c True	c True	c True
d False	d False	d True	d False	d True
e True	e True	e False	e False	e True

Falls in the elderly

Rose Anne Kenny

☐ THE SCOPE OF THE PROBLEM

Falls are a major healthcare and cost priority, associated with considerable mortality, morbidity, reduced functioning and premature nursing home admissions. Falls generally result from multiple, diverse and interacting underlying risk factors and situational causes, many of which are correctable. This interaction is modified by age, disease and the presence of hazards in the environment. Older people frequently do not appreciate the possible consequences of falls or report them to their physician, so falls go undetected until preventable injury and disabilities have occurred.

Both the incidence of falls and the severity of fall-related complications rise steadily after about the age of 60. In the population aged 65 and over approximately 35–40% of community-dwelling, generally healthy elderly people fall annually. After 75 years of age, the rates are higher.

Incidence rates in nursing homes and hospitals are almost three times the community rates for people aged 65 and over (1.5 falls per bed annually). Complication rates are also considerably higher: 10–25% of institutional falls result in fracture, laceration or need for hospital care. Fall-related injuries were found recently to account for 6% of all medical expenditures for people age 65 and older in the US.

A key issue of concern is not simply the high incidence of falls in elderly people, since young children and athletes have an even higher incidence, but rather the combination of high incidence and high susceptibility to injury. This stems from a high prevalence of comorbid diseases (eg osteoporosis) and age-related physiological decline (eg slowed reflexes) that make even a relatively mild fall particularly dangerous. Falls are the most frequently cited reason for residential care and nursing home admissions. Fear of falling and the post-fall anxiety syndrome are also well recognised as negative consequences of falls. The loss of self-confidence to ambulate safely can result in self-imposed functional limitations and increase the requirement for social services input.

☐ RISK FACTORS FOR FALLING

The principal risk factors for falling have been identified in a number of studies and can be classified [1] as either:

- ☐ intrinsic (eg lower extremity weakness, poor grip strength, balance disorders, functional and cognitive impairment, visual deficits) or

☐   extrinsic (eg polypharmacy and environmental factors such as poor lighting, loose carpets, lack of bathroom safety equipment).

The risk of falling dramatically increases as the number of risk factors increases.

☐ OVERLAP BETWEEN THE SYMPTOMS OF FALLS AND SYNCOPE

Recent studies have identified a possible overlap between symptoms of falls and syncope in older adults. In some series, up to 20% of cardiovascular syncope in older adults (over 70 years) present as falls. This particularly applies to carotid sinus syndrome and orthostatic hypotension. The carotid sinus is located at the bifurcation of the internal and external carotid artery. It is the dominant modulator of heart rate and blood pressure homeostasis during postural change and other activities. A hypersensitive response is rare before the age of 50 but increases in prevalence with advancing years. It is characterised by three seconds or longer of asystole (cardioinhibitory) and/or a 50 mmHg or more fall in systolic blood pressure (vasodepressor) in response to firm, unilateral massage (for 5–10 seconds) over the point of maximum pulsation at the carotid bifurcation.

Carotid sinus syndrome is characterised by recurrent syncope attributed to either a cardioinhibitory or vasodepressor response. However, up to 20% of older patients with carotid sinus syndrome complain of falls in addition to syncope. Retrospective data show that two-thirds of older patients who were paced for carotid sinus syndrome, and who had complained of falls before pacing, had not experienced falls up to two years after pacing. In another study of older patients with carotid sinus hypersensitivity who complained only of falls and denied syncope, two-thirds lost consciousness during asystole induced by carotid sinus massage. Subsequently, most of them denied witnessed loss of consciousness, thus demonstrating amnesia for loss of consciousness [2]. Carotid sinus hypersensitivity is significantly more prevalent in older adults who have experienced non-accidental falls (ie self-reported falls with no recall for events such as a slip or trip which caused the fall) compared with accidental falls, suggesting a causal association [3].

Thus, one explanation for syncope presenting as falls is amnesia for loss of consciousness. This has been demonstrated in the cardioinhibitory carotid sinus syndrome. Another explanation is that older patients who have gait and/or balance problems may experience balance instability and consequently fall during an episode of bradycardia-induced hypotension. Syncopal episodes are not witnessed in 40–60% of people over 65, thus rendering more difficult a diagnosis of syncope in the absence of an accurate history and witness account.

☐ ASSESSMENT OF AND INTERVENTION FOR FALLS

Multifactorial intervention strategies have been most rigorously studied, and are most effective, among community-dwelling older persons (ie those living in their own homes). The effective components of these strategies are:

☐   gait training and advice on the appropriate use of assistive devices

☐   exercise programmes, with balance training as one component

☐   review and modification of medication, especially psychotropic medication

☐   treatment of postural hypotension

☐   modification of environmental hazards

☐   treatment of cardiovascular disorders, including cardiac arrhythmias.

In long-term care and assisted living settings, multifactorial interventions of benefit in reducing falls are staff education programmes and review and modification of medications, especially psychotropic medications. Surprisingly, although different nursing assessment protocols and intervention strategies are widely implemented in hospital inpatients, there are no randomised controlled trials (RCTs) of single or multifactorial intervention studies for falls in this setting [4].

☐ FALLS IN THE ACCIDENT AND EMERGENCY DEPARTMENT

There are few published studies [5] of the benefit obtained from assessment of and intervention for falls carried out in the accident and emergency (A&E) department, although it is widely accepted that falls and syncope are a major component of emergency activity. Three RCTs have been conducted in the A&E department in Newcastle. Preliminary results from these studies are presented in this chapter. The studies are due to report shortly.

1   *SAFE PACE*: a study, sponsored by National Research and Development, which described the prevalence of carotid sinus hypersensitivity in fallers attending the A&E department. This was followed up with an RCT to determine whether cardiac pacing subsequently reduced falls in these patients.

2   *SAFE COG*: a multifactorial intervention RCT, sponsored by the Alzheimer's Society and Regional Research and Development, in patients with cognitive impairment and dementia who attended A&E because of a fall.

3   *SAFER*: a multifactorial intervention RCT, sponsored by Wellcome, in recurrent fallers who do not have dementia.

SAFE PACE

A total of 71,279 consecutive adults (>50 years) were screened as they attended the A&E department. Falls and syncope were the commonest single reason for attendance (34% and 42% of those over 50 and 65, respectively). The reasons for the falls are shown in Fig. 1.

The prevalence of non-accidental or unexplained falls increased with advancing age (Fig. 2). Carotid sinus hypersensitivity was present in 34% of this group, with half the cases cardioinhibitory. The latter group (mean age 75 years) were randomised to cardiac pacing or no intervention.

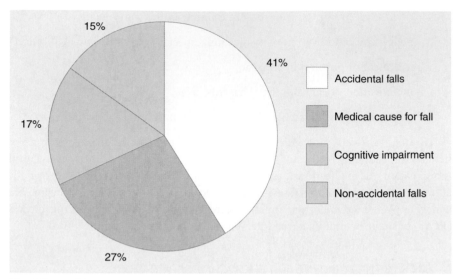

Fig. 1 Types of falls in adults attending the accident and emergency department.

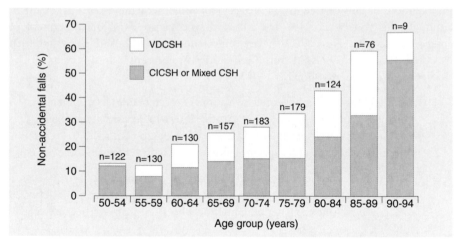

Fig. 2 Prevalence of cardioinhibitory carotid sinus hypersensitivity (CICSH) and vasodepressor CSH (VDCSH) in cognitively normal older adults attending the accident and emergency department because of non-accidental or unexplained falls.

Falls and fall related injuries were significantly reduced (by over 70%) in patients who received pacemakers. At present, patients with non-accidental falls would not be systematically referred from A&E for cardiovascular assessment.

SAFE COG

Of attendees over 64 years, 25% had cognitive impairment and dementia. Risk factors were common in these patients, with an average of four modifiable risk factors per patient (Fig. 3). These included:

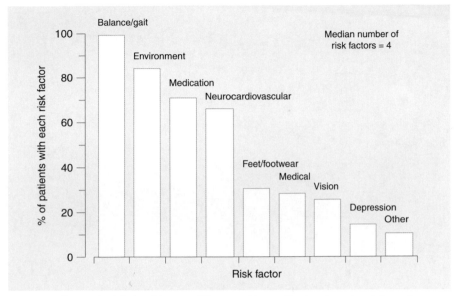

Fig. 3 Risk factors for falls in adults over 65 years with cognitive impairment and dementia.

☐   gait and balance: over 96%

☐   environmental hazards: over 80%

☐   culprit medications: 70%

☐   cardiovascular abnormalities: almost 65% (in particular,
     orthostatic hypotension, carotid sinus hypersensitivity and other
     bradyarrhythmias).

Preliminary data suggest that the patients who benefited most from the intervention were community-dwelling patients with cognitive impairment and dementia who have a cardiovascular abnormality. Many issues were raised about poor compliance with gait and balance training and environmental modifications in these patients. Future studies will address whether better compliance can further modify the risk of falls and what factors determine compliance with specific components of the intervention.

SAFER

In this study, fallers who had recurrent falls but no syncope (two or more falls in the past year, whether accidental or non-accidental) were randomised to multi-factorial intervention, including systematic cardiovascular intervention, or to standard care. Of note, 41% of these patients had carotid sinus hypersensitivity and 38% had orthostatic hypotension, thus emphasising the possible overlap for falls and syncope in patients with recurrent falls – even recurrent accidental falls (Fig. 4).

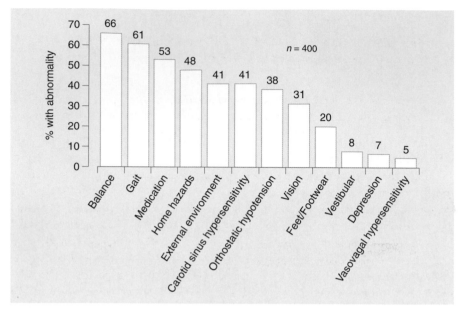

Fig. 4 Risk factors for falls in adults over 65 years attending accident and emergency with recurrent falls.

□ IMPACT OF A DEDICATED FALLS AND SYNCOPE FACILITY ON EMERGENCY BED ACTIVITY

In 1991, a syncope and falls facility for older adults was set up in Newcastle Royal Victoria Infirmary (RVI) in order to focus care pathways in a dedicated day-case facility. Prior to this, there was no day-case activity at the RVI for syncope and falls, and the average length of hospital stay was 10.9 days.

Acute hospital admissions were referred to the facility as inpatients, reviewed within a week, discharged, and either seen as urgent outpatients/day cases within 1–3 weeks or reviewed as non-urgent outpatients/day cases within six weeks. This was in addition to routine and urgent outpatient referrals from general practitioners (GPs), the A&E staff and other specialists. Consultant episodes have increased from 90 in 1991 to 2,400 in 1999.

The activity and performance data for syncope and falls in adults over 65 years for the RVI were compared with 13 peer inner city UK teaching hospitals to determine the impact of the facility on emergency bed occupancy. Syncope and falls were the sixth most frequent reason for acute emergency admissions in over 65 year olds. At the RVI, 35% of activity for syncope and falls was emergency compared with 98% in the other hospitals. The average length of stay for the fewer patients who were admitted was also much shorter at the RVI (2.4 days vs 8.6 days at peer sites). In 1999, the RVI had saved 6,616 bed-days compared with the average length of stay at the other sites, which equates to 18 beds in that year.

There are several possible explanations for the high day-case activity, low emergency activity and shorter length of stay at the RVI:

☐   Inpatient admissions stay a shorter period of time.

☐   Inpatient admissions are reduced locally because GPs and the A&E department have an alternative option of an urgent referral for specialist investigation.

☐   The number of inpatient episodes is reduced because of successful investigation and treatment strategies, resulting in fewer subsequent events.

Each year additional funding is provided to acute hospitals to assist with winter bed pressures. Dedicated rapid access facilities for syncope and falls throughout the UK could have a significant impact on acute bed usage and costs and help to address some of the recurrent pressures within the system. For example, one of the other sites in our study, which had 1,300 episodes for syncope and falls, could make savings of 15,804 bed-days or 43 beds, a saving of £3,160,800 at £200 per bed-day. If the 1991–92 length of stay continued today at the RVI, the annual estimated cost would be £2,405,000. The RVI would have used 12,025 bed-days and require a further 33 beds. It is estimated that the annual running cost of the facility at the RVI is £250,000. At present, over half of the service activity is funded by research funds and manned by research staff. The national service framework for older adults has highlighted falls as a key area for service standards and development. The present data should guide the resourcing of appropriate facilities for day-case management of these common problems.

The staffing necessary to maintain this level of day-case activity is nine consultant, nine junior medical and 25 nursing staff sessions, in addition to database management and secretarial support. Investigations and treatments take place in a dedicated seven-bed cardiovascular laboratory. Expertise and training are required in relevant components of geriatric medicine, cardiology and neurology.

The facility enables concentration of training and resources, and maximises the opportunities for implementing the new practice guidelines for syncope and falls [4,6]. Further research studies are needed of the health economic and health burden benefits of the facility. Resourcing of new facilities, possibly as a component of evolving intermediate care, will afford an ideal opportunity for further research of these health service questions.

☐ SUMMARY

Falls are a major healthcare and cost priority. Previous work has clearly shown benefit for multifactorial intervention strategies for falls in community-dwelling elderly. Emerging data from RCTs in the A&E department in Newcastle confirm that:

☐   falls and syncope are common reasons for attendance

☐   there is a significant overlap between symptoms of falls and syncope, and

☐   there is a clear benefit of detailed cardiovascular assessment in fallers, in particular for carotid sinus hypersensitivity, arrhythmias and orthostatic hypotension.

A dedicated day-case facility for older adults markedly reduces the number of emergency admissions for falls and syncope. It greatly reduces length of stay for admitted patients and allows focused implementation of recommended guidelines for falls and syncope. More widespread development of such units will go some way to alleviate the perpetual resource issues around emergency beds' activity in the UK.

Acknowledgements

I would like to acknowledge the work of the following research fellows on the three studies described: Dr D Andrew Richardson (SAFE PACE), Dr Fiona Shaw (SAFE COG) and Dr John Davison (SAFER).

REFERENCES

1   Rubenstein LZ, Josephson KR. The epidemiology of falls and syncope. In: Kenny RA (ed). *Clinics in Geriatric Medicine.* Philadelphia: WB Saunders (to be published Jan 2002).

2   Kenny RA, Dey AB. Syncope. In: Brocklehurst J, Tallis R, Fillit H (eds). *Textbook of Geriatric Medicine and Gerontology,* 5th edn. Oxford: Oxford University Press, 1998: 455–73.

3   Davies A, Steen N, Kenny RA. Carotid sinus hypersensitivity is common in older patients presenting to an accident and emergency department with unexplained falls. *Age Ageing* 2001; **30**: 289–93.

4   Guideline for the prevention of falls in older persons. American Geriatrics Society, British Geriatrics Society, and American Academy of Orthopaedic Surgeons Panel on Falls Prevention. *J Am Geriatr Soc* 2001; **49**: 664–72.

5   Close J, Ellis M, Hooper R, Glucksman E, *et al.* Prevention of falls in the elderly trial (PROFIT), a randomised controlled trial. *Lancet* 1999; **353**: 93–7.

6   Brignole M, Alboni P, Benditt D, Bergfeldt L, *et al.* Guidelines on management (diagnosis and treatment) of syncope. *Eur Heart J* 2001; **22**: 1256–306.

☐ SELF ASSESSMENT QUESTIONS

1   Carotid sinus hypersensitivity:
(a) Is rare after the age of 50
(b) Can present as falls
(c) Is present if carotid sinus massage induces sinus pauses
(d) Is best treated by AA1 pacing
(e) Is a component of sick sinus syndrome

2   Cardiovascular syncope:
(a) Is a distinct clinical syndrome
(b) Is often associated with amnesia for loss of consciousness
(c) Has a 20% annual incidence in over 75 year olds
(d) Is usually treated by cardiac pacing
(e) Is most often diagnosed by Holter heart rate monitoring

3   Falls in older adults:
(a) Usually result in injury

(b) Are less common in advanced age
(c) Are less common in nursing home settings
(d) Have multiple risk factors
(e) Are more common than in children

4   In patients with cognitive impairment who fall:
(a) Multifactorial interventions are inferior to single interventions
(b) Injuries are frequent
(c) Cardiovascular causes are common
(d) Culprit medications are common
(e) Gait and balance abnormalities are present in over 80%

ANSWERS

1a False	2a False	3a False	4a False
b True	b False	b False	b True
c False	c False	c False	c True
d False	d False	d True	d True
e False	e False	e False	e True

Updates in oncology

Melanoma: King Canute and a rising tide

Anna Stevenson and Martin Gore

□ INTRODUCTION

Malignant melanoma arises from melanocytes and comprises 2% of all cancers, with 5,000 cases newly diagnosed in the UK each year. There were 1,378 deaths from cutaneous melanoma in England and Wales in 1997. The median age of onset is 55–65 years, and amongst 20–34 year olds melanoma is the third most common cancer in women and the fourth most common in men.

Incidence trends

The incidence of melanoma is rising by 3–7% per year in white populations. In the UK, the incidence in 1995 was 6.7 and 8.5 per 100,000 in males and females, respectively, which equates to a lifetime risk of more than one in 200.

The increase in incidence seems to be cohort-related. New data suggest that rates of new cases are declining in the 25–55 year age group, whereas they are still increasing in the over 55 year olds. The reasons for the increased incidence of melanoma are unclear but may be due to:

- □ changes in recreational sun exposure

- □ a rise in the amount of ultraviolet (UV) B irradiation from sunlight due to depletion of stratospheric ozone, or

- □ improvement in early diagnosis.

Mortality trends

Mortality due to melanoma has increased between 1940 and 1990 but the rate of increase has slowed. Reductions in the rise in mortality, especially in women, have occurred in Australia, the Nordic countries and the US. Small decreases have been seen in the UK and Canada in more recent generations, but mortality is still rising in France, Italy and Czechoslovakia. It has been suggested that these three patterns correspond to differences between populations with respect to the promotion of sun protection and early diagnosis. Other factors include changes in the accuracy of reporting procedures, and possibly increased identification of indolent but invasive lesions.

□ AETIOLOGY

It seems likely that both sun exposure and genetic predisposition play important aetiological roles in melanoma. Known risk factors include:

□ a past history or family history of melanoma

□ fair complexion

□ freckling tendency

□ propensity to sunburn

□ time spent outdoors from the age of 10–24 years

□ immunosuppression

□ the presence of clinically atypical moles, congenital melanocytic nevi, or a high number of ordinary melanocytic nevi greater than 2 mm thick.

A 64-fold increased risk for individuals with 50 or more moles greater than or equal to 2 mm across has been reported, and it is thought that 20% of melanomas arise in a pre-existing naevus.

There is an inverse relationship between the incidence of melanoma and the degree of skin pigmentation. Melanoma is 12 and six times more common in white individuals and in those of Hispanic origin, respectively, than in black-skinned races with the same lifestyle.

Sun exposure

Evidence for the role of sunlight is largely epidemiological. People of European descent living in Australia have a significantly higher risk of melanoma than those remaining in Northern Europe. Residence close to the equator in early life is associated with an increased risk of melanoma. Migration studies suggest that moving to an area of more intense sun exposure also increases melanoma risk.

However, there is not a straightforward relationship between sun exposure and melanoma. Several observations argue against UV irradiation being the sole cause of melanoma:

1 The incidence of melanoma does not increase consistently across geographic areas with increasing sunlight.

2 Melanoma more commonly affects white-collar, educated, urban individuals than outdoor or blue-collar workers.

3 Many melanomas occur in relatively young people who have not had years of exposure to sunlight.

4 Melanoma can occur in relatively unexposed sites such as the palms, soles and mucous membranes.

An overview of 29 epidemiological studies suggests an association between melanoma and intermittent sun exposure. This would explain some of the discrepancies listed above. It is likely that the initiation and promotion of carcinogenesis by UV irradiation occur in genetically susceptible subpopulations.

Genetic predisposition

There is a strong family history of melanoma in 5–7% of patients. Many of these patients have the atypical mole syndrome (AMS) with a large number of naevi, some with atypical clinical appearance and dysplastic histological features. The presence of four or more atypical moles is associated with a relative risk of melanoma of 29. Familial cases can also occur in the absence of atypical moles.

Studies of melanoma kindreds suggest linkage to at least three independent loci, namely 9p21–22, 1q36 and 6p21–23. The tumour suppresser gene *INK4α* maps to 9p21–22. Inactivating germline mutations have been detected in this gene which affect one or both of the alternative transcripts encoding p16 (a cyclin-dependent kinase inhibitor) and p14ARF. Although p16 testing is possible, it is not currently recommended outside the investigational setting. Only a minority of familial melanoma families have been shown to have p16 mutations and in these families the penetrance of the gene is not yet known.

□ PRIMARY PREVENTION AND SCREENING FOR MELANOMA

Primary prevention

Despite lack of a clear understanding of the role of sunlight in melanoma carcinogenesis, there is enough epidemiological and laboratory evidence to support reducing sunlight exposure as a primary prevention strategy. This can be achieved via the use of protective clothing, shade and sunscreen lotion with a sun protection factor of at least 15. The last measure is thought to be particularly important in children.

Primary prevention of melanoma has been pioneered by Marks and Hill in Australia, where prevention programmes have been running for almost 20 years. These programmes have resulted in a large shift in knowledge, attitudes and beliefs about sunlight exposure and tanning and a major shift in behaviour [1]. In the UK, a study of 'Sun Awareness Week' in 1995 showed significant improvements in attitudes and behaviour scores [2].

Screening

Detection and treatment of melanoma early in its course are critical for improving outcome. In one study, the majority of patients detected their own melanoma (57%), with females more likely to self-detect than males (69% vs 47%; $p < 0.0001$). Physicians detected melanoma in 16% of patients, followed by the partner in 11%. Only 15% of patients with a past history of melanoma perform self-examinations, but even this low level is associated with a reduction in mortality.

Screening and education programmes dramatically increase the proportion of melanomas diagnosed as 'thin'. In Scotland, the percentage of tumours detected less than 1.5 mm thick rose from 38% in 1979–1984 to 54% in 1985–1989.

Patients at risk should be referred to a specialist clinic, for example, those with:

☐ a previous primary melanoma

☐ a large numbers of moles, some of which are clinically atypical

☐ a strong family history of melanoma (more than three cases in the extended family, two cases with AMS or multiple primary tumours in an individual).

☐ DIAGNOSIS

Melanoma can be located anywhere on the body but most commonly occurs on the lower limbs in women and the trunk in men. There is a seven-point checklist for naevi for use by both patients and general practitioners. Major signs are change in size, shape or colour of a lesion, and minor signs include inflammation, crusting, bleeding, sensory change (eg itch) and diameter above 5 mm. Any significant change in a pigmented lesion should be considered as an indication for excision biopsy.

☐ STAGING AND PROGNOSIS

The American Joint Committee on Cancer (AJCC) Staging has proposed a new classification system with staging ranging from 0 to IV [3]. Tumour stage at presentation is the most significant determinant of prognosis (Fig. 1) [4]. Most melanomas are diagnosed at stages I and II, and within these stages the most important prognostic factor is tumour thickness (Table 1). Breslow thickness,

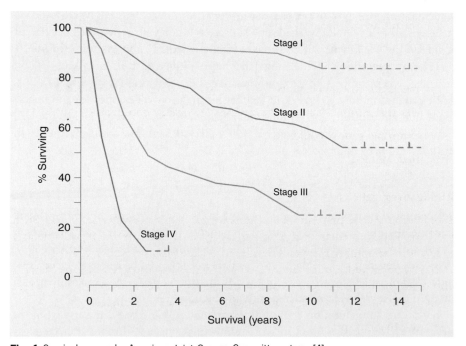

Fig. 1 Survival curves by American Joint Cancer Committee stage [4].

Table 1 Recommended excision margins for the treatment of primary melanoma.

	Margins	
Breslow thickness (mm)	**Minimum (cm)**	**Maximum (cm)**
Melanoma *in situ*	Complete histological excision	0.5
<1.0	1.0	1.0
1–4	1.0	1.0–2.0
≥4	1.0	2.0–3.0

defined as the total vertical height of the invasive lesion, defines subgroups with significantly different survival rates. Correlation between Breslow thickness and survival is better than Clark's level and survival. Clark's level classifies primary tumours according to histological depth of dermal invasion.

Survival

The majority of patients present with early stage disease and surgical excision of the primary melanoma achieves cure rates of at least 90%. Thin melanomas (<1 mm) are rarely associated with relapse, but patients with thick primaries (>4 mm) or melanoma metastatic to regional lymph nodes are at high risk of relapse and have a mortality of 50–90%.

The median survival of patients with metastatic melanoma is six months. Shorter survival has been observed to correlate with:

☐ the number of metastatic sites

☐ an Eastern Oncology Cooperative Group (ECOG) performance status of 1 or more

☐ metastatic disease in the gastrointestinal tract, liver, pleura or lung

☐ elevated serum lactate dehydrogenase and alkaline phosphatase

☐ abnormal platelet count, and

☐ male gender.

Staging investigations

Examination should concentrate on the skin, lymph nodes, central nervous system and liver. The most common first site of relapsed disease is in the regional lymph nodes, and the number of involved nodes correlates with survival (Fig. 2) [4].

No staging investigations are necessary for patients with stage I disease. Patients with moderate or high risk of recurrent disease (AJCC stage IIa and above) should be managed in a specialist centre and staging investigations include:

☐ full blood count

☐ biochemistry including liver enzymes

☐ chest X-ray, and

☐ ultrasound scan of the liver.

Further investigations should be undertaken only as clinically indicated.

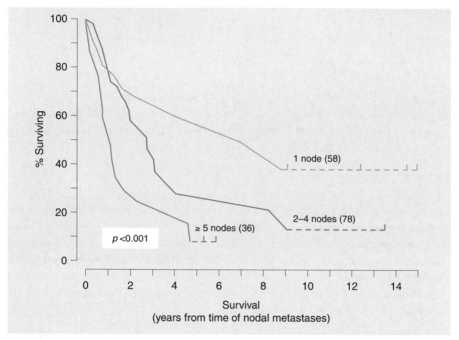

Fig. 2 Survival for American Joint Cancer Committee stage III melanoma patients according to the number of involved lymph nodes [4].

☐ TREATMENT

The mainstay of treatment of primary cutaneous melanoma or of skin or lymph node metastases is surgical excision. Currently, there is no role for adjuvant therapy outside the clinical trial setting, but different adjuvant options are being tested (see below). Recurrent local disease may be treated with surgery, isolated limb perfusion with chemotherapeutic agents, laser therapy or occasionally radiotherapy. Treatment of distant metastatic disease should be regarded as palliative. Studies are underway looking at the roles of biochemotherapy, vaccines and gene therapy in loco-regional (ie for limb melanoma, within the limb or in the regional draining lymph nodes, and for trunk or abdominal wall melanoma, at the excision site or in the regional draining lymph nodes) and metastatic disease.

Treatment of primary cutaneous melanoma

Suspicious skin lesions should be treated with a full thickness excision biopsy with a margin of 2 mm of normal skin. Shave and curette biopsy is absolutely contraindicated. If the diagnosis is confirmed, a subsequent re-excision with wider margins is required (Table 1).

Lymph node dissection

Therapeutic lymph node dissection (LND) is indicated in cases of confirmed regional lymph node involvement in the absence of distant metastases. In a patient with *suspected* lymph node involvement, the initial investigation of choice is fine-needle aspiration, not lymph node excision biopsy because the latter compromises the efficacy of subsequent LND. LND in melanoma should be approached as a way of curing patients with potentially regionally limited disease. Elective LND (ELND) involves lymphadenectomy in the absence of evidence of regional lymph node involvement. Two large randomised trials comparing ELND with observation showed no survival advantage. There is currently no role for ELND outside the trial setting.

Sentinel node biopsy

Sentinel node biopsy was developed as a means of identifying the first lymph node draining the skin in which a melanoma arises. The sentinel lymph node can be identified in over 95% of cases using intradermal radioactive colloid and methylene blue. By examining the excised node it can be determined whether a patient has regional lymph node disease. The indications for its use are not yet fully established, as it is not known whether it has any effect on outcome for the patient.

☐ FOLLOW-UP

Patients with *in situ* melanoma need be reviewed only once after complete excision to confirm adequate excision and to give appropriate education. All patients with invasive melanoma should be followed up on a three-monthly basis for the first three years. Thereafter, patients in whom the melanoma is less than 1 mm thick may be discharged, but the remainder should be reviewed six-monthly for the next two years. Overall, 80% of recurrences occur within the first three years, but a few patients (<8%) have recurrences 5–10 years after the initial surgery.

☐ ADJUVANT TREATMENT

Randomised trials of adjuvant chemotherapy, whether delivered locally (isolated limb perfusion) or systemically, have not shown survival improvement in patients who are at high risk of relapse. Trials using non-specific immune therapies such as *Corynebacterium parvum* transfer factor, levamisole and BCG are similarly negative. Interferon (IFN) and vaccines have also been investigated as possible adjuvant treatments.

Interferon

Three of the six randomised trials investigating the use of low-dose IFN showed an impact on disease-free survival, but none improved overall survival (Table 2). High-dose IFN has been investigated in four randomised studies, three using the

Table 2 Randomised trials of adjuvant interferon (IFN).

| | | Survival | |
Trial	No. of patients	Disease-free	Overall
High-dose IFN			
ECOG 1684	287	+	+
ECOG 1690	427	+	−
ECOG 1694	880	+	+
NCCTG	262	+	−
Low-dose IFN			
Austrian	311	+	−
French	499	+	−
EORTC 18871	830	−	−
Scottish	100	+	−
ECOG 1690	427	−	−
WHO 16	444	−	−

+ = statistically significant advantage for IFN; − = no advantage for IFN.
ECOG = Eastern Cooperative Oncology Group; EORTC = European Organisation for Research and Treatment of Cancer; NCCTG = North Central Cancer Treatment Group; WHO = World Health Organization.

so-called Kirkwood schedule (20 MU/m^2 intravenously five times per week for four weeks, followed by 10 MU/m^2 subcutaneously three times per week for 48 weeks) [5] and one using 20 MU/m^2 three times a week for 12 weeks. All patients showed a significant disease-free survival benefit.

There is still discussion over the significance of these results. Some have argued that the first study (ECOG 1684) only just reached statistical significance on a two-tail test and that the third study (ECOG 1694), which randomised patients to vaccination or high-dose IFN, was closed too early by the Data Monitoring Committee for meaningful interpretation to be possible. Considerable discussion has also taken place around the results of the second study (ECOG 1690) because the investigators suggested that patients on the observation arm who relapsed were 'rescued' by further therapy, particularly high-dose IFN.

IFN toxicity is dose-dependent. At high dose, limiting toxicities include fever, fatigue, anaemia, myalgia, weight loss and detriments in performance status. In ECOG 1684 there was significant toxicity, requiring dose reduction or discontinuation of treatment in over half the patients and there were two treatment-related deaths.

Adjuvant interferon-alpha

A preliminary analysis of a recent overview of adjuvant IFN-alpha [6] has shown a statistically significant benefit for IFN in terms of both disease-free and overall survival.

The results of three studies are awaited:

1   ECOG 1697, which uses only one month of high-dose IFN.

2   The European Organisation for Research and Treatment of Cancer (EORTC) trial 18952, which compares two intermediate-dose schedules.

3   Adjuvant Interferon in Melanoma (high risk) (AIM High), a further study of low-dose IFN.

Since the publication of ECOG 1684, high-dose IFN-alpha has commonly been used in the US in patients at high risk of recurrence. Most groups in Europe feel that confirmatory data are required before high-dose IFN could become standard adjuvant therapy.

Vaccines

Melanoma is one of the most immunogenic solid tumours and, as a result, has served as the major model for tumour vaccine development in both the laboratory and the clinic. Vaccines may be either cell-derived (autologous or allogeneic) or recombinant. The aim of vaccination therapy is to induce a specific host response to tumour antigens. Toxicity is generally low and usually confined to local irritation at the injection site. Vaccines are likely to be most effective in the presence of minimal tumour bulk or in the adjuvant setting.

None of the four randomised trials of vaccination as adjuvant therapy shows a survival benefit for vaccination (Table 3) (for review, see [7]), but three of them demonstrated a significant benefit in those patients who showed an immune response to the vaccination.

Substantial evidence now indicates that immune responses to human tumour antigens occur *in vivo*, and that such responses may be associated with improved prognosis. It is hoped that continued advances will lead to significant changes in the treatment of melanoma in the next decade.

☐ METASTATIC DISEASE

Patients with metastatic melanoma have a poor prognosis, with a median survival of six months and five-year survival rates below 4%. The aim of current therapy is palliation rather than cure. All patients should have access to a palliative care team

Table 3 Randomised trials of adjuvant vaccine therapy in melanoma (reviewed in [7]).

Vaccine	No. of patients	Overall survival
Melanoma cell	134	No difference
GM2	122	No difference
Shed antigen	38	No difference
Vaccinia lysate	250	No difference

providing expertise in symptom control and psychosocial support. There is no consistent randomised evidence for a significant improvement in overall survival with any systemic therapy but responses to treatment can result in good palliation. Where possible, patients should be offered participation in clinical trials. Withholding treatment may be a valid option in the presence of slow-growing asymptomatic metastases, and deferment of treatment allows quality of life to be maintained. The strongest predictors of outcome are:

☐   performance status

☐   disease-free interval

☐   number of organs involved, and

☐   absence of liver involvement.

Chemotherapy

The single most active drug is dacarbazine (DTIC), with best response rates of 15–20% [7]. It is well tolerated when given with a 5-hydroxytryptamine-3 receptor antagonist. Response rates of 10–15% are observed with platinum compounds, vinca alkaloids, nitrosoureas and the taxanes. The nitrosourea fotemustine readily penetrates the blood-brain barrier, and response rates of up to 24% have been reported in patients with brain metastases. Temozolomide is an oral pro-drug of DTIC; it was shown to be equally effective in a randomised comparison against DTIC in 305 patients.

The median duration of response with single-agent chemotherapy is 6–10 months and complete responses are uncommon. Patients with skin, subcutaneous tissue and lymph node involvement respond most frequently (25–35%), while only 15% of those with lung metastases respond and only 5–10% of those with bone, liver and brain metastases.

Randomised trials have shown no benefit for combination chemotherapy over single-agent treatment in terms of response rate or survival, both disease-free and overall.

Immunotherapy

The host immune response is thought to play an important role in the natural history of melanoma for several reasons:

☐   there are documented cases of spontaneous remission

☐   activated lymphocyte populations have been described in tumour tissue, and

☐   the observation that vitiligo is a favourable prognostic factor for overall survival.

As a result, there has been considerable interest in the use of biological response modifiers such as IFN-alpha and interleukin (IL)-2, biochemotherapy (the combination of immunotherapy with chemotherapy) and vaccines.

Interferon-alpha

IFN-alpha has a role in promoting tumour cell differentiation and in enhancing the expression of major histocompatibility cell (MHC) I and II and hence tumour-associated antigens. It also has immunomodulatory effects via the activation of natural killer (NK) cells, cytotoxic T lymphocytes (CTL) and macrophages. Furthermore, it is also anti-angiogenic. An overview of 11 trials (315 patients) using IFN-alpha as a single agent in metastatic melanoma showed a response rate of 15% (range 0–27%) [8]. Responses were seen in both previously treated and untreated patients and there was no cross-resistance with chemotherapy. A third of responses were complete, several of which were durable, but median survival was only eight months. Toxicity of IFN-alpha is manageable and usually limited to nausea, flu-like symptoms (fever, chills, myalgia, anorexia, headache) and lethargy. Rare toxicities include pancytopenia, abnormal liver function tests and neuropsychiatric symptoms.

Interleukin-2

IL-2 is an immunostimulatory cytokine with antitumour effects mediated indirectly via activation of NK cells and specific cytotoxic T cells, lymphokine-activated killer cells. An overview of 15 trials (540 patients) reported an overall response rate of 15% (range 3–50%), with only 2% of patients achieving complete remission [9]. In contrast to chemotherapy, responses are seen with similar frequency in patients with and without visceral metastases.

The toxicity of IL-2 depends on the dose and route of administration, and includes flu-like symptoms, hypotension, vascular leak syndrome and renal, gastrointestinal and haematological toxicities. Hospitalisation for treatment is required, but even high doses can be administered safely with supportive care anticipating these toxicities.

Monocytes and macrophages in the tumour microenvironment induce anergy to IL-2 and apoptosis in tumour-infiltrating lymphocytes (TILs). Histamine dihydrochloride (maxamine) protects T cells and NK cells against monocyte- and macrophage-induced apoptosis and may restore reactivity to IL-2. A phase III study of maxamine plus IL-2 versus IL-2 alone suggested a significant survival advantage for the combination, with a median survival of 355 days and 187 days, respectively ($p = 0.0033$). Confirmatory data are awaited.

IFN-alpha and IL-2 have been used in combination because of their different mechanisms of action and experimental evidence suggesting synergy, but no clear advantage for the combination has been observed.

Biochemotherapy

Chemotherapy and immunotherapy have different mechanisms of action and different toxicity profiles. A number of preclinical studies have indicated additive or synergistic effects for the combination of these two approaches. Five randomised trials have investigated the combination of IFN-alpha with chemotherapy using single-agent DTIC, but only one of them suggested a significant improvement in response or survival with the addition of IFN-alpha.

A recent phase III study in which 105 patients with advanced melanoma were randomised to receive either IFN-alpha and DTIC or combination chemotherapy there was no significant difference in response rate (17.3% vs 26.4%) or for one-year or median overall survival. IFN-alpha has also been added to a number of combination chemotherapy regimens, without significant improvement in response or survival over combination chemotherapy alone.

Fewer trials have looked at the combination of IL-2 and chemotherapy and the regimens and doses vary enormously. A meta-analysis of 19 trials (523 patients) found a response rate of 22% with a median survival of 9.5 months – not significantly different from that seen with chemotherapy or immunotherapy alone.

The term 'biochemotherapy' has recently come to describe a combination of both IFN-alpha and IL-2 with chemotherapy. The most effective biochemotherapy regimens appear to be those containing cisplatin. One of the earliest phase II trials of biochemotherapy, using cisplatin, IL-2 and IFN-alpha, showed a response rate of 54% and a complete remission rate of 13%. Other single-arm studies showed similar promising results. The most notable finding from these phase II studies is that of durable complete responses. However, these regimens are toxic, with patients suffering myelosuppression, gastrointestinal toxicity, capillary leak syndrome, cardiac toxicity and autoimmune phenomena.

Five prospective randomised trials of biochemotherapy in metastatic melanoma have been published (Table 4) [10–14]. An EORTC study has suggested a benefit for the addition of cisplatin to IL-2 and IFN-alpha in terms of response rate (33% vs 18%, $p = 0.04$) and progression-free survival (92 days vs 53 days, $p = 0.02$). Other trials have failed to demonstrate a convincing advantage for biochemotherapy.

Table 4 Randomised studies of biochemotherapy in metastatic melanoma.

Ref.	No. of patients	Regimen	Response rate (%)	Survival (months)
10	65	BCDT ± IL-2 + IFN-α	27 vs 22	No difference
11	102	CDT ± IL-2 + IFN-α	44 vs 27	No difference
12	92	DT + IL-2 + IFN	13	No difference
		CVDT + IFN	35	No difference
		CVDT + IFN + IL-2	37	
13	138	IL-2 + IFN ± cisplatin	15 vs 36 ($p = 0.01$)	No difference
14	118	CD + IFN-α ± IL-2	28 vs 22	Final analysis awaited

BCDT = carmustine (BCNU), cisplatin, dacarbazine (DTIC) and tamoxifen; CD = cisplatin and dacarbazine; CDT = cisplatin, dacarbazine and tamoxifen; CVDT = cisplatin, vindesine, dacarbazine and tamoxifen; DT = dacarbazine and tamoxifen; IFN = interferon; IL = interleukin.

□ VACCINES

Vaccine therapy has been examined in metastatic melanoma as well as adjuvant therapy. Melacine, a vaccine using allogeneic melanoma lysates and the novel adjuvant, detox (a 'detoxified' bacterial endotoxin), has been administered with cyclophosphamide in a randomised comparison with combination chemotherapy (DTIC, cisplatin, carmustine and tamoxifen). The response rates and survival were not significantly different, but melacine was associated with fewer and milder side effects.

Genetic modification of both autologous and allogeneic melanoma cells has been used to generate vaccines that overexpress a number of immunomodulatory agents, including IL-2, IFN-gamma and granulocyte-macrophage colony stimulating factor. As in the adjuvant setting, some studies have shown a significant treatment benefit in those patients demonstrating a host response. For example, autologous cells from 12 patients with metastatic disease were genetically engineered using recombinant retroviruses to secrete IL-2. No clinical responses were seen, but there were delayed type hypersensitivity (DTH) or CTL responses in five patients and significant improvement in the median disease-free survival in this group (7 months vs 1 month, $p = 0.005$) [15].

A number of peptide antigens recognised by T cells have been identified. These are HLA-restricted and are either tumour-specific (melanoma antigen genes, eg MAGE, BAGE and CAGE) or differentiation antigens (tyrosinase, glycoprotein (gp) 100 and melanoma antigen recognised by TIL cells (MART-1). In a trial reported by the National Cancer Institute, patients with stage IV melanoma were vaccinated with a single modified gp100 with or without IL-2 [16]. The combination produced responses in 42% of patients with metastatic disease, a significant improvement over results from trials of high dose IL-2 alone. Interestingly, clinical responses were not dependent on generation of a CTL response.

Another technique involves the use of dendritic cells. These antigen presenting cells are extracted from peripheral blood and exposed *in vitro* to peptides prior to injection back into the patient. Responses, including some durable complete responses, were seen in five of 16 patients with advanced melanoma in one trial. In addition, DTH responses to vaccination in this study correlated with clinical response.

□ CONCLUSIONS

Melanoma is an increasing public health problem. Continued work is needed to analyse trends in incidence and mortality in order to assess the efficacy of primary prevention and screening campaigns. Emphasis should be placed on preventing the disease and diagnosing it while it is curable. Primary prevention and education campaigns should encourage a reduction in sunlight exposure and the avoidance of sunburn, especially in children. Surveillance should be targeted at high-risk populations.

An increasing number of active agents, both chemotherapeutic and immunomodulatory, are becoming available, but this has yet to be translated into any survival benefit either in the adjuvant or metastatic setting. It is unlikely that immunotherapy alone will be effective in the treatment of patients with bulky metastatic disease. Its role will probably be in the adjuvant setting.

Currently, there is no standard adjuvant treatment, but trials of vaccines and IFN are ongoing. Single-agent DTIC remains the gold standard treatment for patients with metastatic melanoma, and is therefore the agent against which new treatments should be compared.

REFERENCES

1   Marks R. Two decades of the public health approach to skin cancer control in Australia: why, how and where are we now? Review. *Australas J Dermatol* 1999; **40**: 1–5.

2   Fleming C, Newell J, Turner S, Mackie R. A study of the impact of Sun Awareness Week 1995. *Br J Dermatol* 1997; **136**: 719–24.

3   Balch CM, Buzaid AC, Atkins MB, Cascinelli N, *et al*. A new American Joint Committee on Cancer staging for cutaneous melanoma. *Cancer* 2000; **88**: 1484–91.

4   Albino AP, Reed JA, McNutt NS. Malignant melanoma. In: Devita VT, Hellman S, Rosenberg SA (ed). *Cancer Principles and Practice of Oncology*. Philadelphia: Lippencott-Raven, 1997: 1935–2012.

5   Kirkwood JM, Strawderman MH, Ernstoff MS, Smith TJ, *et al*. Interferon alfa-2b adjuvant therapy of high-risk resected cutaneous melanoma: the Eastern Cooperative Oncology Group Trial EST 1684. *J Clin Oncol* 1996; **14**: 7–17.

6   Hancock BW, Harris S, Wheatley K, Gore M. Adjuvant interferon-alpha in malignant melanoma: current status. Review. *Cancer Treat Rev* 2000; **26**: 81–9.

7   Chowdhury S, Vaughan MM, Gore ME. New approaches to the systemic treatment of melanoma. Review. *Cancer Treat Rev* 1999; **25**: 259–70.

8   Legha SS. The role of interferon alfa in the treatment of metastatic melanoma. Review. *Semin Oncol* 1997; **24**(1 Suppl 4): S24–31.

9   Philip PA, Flaherty L. Treatment of malignant melanoma with interleukin-2. *Semin Oncol* 1997; **24**(1 Suppl 4): S32–8.

10 Johnston SR, Constenla DO, Moore J, Atkinson H, *et al*. Randomized phase II trial of BCDT (carmustine (BCNU), cisplatin, dacarbazine (DTIC) and tamoxifen) with or without interferon alpha (IFN-alpha) and interleukin (IL-2) in patients with metastatic melanoma. *Br J Cancer* 1998; **77**: 1280–6.

11 Rosenberg S, Yang J, Schwartzentruber D, Hwu P, *et al*. Prospective randomized trial of the treatment of patients with metastatic melanoma using chemotherapy with cisplatin, dacarbazine, and tamoxifen alone or in combination with interleukin-2 and interferon alfa-2b. *J Clin Oncol* 1999; **17**: 968–75.

12 Sertoli M, Queirolo P, Bajetta E, DelVecchio M, *et al*. Multi-institutional phase II randomized trial of integrated therapy with cisplatin, dacarbazine, vindesine, subcutaneous interleukin-2, interferon alpha2a and tamoxifen in metastatic melanoma. BREMIM (Biological Response Modifiers in Melanoma). *Melanoma Res* 1999; **9**: 503–9.

13 Keilholz U, Goey SH, Punt CJ, Proebstle TM, *et al*. Interferon alfa-2a and interleukin-2 with or without cisplatin in metastatic melanoma: a randomized trial of the European Organization for Research and Treatment of Cancer Melanoma Cooperative Group. *J Clin Oncol* 1997; **15**: 2579–88.

14 Keilholz U, Punt C, Gore M, Kruit W, *et al*. Dacarbazine, cisplatin and interferon alpha with or without interleukin-2 in advanced melanoma: interim analysis of EORTC trial 18951. *Proc Am Soc Clin Oncol* 1999; **18**: 2043(abstract).

15 Palmer K, Moore J, Everard M, Harris JD, *et al*. Gene therapy with autologous, interleukin 2-secreting tumor cells in patients with malignant melanoma. *Hum Gene Ther* 1999; **10**: 1261–8.

16 Rosenberg SA, Yang JC, Schwartzentruber DJ, Hwu P, *et al*. Immunologic and therapeutic evaluation of a synthetic peptide vaccine for the treatment of patients with metastatic melanoma. *Nat Med* 1998; **4**: 321–7.

☐ SELF ASSESSMENT QUESTIONS

1   Known risk factors for melanoma include:
    (a) Family history of melanoma
    (b) Propensity to sunburn
    (c) Immunosuppression
    (d) The presence of leg ulcers
    (e) The presence of atypical moles

2   In melanoma, the following treatment strategies are recommended:
    (a) Shave and curette biopsy of the primary lesion for initial histology
    (b) Re-excision with wide margins following a positive biopsy
    (c) Fine-needle aspiration to confirm suspected lymph node involvement
    (d) Elective lymph node dissection
    (e) Adjuvant isolated limb perfusion

3   Regarding chemotherapy and the treatment of metastatic melanoma:
    (a) Single-agent dacarbazine (DTIC) improves disease-free and overall
         survival
    (b) DTIC has response rates of 15–20% and is poorly tolerated
    (c) The taxanes have activity in melanoma
    (d) Overall survival is improved by the use of combination chemotherapy
         compared with single-agent DTIC
    (e) Patients with skin metastases respond more frequently than those with
         liver metastases

4   Regarding immunotherapy in metastatic melanoma:
    (a) Interferon (IFN)-alpha promotes tumour cell differentiation
    (b) The response rate to single agent IFN-alpha is 50–60%
    (c) IFN-alpha can cause neuropsychiatric symptoms
    (d) Immunotherapy works best in patients with bulky disease
    (e) Immunotherapy cannot be used after chemotherapy because of cross-
         resistance

5   Regarding the use of vaccines in melanoma:
    (a) Vaccines may be cell-derived or recombinant
    (b) Vaccines are generally toxic and poorly tolerated
    (c) Vaccines are probably most effective in the presence of minimal tumour
         bulk or in the adjuvant setting
    (d) Benefit following vaccination usually depends on the generation of a host
         immune response
    (e) Randomised trials of vaccination in the adjuvant setting consistently show
         an overall survival benefit for vaccination

ANSWERS

1a True	2a False	3a False	4a True	5a True
b True	b True	b False	b False	b False
c True	c True	c True	c True	c True
d False	d False	d False	d False	d True
e True	e False	e True	e False	e False

Growth hormone antagonism: a paradigm shift in the treatment of acromegaly

Susannah Rowles, Craig Parkinson and Peter Trainer

☐ INTRODUCTION

Acromegaly is characterised by a distinct phenotype (Fig. 1) and in virtually all cases is the result of excess growth hormone (GH) secretion from a pituitary adenoma. While the consequent disfigurement is recognised, it is less well appreciated that the

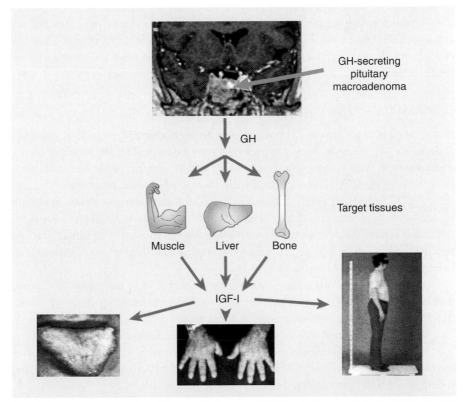

Fig. 1 Cartoon representation of the growth hormone (GH)/insulin-like growth factor (IGF) axis. GH regulates IGF-I generation in multiple target organs. IGF-I, which has autocrine, paracrine and endocrine actions, is responsible for many of the manifestations of acromegaly. The liver is the main source of circulating IGF-I. In the example shown, a pituitary macroadenoma is the source of GH secretion. Macroglossia, soft tissue thickening of the hands and gigantism are illustrated [1].

consequence of long-term elevation of circulating GH levels is premature death. Improvements in biochemical and radiological techniques mean that acromegaly is now diagnosed with increasing frequency, but it remains a rare condition with an estimated incidence of 3–4 per million and a prevalence of 55–59 per million [2].

Over 70% of patients with acromegaly have a pituitary macroadenoma (>1 cm diameter) which, in addition to secreting excess GH, may produce visual field defects and cranial nerve palsies by upward extension to compress the optic chiasm or lateral growth into the cavernous sinuses. Compression of the normal pituitary tissue often leads to hypopituitarism, a condition itself associated with increased mortality and morbidity.

GH is synthesised and secreted in a pulsatile manner by the somatotroph cells in the anterior lobe of the pituitary gland. Insulin-like growth factor-I (IGF-I) is secreted in response to GH stimulation in various tissues, including liver, muscle and bone. Much of the action of IGF-I may be autocrine or paracrine, but circulating IGF-I, which is predominately hepatic in origin, is also important. Most of the actions of GH can be attributed to IGF-I, but those not mediated by IGF-I are still consequent upon GH inducing GH receptor dimerisation with alternative genes being induced.

☐ MORBIDITY AND MORTALITY

In a retrospective analysis of 151 patients diagnosed at an average age of 41 years, life expectancy was shortened by approximately one decade [3]. As in other series, cardiovascular causes accounted for most of the deaths, with elevated post-treatment serum GH levels associated with a worse prognosis. A survey of the case records of 1,362 patients with acromegaly [4] found increased mortality as a result of cardiovascular, cerebrovascular and respiratory disease in patients with post-treatment serum GH levels above 5 mU/l. The overall incidence of cancer was not elevated, although colon cancer related mortality was higher than expected in patients with serum GH levels above 5 mU/l.

Bates *et al* [3] reported a relative mortality ratio of 2.68 in patients with elevated post-treatment serum GH levels, but mortality rates were normal in patients with post-treatment serum GH levels below 5 mU/l. More recent data from Swearingen *et al* [5] also suggest that normalisation of serum IGF-I restores life expectancy to normal.

Therefore, although there are several aims of treatment (Table 1), the primary goal is the reduction of mean circulating GH concentrations to below 5 mU/l and reduction of IGF-I into the age-related reference range.

☐ TREATMENT

Three treatment modalities are employed in the management of acromegaly:

1   Surgery.

2   Radiotherapy.

3   Pharmacological intervention.

Table 1 Aims of treatment.

- Reduction of serum growth hormone to below 5 mU/l
- Reduction of insulin-like growth factor-I into age-related reference age
- Removal – or at least debulking – of tumour mass
- Relief of symptoms and soft tissue swelling
- Prevention of further skeletal deformity
- Preservation of pituitary function

Surgery

Transsphenoidal surgery remains the primary mode of therapy for acromegaly. Several variables influence the outcome but a critical factor is the choice of pituitary surgeon. In the best centres the biochemical remission rate for microadenomas (<1 cm) is about 90% [6], while in the worst published series it is only 39% [7]. Even in the hands of an expert pituitary surgeon the 'cure' rate falls to less than 30% for macroadenomas [7]. Pre-operative serum GH levels, together with tumour size and position (ie cavernous sinus invasion), are other important determinants of outcome.

Radiotherapy

Radiotherapy is largely restricted to patients in whom surgery has not lowered serum GH and IGF-I levels into the target range or who are unfit for operation. Three-field multifraction conventional pituitary radiotherapy (4,500 cGy in 25 fractions over 5 weeks) has been used since the 1960s and is highly effective, although it may take many years to lower serum GH to below 5 mU/l and invariably causes hypopituitarism. Pretreatment serum GH is the best predictor of the rapidity of GH biochemical remission, with a 50% reduction in serum GH anticipated in the first two years following treatment [8]. Stereotactic radiotherapy, namely, the gamma knife and linear accelerator, are being developed but few data are available.

Pharmacological intervention

Most GH-secreting pituitary tumours are macroadenomas. Since radiotherapy can take many years to control serum GH levels, there is a need to control GH secretion meanwhile.

The dopamine agonist bromocriptine was the first effective medical treatment for acromegaly but, at best, will normalise GH and IGF-I levels in only 10% of patients. Cabergoline is a more potent, longer acting and better-tolerated dopamine agonist that normalises serum IGF-I in up to 39% of patients [9].

The introduction of the somatostatin (SMS) analogue octreotide in the early 1990s represented a major advance in the treatment of acromegaly. SMS, as a 14- and N-terminal extended 28 amino acid peptide, is widely distributed in the body, predominantly within the central nervous system and gastrointestinal (GI) tract. It is an important inhibitor of hormone secretion, including GH, thyroid-stimulating hormone, insulin, glucagon and many other hormones. At least five subtypes of somatostatin receptor have been identified, with types 2 and 5 the most important for the regulation of GH secretion. The two commercial analogues, octreotide and lanreotide, are eight amino acid peptides with greater specificity for inhibiting GH secretion and a longer half-life than native SMS.

Pretreatment serum GH levels and tumour SMS receptor status are the most important determinants of efficacy of SMS therapy, highlighting the importance of adequate tumour debulking at initial pituitary surgery. SMS is reported to lower GH and IGF-I into the target range in up to 60% of patients [10]. Although generally well tolerated, GI side effects can be troublesome, particularly on initiation of therapy. Up to 50% of patients develop gallstones, although these are rarely symptomatic. Octreotide is available both as a thrice daily subcutaneous injection and as a monthly intramuscular (IM) depot injection, while lanreotide is given as a fortnightly IM injection.

☐ GROWTH HORMONE RECEPTOR ANTAGONISTS

An understanding of the interaction between GH and its receptor is necessary to comprehend the mechanism of action of the GH receptor antagonist.

Human GH is a linear 191 amino acid chain, with a secondary structure maintained by two disulphide bonds and containing two separate sites for receptor binding (Fig. 2). In a sequential process, GH first binds via site 1 to a GH receptor and, subsequently, via site 2 to a second identical GH receptor. This results in the functional GH receptor dimerisation necessary for GH signal transduction (Fig. 3) [11].

A GH receptor antagonist that blocks functional receptor dimerisation is created by substitution of an arginine for glycine in position 120 of the third α-helix of GH (corresponding to site 2) that sterically hinders binding of the second receptor.

☐ PEGVISOMANT

Pegvisomant is a recombinant protein of human DNA origin, identical in sequence to GH except for eight amino acid substitutions within site 1, which give it a substantially higher affinity for the GH receptor at site 1 than native GH, and one substitution at position 120 (glycine to arginine) (Fig. 4). It has been conjugated with polyethylene glycol polymers to increase its hydrodynamic volume and thereby slow systemic clearance. This has the dual advantages of increasing the half-life of the protein from 11 minutes to more than 70 hours and reducing its immunogenicity [12].

GH receptor antagonist therapy does not attempt to inhibit GH secretion, so GH level cannot be used as a measure of disease activity in patients receiving pegvisomant. Furthermore, the high homology with wild-type GH means that pegvisomant is detected by conventional GH assays. Serum IGF-I is the preferred measure of disease activity in patients on pegvisomant therapy and the goal of treatment is reduction of serum IGF-I into the age-related reference range.

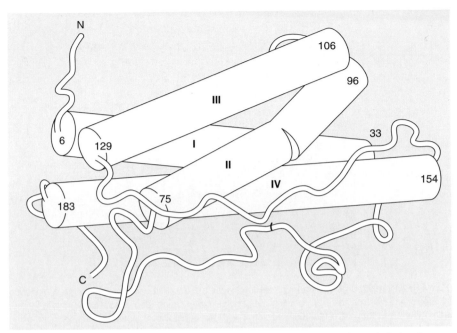

Fig. 2 Structure of growth hormone. It is a 191 amino acid peptide with a four α-helix bundle core (shown as cylinders) and two disulphide bonds (not shown). The third α-helix is crucial for the growth stimulating activity.

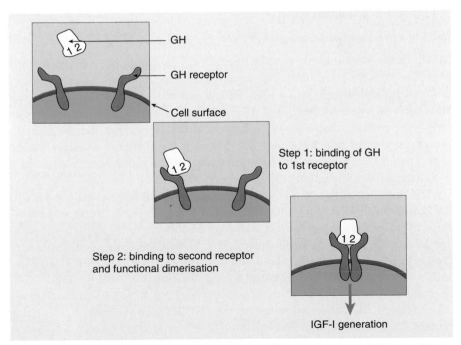

Fig. 3 Mechanism of growth hormone (GH) binding and signal transduction. GH has two binding sites, each of which binds identical cell surface receptors. Binding of both sites causes functional GH receptor dimerisation (IGF = insulin-like growth factor).

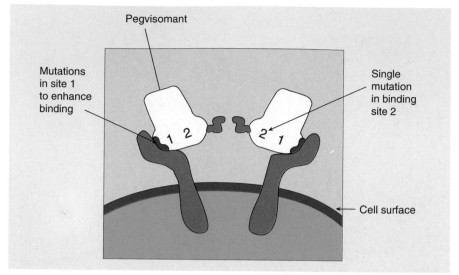

Fig. 4 Pegvisomant, a growth hormone (GH) analogue of 191 amino acids with a single substitution at position 120 (gly to arg) to inhibit functional dimerisation and insulin-like growth factor-I generation. A further eight mutations at site 1 give the antagonist a kinetic advantage over GH in site 1 binding.

Studies with pegvisomant

Reduction in serum insulin-like growth factor-I

In an initial randomised, placebo-controlled, double-blind, six-week study pegvisomant was administered once weekly to 46 patients with acromegaly in two doses (30 mg and 80 mg). Serum IGF-I fell significantly (15% and 30% on the lower and higher doses, respectively), but disappointingly normalisation was achieved in only three patients. Subsequently, pharmacokinetic modelling indicated that a dosing interval of one week was not sufficient to maintain adequate plasma concentrations of pegvisomant between doses and all subsequent studies have involved daily administration [13].

The landmark study indicating the efficacy of pegvisomant treated 112 patients for 12 weeks with daily pegvisomant at doses of 10 mg, 15 mg or 20 mg, or placebo. Prior to randomisation, serum IGF-I was at least 30% above the upper limit of the age-related reference range in all patients (Fig. 5). In all three pegvisomant-treated groups there was a statistically significant, dose-dependent decrease in serum IGF-I within two weeks which was sustained for the duration of the study. Serum IGF-I normalised in 54%, 81% and 89% of patients receiving 10 mg, 15 mg and 20 mg daily, respectively. Other measures of the GH/IGF axis, namely IGF binding protein 3, acid labile subunit and free IGF-I, demonstrated similar dose-dependent improvements. In addition, patient well-being (Fig. 6), specifically perspiration, fatigue and soft tissue swelling, improved in a dose-dependent manner. Subjective improvement in soft tissue swelling was objectively confirmed in the 15 mg and

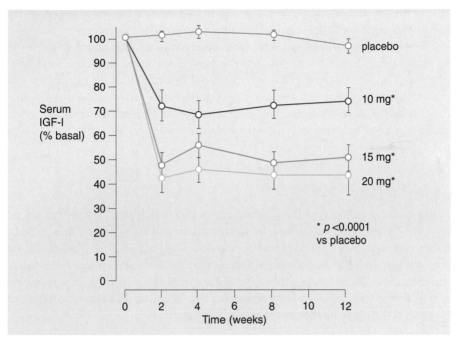

Fig. 5 The change in serum insulin-like growth factor-I (IGF-I) as a percentage of basal in patients with acromegaly treated with daily pegvisomant or placebo (mean change ± SEM).

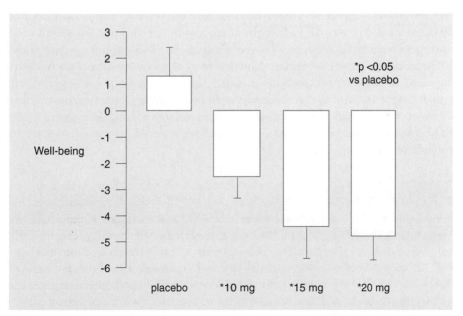

Fig. 6 Improvement in well-being (fall in symptom score) after 12 weeks of daily pegvisomant (mean change ± SEM).

20 mg treatment groups by a reduction in the size of the ring finger of the non-dominant hand using standardised European jewellers' rings.

In a subsequent open-label extension dose titration study using doses up to 40 mg per day, serum IGF-I fell into the age-related reference range in 97% of patients. The fall in serum IGF-I was mirrored by an increase in circulating GH measured using an assay that does not detect pegvisomant. This rise occurred during the first two weeks of treatment and remained constant thereafter, and may reflect either increased secretion or reduced clearance of GH, or both. Further study is needed of the mechanisms involved [14].

Tolerability of pegvisomant

Pegvisomant has been well tolerated in placebo-controlled studies, with no difference in reported side effects between placebo and active limbs. Two patients developed significant asymptomatic elevation of hepatic transaminases on pegvisomant. In both cases liver function returned to normal on discontinuation of treatment. The disturbance in liver function recurred in one patient on undergoing a rechallenge with 10 mg of pegvisomant. The aetiology is unknown, but liver function will need to be monitored in future patients.

Tumour bulk reduction

Pegvisomant, unlike all other treatment modalities for acromegaly, does not act on the pituitary and will not induce tumour shrinkage. Concerns have been raised that the elevation of serum GH during treatment with pegvisomant may be indicative of tumour growth. All patients on pegvisomant have had pituitary magnetic resonance scans performed by a single radiologist at six-month intervals to allow monitoring of tumour volume. No change has been observed in mean tumour volume in the 92 patients who have had pegvisomant for more than six months. Two tumours increased in size, but the available evidence suggests that both were aggressively growing tumours prior to commencing pegvisomant therapy. However, the number of patients studied and the duration of treatment are modest, with the majority having had previous radiotherapy. More data are required on tumour volume in patients receiving pegvisomant.

□ CONCLUSIONS

Acromegaly is associated with increased morbidity and mortality. If untreated, the premature mortality is significant. Evidence suggests that such mortality is significantly reduced by decreasing serum GH to below 5 mU/l and IGF-I levels to those of an age-matched population. Surgery, radiotherapy and available medical therapies are all directed at the pituitary and their efficacy is dependent on tumour characteristics. For surgery, the choice of surgeon is crucial to the prospects of a successful outcome.

In contrast, the GH receptor antagonist pegvisomant blocks GH action and reduces serum IGF-I by preventing functional GH receptor dimerisation. Clinical studies have demonstrated that pegvisomant is a highly effective new medical therapy for acromegaly, with normalisation of IGF-I levels in up to 97% of patients and corresponding improvement in patient well-being. It is incumbent on those using pegvisomant to demonstrate that long-term suppression of GH action, as evidenced by normalisation of serum IGF-I, is associated with improvement in morbidity and mortality.

REFERENCES

1   Wass JAH. Acromegaly. In: Besser M, Turner MO, Reichlin S, Wass JAH, Sonksen PH (eds). *Slide Atlas of Clinical Endocrinology*, 2nd edn. Wolfe Publishing, Mosby-Year Book Europe Limited, 1994, Ch 3.

2   Melmed S, Ho K, Klibanski A, Reichlin S, Thorner M. Recent advances in pathogenesis, diagnosis and management of acromegaly. Review. *J Clin Endocrinol Metab* 1995; 80: 3395–402.

3   Bates AS, Van't Hoff W, Jones JM, Clayton RN. An audit of outcome of treatment in acromegaly. *Q J Med* 1993; 86: 293–9.

4   Orme SM, McNally RJ, Cartwright RA, Belchetz PE. Morbidity and cancer incidence in acromegaly: a retrospective cohort study. United Kingdom Acromegaly Study Group. *J Clin Endocrinol Metab* 1998; 83: 2730–4.

5   Swearingen B, Barker FG 2nd, Katznelson L, Biller BM, *et al*. Long-term mortality after transsphenoidal surgery for acromegaly. *J Clin Endocrinol Metab* 1998; 83: 3419–26.

6   Sheaves R, Jenkins P, Blackburn P, Huneidi AH, *et al*. Outcome of transsphenoidal surgery for acromegaly using strict criteria for surgical cure. *Clin Endocrinol (Oxford)* 1996; 45: 407–13.

7   Lissett C, Peacey SR, Laing I, Tetlow L, *et al*. The outcome of surgery for acromegaly: the need for a specialist pituitary surgeon for all types of growth hormone (GH) secreting adenoma. Review. *Clin Endocrinol (Oxford)* 1998; 49: 653–7.

8   Van der Lely AJ, de Herder WW, Lamberts SW. The role of radiotherapy in acromegaly. Review. *J Clin Endocrinol Metabol* 1997; 82: 3185–6.

9   Abs R, Verhelst J, Maiter D, van Acker K, *et al*. Cabergoline in the treatment of acromegaly: a study in 64 patients. *J Clin Endocrinol Metab* 1998; 83: 374–8.

10   Barkan AL. Acromegaly: diagnosis and therapy. Review. *Endocrinol Metab Clin North Am* 1989; 18: 277–310.

11   de Vos AM, Ultsch M, Kossiakoff AA. Human growth hormone and extracellular domain of its receptor: crystal structure of the complex. *Science* 1992; 255: 306–12.

12   Parkinson C, Trainer PJ. Growth hormone receptor antagonists therapy for acromegaly. Review. *Baillières Best Pract Res Clin Endocrinol Metab* 1999; 13: 419–30.

13   Thorner MO, Strasburger CJ, Wu Z, Straume M, *et al*. Growth hormone (GH) receptor blockade with a PEG-modified GH (B2036-PEG) lowers serum insulin-like growth factor-I but does not acutely stimulate serum GH. *J Clin Endocrinol Metab* 1999; 84: 2098–103.

14   Trainer PJ, Drake WM, Katznelson L, Freda PU, *et al*. Treatment of acromegaly with the growth hormone-receptor antagonist pegvisomant. *N Engl J Med* 2000; 342: 1171–7.

☐ SELF ASSESSMENT QUESTIONS

1   Patients with acromegaly may present with:
(a) Hypotension
(b) Sleep apnoea
(c) Gigantism in over 20% of cases
(d) Bitemporal hemianopia
(e) Amenorrhoea

2   In acromegaly:
   (a) Untreated acromegaly reduces life expectancy by 10 years
   (b) Insulin-like growth factor (IGF) binding protein-2 is consistently elevated
   (c) Somatostatin analogue treatment lowers serum growth hormone (GH) to below 5 mU/l in 90% of patients
   (d) Pegvisomant increases circulating GH levels
   (e) Conventional assays can distinguish GH from pegvisomant

3   IGF-I:
   (a) Is a peptide
   (b) Is synthesised by the somatotroph cells of the anterior pituitary gland
   (c) Levels are reduced in patients treated with pegvisomant
   (d) Acts by inducing receptor dimerisation
   (e) Has a circadian rhythm

4   Pegvisomant:
   (a) Is a potent GH antagonist in rats, mice and rabbits
   (b) Acts by inhibiting functional GH receptor dimerisation
   (c) Has a half-life of 11 minutes
   (d) Is administered as a continuous intravenous infusion
   (e) Causes rapid tumour shrinkage in the majority of patients

5   In clinical trials of pegvisomant in patients with active acromegaly:
   (a) Irreversible liver damage occurred in two patients
   (b) There was a dose-related improvement in patient well-being
   (c) Circulating GH levels were used as the primary marker of drug efficacy
   (d) Serum IGF-I normalised in 90% of patients receiving 20 mg/day
   (e) Soft tissue swelling improved

ANSWERS

1a False	2a True	3a True	4a False	5a False
b True	b False	b False	b True	b True
c False	c False	c True	c False	c False
d True	d True	d False	d False	d True
e True	e False	e False	e False	e True

Curing colorectal cancer

Rachel Midgley, Simon Grumett and David Kerr

☐ INTRODUCTION

The title of this chapter, 'Curing colorectal cancer', is provocative – very much the province of the surgeons who remind us frequently, if good-naturedly, that they offer cure whereas medical oncologists more traditionally offer palliation, improved quality of life and perhaps life prolongation. Increasing use of adjuvant chemotherapy following apparently curative resection suggests, however, that chemotherapy might contribute to cure. Furthermore, colorectal cancer (CRC) is a sufficiently common disease to consider the role of chemotherapy in both the advanced and the adjuvant setting.

☐ CHEMOTHERAPY FOR ADVANCED COLORECTAL CANCER

The role of chemotherapy in the advanced setting is summarised in Table 1. In the situation of a patient with advanced disease it is imperative carefully to evaluate the cost-benefit ratio of chemotherapy individually. Objective and rigorous assessment of the following factors is essential when evaluating the worth of a new drug or specific regimen in a clinical trial:

☐ *Costs* in terms of toxicity, hospital attendance/admissions and finance. The major dose-limiting toxicities of the common CRC chemotherapy regimens are mucositis, diarrhoea (this can usually be controlled by loperamide), plantar-palmar erythema and mild myelosuppression.

☐ *Benefits* measured by months of life gained and palliation of symptoms or improved quality of life. A randomised trial almost 10 years ago established that chemotherapy with 5-fluorouracil (5-FU)-based regimens improved median survival from five to 10 months when compared with best supportive care for patients with metastatic colorectal cancer [1]. There is also evidence of improvement in quality of life in responding patients.

5-Fluorouracil

5-FU has been the mainstay of colorectal cancer chemotherapy for over 40 years. It is an anti-metabolite and a prodrug which is converted into its active form,

Table 1 Chemotherapy for advanced colorectal cancer.

• Infusional 5-fluorouracil regimens, biomodulated with folinic acid, are the gold standard first-line therapy
• Irinotecan has demonstrated activity as a second-line agent, and there are now compelling data to recommend it in first-line treatment for advanced colorectal cancer
• Response rates and progression-free survival data with oxaliplatin are promising, but there is insufficient overall survival data to recommend its first-line use
• Trials are underway to establish optimal combinations and their most efficient sequencing

fluorodeoxyuridine monophosphate (FdUMP), within the cell. This metabolite binds to the enzyme thymidylate synthase (TS), blocking its action and preventing pyrimidine, and therefore DNA, synthesis (Fig. 1). 5-FU can also be falsely incorporated into RNA, interfering with protein synthesis. Interestingly, there is a degree of genetic polymorphism governing the enzyme (dihydropyrimidine dehydrogenase) that inactivates FdUMP. Approximately 1–2% of the Caucasian population exhibit severely depressed levels of this enzyme. These individuals retain exaggerated and prolonged plasma levels of FdUMP, leading to augmented toxicity such as prolonged neutropenia and complete alopecia.

As the major effect of 5-FU is disruption of DNA replication, the drug is largely S-phase-specific, which may have implications with respect to efficacy of particular regimens. Given the small number of cells in S phase at any one time, it is

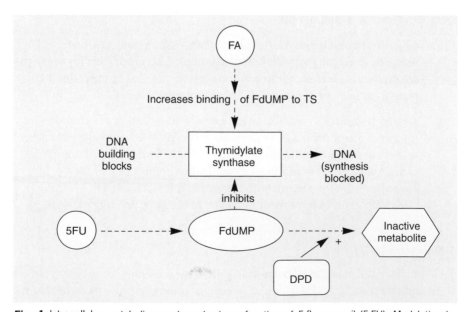

Fig. 1 Intracellular metabolism and mechanism of action of 5-fluorouracil (5-FU). Modulation by folinic acid (FA) (FdUMP = fluorodeoxyuridine monophosphate; DPD = dihydropyrimidine dehydrogenase; TS = thymidylate synthase).

theoretically compelling to suggest that infusional regimens will have a greater 'hit' against cycling cells than bolus regimens. Indeed, a meta-analysis in advanced CRC, comparing infusional 5-FU and bolus 5-FU treatment given on five consecutive days every four weeks (Mayo regimen), found that infusional therapy delivered a higher response rate (32.6% vs 14.5%) and prolonged progression-free survival (27.6 weeks vs 22 weeks), but only a negligible improvement in median survival [2].

de Gramont regimen

At present, the Mayo regimen remains more common in the US, whereas infusional therapy, such as the de Gramont regimen [3], is more commonly used in Europe. The de Gramont regimen comprises a two-hour intravenous (iv) infusion of folinic acid (FA) at a dose of 200 mg/m^2, followed by a 400 mg/m^2 iv bolus of 5-FU and, finally, a 22-hour iv infusion of 5-FU at a dose of 600 mg/m^2. This is repeated on day 2, and the cycle is repeated every 14 days.

The CR06 clinical trial [4], sponsored by the Medical Research Council (MRC), compared the de Gramont regimen against the Lokich regimen [4] (continuous infusion of 5-FU at a dose of 300 mg/m^2/day, 21-day cycle) and raltitrexed, a TS inhibitor, given as a three-weekly bolus injection (Fig. 2). There was no difference in overall survival or response rate, but there was a poorer quality of life and an excess of treatment-related deaths in the raltitrexed arm. The Lokich regimen incurred an increased rate of palmar-plantar erythema and desquamation.

The de Gramont regimen is well tolerated and allows the patient to be free of infusion for 12 of every 14 days. It has become the gold standard for 5-FU-based chemotherapy for advanced CRC in Europe. However, it is imperative to stress that, unless patients want to be confined to hospital for the duration of their chemotherapy, a prerequisite for infusional therapy is central line insertion, with all the incumbent risks of infection and thrombophlebitis.

In addition to the benefits derived from infusional administration, the de Gramont regimen employs a further mechanism to augment the efficacy of 5-FU:

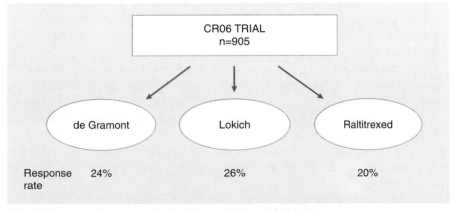

Fig. 2 Design and results of the Medical Research Council CR06 trial.

biomodulation with FA. Addition of FA increases the pool of reduced folate in the cell and stabilises the FdUMP/TS complex. Studies have shown that the addition of FA to bolus 5-FU improves response rates (23% vs 11%) and slightly increases toxicity, especially mucositis and diarrhoea, but have not demonstrated an overall statistically significant survival benefit in the advanced setting compared with single agent 5-FU [5].

Intrahepatic arterial chemotherapy

The rationale for giving chemotherapy via the hepatic artery has an anatomical and pharmacological basis. It has been known for many years that micrometastases within the liver derive their blood supply from the hepatic artery, whilst normal hepatocytes derive theirs predominantly from the portal vein. Also, a number of chemotherapeutic drugs are largely metabolised during their first pass through the liver. Hence, relatively high doses of drug can be administered directly to the liver, while still keeping systemic exposure low. Randomised trials comparing hepatic arterial infusion with systemic therapy have given conflicting results, but many have suffered from poor design. Most have confirmed a higher response rate, but have lacked evidence of improved survival.

The problem of dose imbalance between the systemic and intrahepatic arms of such trials has been addressed by the UK MRC group. In the CR05 trial, the systemic spillover and plasma levels of 5-FU were specifically designed to be the same in both arms. The results of this trial are awaited, but at present the insertion of a hepatic portocath, with the attendant risks of thrombosis and hepatic arteritis, cannot be advocated outside of a formal clinical trial.

Novel agents

Irinotecan

Irinotecan (CPT-11) is a potent inhibitor of topoisomerase I, an enzyme essential for DNA supercoiling. Early phase III randomised studies have shown that, for patients whose advanced colorectal cancer has become resistant to treatment with 5-FU, response rates of up to 15% are achievable with single agent irinotecan, resulting in a statistically significant overall survival benefit when compared with best supportive care alone [6].

Both the translation of irinotecan into the first-line setting and its use in combination with 5-FU were initially hampered by reservations about toxicity. It can be a difficult drug for patients to tolerate, with approximately one-quarter to one-third of patients suffering grade 3 or 4 diarrhoea. Neutropenia, nausea and alopecia are also frequently reported. However, more recently, with greater experience of the drug and an evolving ability to deal with the toxicities, there has been increasing interest in the use of irinotecan in combination with 5-FU as first-line palliative CRC therapy.

Two recent large randomised phase III studies have shown that triple therapy with infusional 5-FU/FA/irinotecan gives better response rates, increased median time to progression and increased median survival compared with single or double agent combinations (Table 2) [7,8]. As a result, it is felt by many that there is sufficient evidence to support the use of triple therapy as first-line treatment. Unfortunately, irinotecan is not widely and evenly available throughout the UK at present, due to variability in prioritisation by different health authorities.

Table 2 Two large randomised trials of 5-fluorouracil (5-FU)/irinotecan (IR) combination chemotherapy in the first-line treatment of advanced colorectal cancer.

Trial	Douillard *et al* [7]		Saltz *et al* [8]		
No. of patients randomised	387		683		
Randomised comparison	IR/5FU/FA	5FU/FA	IR/5FU/FA	5FU/FA	IR
	Weekly or fortnightly		4 weeks weekly		
Response rates (%)	49	31	39	21	18
	$p < 0.001$		$p < 0.001$		
Time to progression (months)	6.7	4.4	7.0	4.3	4.2
	$p < 0.001$		$p = 0.004$		
Overall survival (months)	17.4	14.1	14.8	12.6	12.0
	$p = 0.031$		$p = 0.04$		
G3/4 diarrhoea (%)	44.4	25.6	22.7	13.2	31.0
G3/4 neutropenia (%)	28.8	2.4	53.8	66.2	31.4

FA = folinic acid.

Oxaliplatin

Oxaliplatin (OX) is a third-generation platinum compound that induces DNA cross-linkages and apoptotic cell death. Unlike related agents cisplatin and carboplatin, it has activity against human colorectal cancer, with a 10–24% response rate as a single agent. There is also evidence that it acts synergistically with 5-FU, the combination achieving response rates of up to 50% when used in first-line therapy. In a recent study 420 patients were randomised to receive 5-FU according to the de Gramont regimen plus or minus oxaliplatin (85 mg/m² fortnightly) as first-line treatment for advanced CRC. Response rates were significantly better in the OX+ arm (57% vs 26%), with an enhanced progression-free survival (39.6 weeks vs 27.8 weeks). There was a trend towards greater overall survival in the OX+ arm, but this did not achieve statistical significance [9]. Oxaliplatin has no renal and only minimal haemato-logical toxicity, but it causes a particular dysasthesia precipitated by cold, as well as a cumulative sensory neuropathy.

Oral 5-fluorouracil analogues

There is growing interest in oral agents such as UFT (a combination of tegafur, a 5-FU prodrug, and uracil). Four multicentre trials in patients with advanced CRC compared oral UFT plus FA or capecitabine with iv 5-FU and demonstrated approximately equal efficacy and similar median survival times. There was less mucositis, neutropenia and alopecia but more hand-foot syndrome with oral agent administration.

Combination of novel agents

The next logical step in the path towards improved effectiveness will probably be combination of the novel agents discussed above. Early unpublished data from the coadministration of capecitabine and irinotecan suggest that this might be a particularly promising combination. Combinations of 5-FU/irinotecan and 5-FU/OX and the relative benefits of particular sequencing of combinations are presently under study in the MRC CR08 trial.

☐ HEPATIC METASTATIC RESECTION

In recent years, the surgeon has again established a potentially curative role in the setting of advanced disease. In approximately 10–15% of patients with stage D disease, the metastases will be small, fewer than three, and anatomically confined to one lobe of the liver. In these circumstances, metastatic resection yields approximately 25% chance of overall survival five years post-metastatectomy, compared with no chance without resection. Interestingly, a recent study by Kemeny *et al* suggests that delivering chemotherapy via a portocath directly to the residual liver for six months post-resection significantly reduces the chances of subsequent hepatic recurrence and improves overall survival [10]. It is also possible that neo-adjuvant chemotherapy prior to resection of metastases might improve resectability and overall survival, although this has not yet been tested in an appropriately powered trial.

☐ ADJUVANT CHEMOTHERAPY FOR COLORECTAL CANCER

Adjuvant chemotherapy in CRC is summarised in Table 3. Little in the way of convincing evidence for the role of the oncologist in curing colorectal cancer has so far been described, but the situation is different in the adjuvant setting. Despite the best efforts of the surgeon in the 80% of colorectal tumours deemed operatively curable, 50% of these patients will subsequently relapse and die of their disease. This

Table 3 Adjuvant therapy of colorectal cancer.

- Bolus 5-fluorouracil/folinic acid adjuvant therapy produces an absolute survival benefit of 6–7% in Dukes C colon cancer
- Adjuvant chemotherapy in Dukes B colon tumours or Dukes B/C rectal tumours is not routinely advocated on present evidence
- Newer drugs such as capecitabine, irinotecan and oxaliplatin are entering adjuvant trials
- Pre-operative radiotherapy is presently the most routinely advocated adjuvant treatment for rectal tumours

---

is because occult tumour cells present at the time of the operation, either locally in the lymph nodes or at distant sites, are too small to be detected by currently available radiological methods.

With chemotherapy, it has become increasingly apparent that macroscopic *prevention* (ie eradicating the cells before they become large functional tumour masses) is more likely to be successful than attempts at macroscopic *cure*. Cytotoxic efficacy is likely to be inversely related to the residual tumour mass. This implies that the earlier adjuvant chemotherapy can be initiated after primary resection, the better the outcome. To date, there has not been an adequately powered trial to test whether early initiation of adjuvant therapy is critical. However, the role of adjuvant chemotherapy in colorectal cancer *is* now well established.

Dukes C colon cancer

After early scepticism and initial disappointment, the tide turned when Moertel *et al* [11] published results suggesting a 33% and 41% reduced risk of death and recurrence, respectively, amongst Dukes C colon patients who received adjuvant 5-FU/levamisole after surgery compared with surgery alone. Levamisole is now believed to contribute little to the cytotoxic effect and has been superseded by FA as in the advanced treatment setting. Three large prospective randomised trials have shown convincing evidence of improved three-year disease-free survival and overall survival in patients treated with 5-FU/FA, with a 25–30% decrease in the odds of dying from colon cancer (or an absolute improvement in survival of 5–6%) compared with controls [13].

Recently, a meta-analysis of updated individual data from all unconfounded randomised studies of adjuvant chemotherapy found that overall there was a 6–7% absolute improvement in survival with chemotherapy compared with surgery alone (standard deviation 2.3, $p = 0.01$). Based on this, it is now advised that six months' bolus treatment with the combination of 5-FU/FA should be accepted as standard adjuvant therapy for patients with Dukes C colon cancer. With publication of the first phase of the Quasar trial [13], it can be firmly stated that low-dose FA is as effective as high-dose, and that levamisole adds absolutely no extra benefit.

Dukes B colon cancer

The role of chemotherapy in Dukes B colon cancer is less certain. It is estimated that for this cohort only two or three patients might be additionally cured for every 100 patients treated. This represents a large investment in terms of finance and toxicity for borderline return, and adjuvant therapy in this setting is not recommended as standard practice. However, the uncertain arm of the Quasar trial, which randomises Dukes B colon patients to chemotherapy or surgery alone in patients for whom the role of adjuvant therapy is genuinely uncertain, will help to resolve this issue. It is likely that a subset of Dukes B patients who have specific bad prognostic factors will benefit from adjuvant therapy. The growing field of proteomics may allow identification of the population most at risk.

Rectal tumours

Adjuvant chemotherapy for rectal tumours is another contentious issue. Because of the anatomical constraints within the pelvis, local recurrence, rather than distant metastasis, has historically been the main problem and the major determinant of outcome. Based upon this, the role of the oncologist has been largely restricted to pre-operative radiotherapy, with the largest trial to date indicating a 61% decrease in local recurrence and an absolute survival benefit of 10% with pre-operative radiotherapy compared with surgery alone. However, with the advent of newer surgical techniques, such as total mesorectal excision and wide lateral excision, the problem of local recurrence is diminishing. It is possible to imagine that adjuvant radiotherapy may become less important and be reserved as a postoperative tool for use when the circumferential resection margins are involved on histological inspection. Such a hypothesis is being tested in the MRC CR07 trial. Chemotherapy for rectal cancer is being assessed in the uncertain arm of the Quasar trial. To date, its combination with radiotherapy in the postoperative setting has been too toxic to allow standard use and its efficacy has not been rigorously established.

☐ CONCLUSIONS AND FUTURE DIRECTIONS

Do oncologists cure colorectal cancer? Certainly, in the setting of advanced disease the major role is palliative, with a short extension of life and alleviation of symptoms, but chemotherapy has a definite role in improving overall survival in the adjuvant setting for Dukes C colon cancer patients. With the translation of newer drugs such as capecitabine and irinotecan into the adjuvant setting, as envisaged over the next decade, cure rates are likely to improve further. Acceptability for patients, in terms of fewer hospital visits and the obvious benefits of oral therapy, may further swing the cost-benefit relationship in favour of chemotherapy.

Other new, exciting therapies predicated on basic science advances such as immunotherapy and gene therapy are now entering phase I trial. These are likely to have the greatest impact in the curable adjuvant setting, where tumour burden is low and biological intervention will have the greatest chance of success.

Finally, much of the advancement in terms of cure is likely to be based on the success of streamlined care between primary care, general physician, site-specialised surgeon and oncologist. The role of the multidisciplinary team in shifting the natural history of the disease so that more patients present with early stage tumours should not be underestimated.

REFERENCES

1   Scheithauer W, Rosen H, Kornek GV, Sebasta C, Depisch D. Randomised comparison of combination chemotherapy plus supportive care with supportive care alone in patients with metastatic colorectal cancer. *Br Med J* 1993; **306**: 752–5.
2   Efficacy of intravenous continuous infusion of fluorouracil compared with bolus administration in advanced colorectal cancer. Meta-analysis Group In Cancer. *J Clin Oncol* 1998; **16**: 301–8.

3   de Gramont A, Bosset JF, Milan C, Rougier P, *et al.* Randomized trial comparing monthly low-dose leucovorin and fluorouracil bolus with bimonthly high-dose leucovorin and fluorouracil bolus plus continuous infusion for advanced colorectal cancer: a French intergroup study. *J Clin Oncol* 1997; **15**: 808–15.

4   Maughan T, James R, Kerr D, Ledermann J, *et al.* Excess treatment related deaths and impaired quality of life shows raltitrexed is inferior to infusional 5FU regimens in the palliative chemotherapy of advanced colorectal cancer (CRC): final results of MRC CR06. *Ann Oncol* 2000: **11** (Suppl 4): 43.

5   Modulation of fluorouracil by leucovorin in patients with advanced colorectal cancer: evidence in terms of response rate. Advanced Colorectal Cancer Meta-Analysis Project. *J Clin Oncol* 1992; **10**: 896–903.

6   Rougier P, Van Cutsem E, Bajetta E, Niederle N, *et al.* Randomised trial of irinotecan versus fluorouracil by continuous infusion after fluorouracil failure in patients with metastatic colorectal cancer. *Lancet* 1998; **352**: 1407–12.

7   Douillard JY, Cunningham D, Roth AD, Navarro M, *et al.* Irinotecan combined with fluorouracil compared with fluorouracil alone as first-line treatment for metastatic colorectal cancer: a multicentre randomised trial. *Lancet* 2000; **355**: 1041–7.

8   Saltz LB, Cox JV, Blanke C, Rosen LS, *et al.* Irinotecan plus fluorouracil and leucovorin for metastatic colorectal cancer. Irinotecan Study Group. *N Engl J Med* 2000; **343**: 905–14.

9   de Gramont A, Figer A, Seymour M, Homerin M, *et al.* Leucovorin and fluorouracil with or without oxaliplatin as first-line treatment in advanced colorectal cancer. *J Clin Oncol* 2000; **18**: 2938–47.

10 Kemeny N, Huang Y, Cohen AM, Shi W, *et al.* Hepatic arterial infusion of chemotherapy after resection of hepatic metastases from colorectal cancer. *N Engl J Med* 1999; **341**: 2039–49.

11 Moertel CG, Fleming TR, Macdonald JS, Haller DG, Laurie JA. Hepatic toxicity associated with fluorouracil plus levamisole adjuvant therapy. *J Clin Oncol* 1993; **11**: 2386–90.

12 Midgley R, Kerr D. Colorectal cancer. Review. *Lancet* 1999; **353**: 391–9.

13 Comparison of fluorouracil with additional levamisole, higher-dose folinic acid, or both, as adjuvant chemotherapy for colorectal cancer: a randomised trial. QUASAR Collaborative Group. *Lancet* 2000; **355**: 1588–96.

☐ SELF ASSESSMENT QUESTIONS

1   Which of the following is true:
(a) 5-fluorouracil (5-FU) is S-phase specific
(b) There is no evidence that chemotherapy improves median survival in colorectal cancer
(c) Oxaliplatin is standard first-line chemotherapy for colorectal cancer
(d) The de Gramont regimen relates to surgery for colon cancer
(e) Patients with Dukes stage C tumours will almost certainly benefit from adjuvant chemotherapy

2   Regarding irinotecan, which of the following is true?
(a) Irinotecan is an inhibitor of thymidylate synthase
(b) Diarrhoea is a common dose-limiting toxicity
(c) Response rates are approximately 55% as second-line therapy for metastatic colorectal cancer
(d) Alopecia rarely occurs
(e) Chemotherapy-induced neutropenia is clinically unimportant

3   Regarding adjuvant chemotherapy for colorectal cancer:
(a) The absolute survival benefit in Dukes C patients is approximately 7%
(b) The absolute survival benefit in Dukes B patients is approximately 15%
(c) Adjuvant chemotherapy for rectal cancer is standard practice
(d) Pre-operative radiotherapy for rectal cancer is standard practice
(e) Infusional 5-FU chemotherapy is the most commonly used adjuvant therapy

4   Regarding the aims of treatment of colorectal cancer:
(a) Metastatic disease is incurable
(b) Median survival for metastatic disease with best supportive care is five months
(c) Five-year survival for patients with Dukes B disease is 50% following surgery
(d) The primary objective of adjuvant therapy is to improve quality of life
(e) Pre-operative radiotherapy for rectal cancer aims to reduce local recurrence

ANSWERS

1a True	2a False	3a True	4a False
b False	b True	b False	b True
c False	c False	c False	c False
d False	d False	d True	d False
e False	e False	e False	e True

Taxoids, a chemotherapeutic breakthrough for breast cancer?

Robert Leonard

□ INTRODUCTION

About 50% of women who present with local breast cancer and are treated by surgery, with or without radiotherapy, will eventually relapse and die from distant metastatic disease. The current paradigm that has directed research and translated into modern practice is that most of these women with apparently localised disease must have undetected microscopic metastatic disease at the time of local treatment.

A succession of hormone and chemotherapy trials during the last 30 years has shown that several therapeutic approaches will substantially reduce the 10–15 year risk of relapse and death. These approaches have been:

- □ hormonal manipulation, classically with the anti-oestrogen tamoxifen

- □ ovarian ablation in premenopausal women, and

- □ polychemotherapy in hormone-insensitive disease.

Some trials show an added benefit for combined chemotherapy and hormone treatment. There is up to 45% risk reduction for tamoxifen (in oestrogen receptor-positive disease) and about 35% for cytotoxic chemotherapy [1,2].

These risk reductions appear to be irrespective of the actual risk of the individual patient. For those at low or moderate risk of relapse, single-agent tamoxifen is adequate treatment, especially in older postmenopausal women. For younger women with risk factors for poor prognosis, even standard polychemotherapy using the cyclophosphamide, methotrexate and 5-fluorouracil (CMF) combination does not result in good long-term survival.

In the last decade or so there have been increasing efforts to find more effective chemotherapy programmes for women with 30–80% risk of relapse. The obvious agents for testing are those with the highest anti-cancer activity, defined by objective measures of cancer response rates in advanced disease. The taxoids are the most promising compounds among the new cytotoxics with anti-breast cancer activity tested in the last decade.

□ THE TAXOIDS

The taxoids are semisynthetic derivatives of natural products of varieties of the yew tree:

☐   Paclitaxel (taxol) is obtained from the bark of the Western Pacific yew tree, *taxus brevifolia.*

☐   Docetaxel (taxotere) comes from the leaves of the European yew, *taxus baccata.*

Their target in the dividing mammalian cell is the tubulin complex formed during cell division, which they stabilise irreversibly thus preventing mitosis.

Preclinical and early clinical trials suggested only limited cross-resistance with anthracyclines. The taxoids were approved in 2000 for the treatment of advanced breast cancer, but limited to the indication of post-anthracycline relapse and the small number of cases of advanced disease where anthracyclines are contraindicated.

This chapter will examine the comparative data on their activity in the licensed indications as well as trials in their unlicensed settings, including adjuvant, neo-adjuvant (sometimes called pre-operative), first-line metastatic disease combined with other cytotoxics and, finally, combined with the antibody against the type 1 growth factor receptor trastuzumab (herceptin) which is expressed in about 20% of breast cancers. The activity of these drugs in advanced breast cancer will be reviewed.

The systematic five-year overview analyses of the Early Breast Cancer Trialists Group, which gathers data on virtually all the randomised trials in breast cancer throughout the world, have demonstrated with increasing clarity the added benefit of anthracyclines in polychemotherapy for poorer risk groups. However, the drugs are more toxic and they cost considerably more than standard CMF.

Three years ago the American Intergroup and Cancer and Leukemia Group B (CALGB) groups reported a trial in which the novel cytotoxic agent paclitaxel was added to an anthracycline-based regimen. The early results are impressive and will be discussed below, together with the effect of this agent and the related drug, docetaxel, in advanced disease.

In June 2000 the National Institute for Clinical Excellence pronounced on the proven efficacy of these agents in advanced breast cancer after anthracycline failure. The current research effort has two objectives:

1   To define the true added benefit of both paclitaxel and docetaxel in the first-line treatment of relapsed breast cancer.

2   To evaluate the added impact of the taxoids as part of the adjuvant treatment of early-stage breast cancer.

☐ TAXOIDS AND ADVANCED BREAST CANCER

Although advanced breast cancer has a variable natural history, it is considered to be incurable and the treatment offered is usually palliative. However, when drug therapy is considered an option, an agent that maximises survival time [1,2] and has predictable and manageable side effects should be selected.

Typical response rates to the alkylating agent/antimetabolite combination CMF are about 30–40% in relapsed breast cancer. Duration of response is brief, typically only 4–6 months after completing a 4–5 month treatment period. The response rates for the anthracyclines are higher at around 50–70% if used in combined chemotherapy regimens but the response duration is no better.

More patients will derive symptomatic benefit than the objective responses suggest, but there is always the problem of toxic side effects, mainly fatigue, a degree of nausea for several days after each 3–4 weekly pulse, hair loss and possibly neutropenic sepsis. Sometimes altered taste sensation or mouth ulcers are prominent. Other side effects are variable, and there may be few or none.

The aim of treatment is to balance the risks and toxicities of potent cytotoxic agents against the undoubted benefits of relieving unpleasant symptoms, reducing the burden of possibly life-threatening metastases, and providing the patient with hope by sometimes substantially extending her survival.

The increasing use of powerful combination chemotherapy in the postoperative setting reduces the options for treatment of those patients who relapse. Several new classes of cytotoxic agent have become available in the last decade, amongst which the taxoids have shown considerable anti-cancer effects in breast cancer.

In the UK, standard adjuvant or first-line therapy for advanced breast cancer usually involves an anthracycline or alkylating agent. Following relapse, patients with active disease progression may undergo second-line chemotherapy. The three major second-line chemotherapy options licensed for use in the UK are the taxoids, docetaxel and paclitaxel, and the vinca alkaloid, vinorelbine. A fourth agent under active investigation is the oral fluoropyrimidine, capecitabine, which does not have a licence and has not been used in comparator analyses.

Literature search

No head-to-head phase III randomised controlled trials comparing the three licensed agents have been published, and there is insufficient evidence to guide a choice between the best 'salvage' chemotherapy regimens in patients with advanced breast cancer. In an attempt to compensate for this deficit, a systematic review was carried out of the published literature on the efficacy and safety profiles of docetaxel, paclitaxel and vinorelbine, according to the dosing schedules licensed in the UK.

The design of the literature search followed the Cochrane Collaboration methodology and included the following databases:

- [ ] EMBASE (1974 to 18 August 1999)

- [ ] EMBASE Alert (for the most recent period to 18 August 1999)

- [ ] HealthStar (1975 to 18 August 1999)

- [ ] CancerLit (1986 to 18 August 1999)

- [ ] MEDLINE (1985 to July 1999).

In addition, the bibliographies of review articles were examined in an attempt to discover further publications that had not been recovered by the electronic search strategy.

The trials

All but five of the 275 papers identified in the literature search were excluded for one or more reasons (eg review article, did not meet inclusion criteria, etc.). The five papers (docetaxel (3), paclitaxel (1), vinorelbine (1)) which were included in the evaluation reported on phase III clinical trials with study populations and dosing schedules according to the UK licensed indications [3–7]. They all described randomised multicentre trials that were unblinded or for which the publication did not specify blinding [8] and compared:

- [ ] docetaxel with doxorubicin [3]

- [ ] docetaxel with mitomycin plus vinblastine [4]

- [ ] docetaxel with sequential methotrexate and 5-fluorouracil [5]

- [ ] single-agent paclitaxel at two different doses (the UK licensed dose of 175 mg/m^2 and an unlicensed dose of 135 mg/m^2) in anthracycline-pretreated and anthracycline-naïve patients [6], and

- [ ] vinorelbine with melphalan [7].

The studies were evaluated for tumour response to medication (overall, complete and partial), time to disease progression, and survival – all of which are considered important efficacy outcomes for anti-cancer agents. There was sufficient tumour response data from the phase III trials to permit the use of meta-analysis, but the limited data for time to disease progression and survival necessitated qualitative assessment.

Tumour response rates

In all the trials, tumour response to medication was classified according to World Health Organization criteria [8]. Complete response (no detectable tumour, including bone) and partial response ($\geq$50% reduction) were confirmed by a second evaluation at least four weeks later.

Review of the trials comparing docetaxel with standard therapies showed that docetaxel demonstrated significant superiority in terms of overall tumour response rate compared with mitomycin plus vinblastine (p <0.0001), methotrexate plus 5-fluorouracil (p <0.001) or doxorubicin (p = 0.012). Docetaxel is the first agent to show superiority over doxorubicin for the treatment of advanced breast cancer. An increased overall response rate was obtained with paclitaxel at a dose of 175 mg/m^2 compared with the lower dose of 135 mg/m^2.

Safety

The trials comparing docetaxel with standard therapies showed that docetaxel has a safety profile typical of that of an effective chemotherapeutic agent. There were no major safety concerns when docetaxel was compared with mitomycin plus vinblastine. Neutropenia of severity grade 3/4, febrile neutropenia and grade 3/4 infections occurred more frequently with docetaxel ($p \leq 0.05$), while the incidence of thrombocytopenia was significantly higher for mitomycin plus vinblastine (overall $p < 0.001$; grade 3/4 $p = 0.004$).

The comparison with doxorubicin favoured docetaxel. Of particular note was the unpredictable, irreversible cardiotoxicity seen with doxorubicin that resulted in four deaths [3]. Clinical congestive heart failure was observed in six patients receiving doxorubicin at cumulative doses below 460 mg/m². The relatively high incidence of adverse events with docetaxel in this trial may have been due to the inclusion of patients with grossly elevated liver enzymes. The decision to include patients with compromised liver function was made so that the study population was similar to that encountered in the clinical setting.

Haematological adverse events were the most frequent toxicities seen with vinorelbine (granulocytopenia) and melphalan (thrombocytopenia and granulocytopenia). Comparable phase III safety profile data were not available for paclitaxel because the adverse event data for the anthracycline-pretreated and anthracycline-naïve patients were combined.

The meta-analysis of the safety profile data extracted from the phase III trials with docetaxel and vinorelbine showed that docetaxel was associated with a higher incidence of side effects.

The most active agent in patients with second relapse appears to be docetaxel which has a single-agent activity probably even higher than that of doxorubicin, hitherto the gold standard drug with the highest activity against advanced breast cancer. It is, however, accompanied by considerable toxicity for older, less fit patients and may be contraindicated in patients with impaired liver function – a common problem due to breast cancer metastases.

For these patients and possibly others, who may benefit from lower doses of drug and more frequent monitoring, weekly paclitaxel may have an advantage. There appears to be a lower risk of dangerous toxicity whilst the anti-cancer activity in early trials (published only in abstract form) is impressive [9].

☐ CURRENT STATUS OF TAXOIDS

A major international trial of combination chemotherapy compared doxorubicin plus docetaxel against most commonly used anthracycline combination regimen for relapsed breast cancer, doxorubicin and cyclophosphamide. The benefit for the taxoid combination was clear in terms of measurable response rates, duration of response but, at the time of reporting, not of survival. The results for paclitaxel are less convincing in this setting. To date, the activity of combined paclitaxel and anthracycline looks similar to anthracycline/cyclophosphamide.

Although the evidence strongly favours docetaxel as the more active of the two agents in the 21-day schedule either alone or combined with other cytotoxic agents, it is sometimes a difficult drug to use in older or sicker patients, especially those with impaired liver function. There is growing interest in the use of weekly therapy at lower doses, and currently experience with paclitaxel is impressive in phase II non-randomised trials [10]. These trials, however, need to be extended and reported in full and should probably be supported by some randomised controlled trials comparing this weekly therapy against a standard comparator such as one of the oral fluoropyrimidines or vinorelbine in the setting of palliative therapy for second or third relapse.

There is no doubt that, true to the traditions of new anti-cancer agents, the impetus is to move the use of taxoids to earlier stages of breast cancer. They are currently under test in the UK in randomised trials after initial relapse and in the adjuvant and even the neo-adjuvant settings [10,11].

The adjuvant setting

There are no fully published reports of the taxoids in the adjuvant setting because the true impact of a new treatment must of necessity take some years to be revealed in terms of long-term disease-free survival and change in overall survival. Nevertheless, medium-term follow-up of at least one major American trial involving the use of paclitaxel looks encouraging and is influencing current trial design in the UK and the rest of Europe [10]. For patients with high-risk disease, cytotoxic chemotherapy provides the main chance of extending survival free of recurrence. Trials are underway to see whether the taxoids can provide a major benefit for patients in this category who have multiple axillary lymph node involvement.

The neo-adjuvant setting

In the neo-adjuvant setting drug treatment is given after diagnosis but before primary surgery. The aim is to reduce the tumour mass in the breast, making breast-conserving surgery possible, and theoretically to attack the micrometastases earlier than in the more typical postoperative phase. So far, there has been no demonstrable gain in survival or relapse-free survival from neo-adjuvant chemotherapy, but in general the cancer reduction rates have been impressive for the taxoids in early trials.

A trial of neo-adjuvant chemotherapy in Aberdeen has suggested that a substantial improvement in the rate of pathological eradication of invasive cancer in the breast can be obtained by sequencing anthracycline combination chemotherapy with docetaxel [11]. It remains to be seen whether this promising observation translates into higher rates of long-term disease-free survival in this group of patients whose large or inoperable cancers demand this sort of approach.

☐ TAXOIDS AND TRASTUZUMAB

A large international trial has recently produced the unusual result of a substantial survival benefit as well as a major response improvement when either anthracycline chemotherapy or paclitaxel was combined with the humanised monoclonal antibody trastuzumab (herceptin) [12] (Table 1). The significant, though reversible, cardiac toxicity seen with the anthracycline/trastuzumab combination needs further study, but the taxoid results are encouraging further development of trastuzumab/taxoid therapy for poor-risk, Her2 protein-overexpressing cancers both in advanced disease and in the adjuvant setting.

Table 1 Anticancer activity of taxoids.

	Objective response rates (%)				
	After anthracycline failure	Combined with anthracyclines	As weekly therapy	In combination with trastuzumab	Main toxicities*
Paclitaxel	25–30	40	50	60**	Neurotoxic Mild myelotoxicity
Docetaxel	35–50**	60	NA	NA	Myelotoxic Mild neurotoxicity

* Both agents require premedication with corticosteroids to minimise idiosyncratic/allergic reactions.
**Survival benefit seen compared with standard therapy in randomised controlled trial.
NA = not applicable.

☐ CONCLUSIONS

The small number of phase III trials retrieved by the search strategy highlights the paucity of high quality clinical evidence available on the taxoids and other new agents in patients with advanced breast cancer. The largest amount of high quality data is available for docetaxel. According to the currently available clinical evidence, the clinical implication of this systematic review and meta-analysis is that docetaxel is the most effective chemotherapeutic agent for the treatment of advanced breast cancer after failure of previous therapy with an anthracycline or alkylating agent. Docetaxel is the first agent to show superiority over doxorubicin in patients with advanced breast cancer. Similarly, docetaxel showed a significantly higher overall response rate than paclitaxel. The safety profile of the taxoids is both predictable and manageable.

The true added benefit for the agents at any stage will have to be unarguable as they will certainly add a significant new cost to the already overstretched and under-resourced drug budgets of UK cancer centres. The typical cost for a single pulse of the taxoids is in the range of £1,200–1,500 (3–4 times that of the anthracyclines). Against this should be balanced:

☐ the potential economic impact of effective treatment relieving the health service of palliative care costs in hospital and the community

☐ the economic benefits of returning patients to active productive lives for a time after treatment, and

☐ the immeasureable benefit to patients whose hope of fruitful lives extended may be considerably enhanced.

REFERENCES

1 Cancer Guidance Sub-Group of the Clinical Outcomes Group. Improving outcomes in breast cancer: guidance for purchasers, the research evidence. Leeds: NHS Executive, 1996.
2 Fossati R, Confalonieri C, Torri V, Ghislandi E, *et al.* Cytotoxic and hormonal treatment for metastatic breast cancer: a systematic review of published randomized trials involving 31,510 women. *J Clin Oncol* 1998; **16**: 3439–60.

3   Chan S, Friedrichs K, Noel D, Pinter T, *et al*. Prospective randomized trial of docetaxel versus doxorubicin in patients with metastatic breast cancer. The 303 Study Group. *J Clin Oncol* 1999; 17: 2341–54.

4   Nabholtz JM, Senn HJ, Bezwoda WR, Melnychuk D, *et al*. Prospective randomized trial of docetaxel versus mitomycin plus vinblastine in patients with metastatic breast cancer progressing despite previous anthracycline-containing chemotherapy. 304 Study Group. *J Clin Oncol* 1999; 17: 1413–24.

5   Sjöström J, Blomqvist C, Mouridsen H, Pluzanska A, *et al*. Docetaxel compared with sequential methotrexate and 5-fluorouracil in patients with advanced breast cancer after anthracycline failure: a randomised phase III study with crossover on progression by the Scandinavian Breast Group. *Eur J Cancer* 1999; 35: 1194–201.

6   Nabholtz JM, Gelmon K, Bontenbal M, Spielmann M, *et al*. Multicenter, randomized comparative study of two doses of paclitaxel in patients with metastatic breast cancer. *J Clin Oncol* 1996; 14: 1858–67.

7   Jones S, Winer E, Vogel C, Laufman L, *et al*. Randomized comparison of vinorelbine and melphalan in anthracycline-refractory advanced breast cancer. *J Clin Oncol* 1995; 13: 2567–74.

8   Miller AB, Hoogstraten B, Staquet M, Winkler A. Reporting results of cancer treatment. *Cancer* 1981; 47: 207–14.

9   Fornier M, Seidman AD, Esteva FJ, Theodoulou M, *et al*. Weekly herceptin plus 1 hour taxol: Phase 2 study I HER2 overexpressing and non-overexpressing metastatic breast cancer. *Proc Am Soc Clin Oncol* 1999; 482: 126a.

10   Henderson IC, Berry D, Demetri G, Cirrincione C, *et al*. Improved disease-free survival and overall survival from addition of sequential paclitaxel but not from escalation of doxorubicin dose level in adjuvant chemotherapy of patients with node positive primary breast cancer. *Proc Am Soc Clin Oncol* 1998; 390: 111a.

11   Hutcheon A, Ogston KL, Heys SD, Smith IC, *et al*. Primary chemotherapy in the treatment of breast cancer: significantly enhanced clinical and pathological response with docetaxel. *Proc Am Soc Clin Oncol* 2000; 317: 83a.

12   Norton L, Slamon D, Leyland-Jones B, Wolter J, *et al*. Overall survival advantage to simultaneous chemotherapy plus humanised anti HER2 antibody herceptin in HER2 overexpressing metastatic breast cancer. *Proc Am Soc Clin Oncol* 1999; 483: 127a.

□ SELF ASSESSMENT QUESTIONS

1   The risk of relapse and death from breast cancer following surgery for localised disease is reduced by the following endocrine manipulations:

    (a) Ovarian suppression in premenopausal women

    (b) Ovarian suppression in postmenopausal women

    (c) Tamoxifen, but only for postmenopausal women

    (d) All postmenopausal women, regardless of hormone receptor status, benefit from antihormone therapy

    (e) All women who are hormone receptor-positive should be considered for antihormone therapy

2   Chemotherapy used as adjuvant treatment following surgery for localised disease:

    (a) Polychemotherapy should be considered for younger patients with poor risk factors

    (b) The impact of effective polychemotherapy is higher than the impact of tamoxifen in general

(c) Anthracycline chemotherapy should be standard treatment for the poorest risk patients

(d) The taxoids have shown a clear added benefit in treating poor risk patients in the adjuvant setting

(e) Some of the effect of chemotherapy in younger patients may be due to induction of premature menopause

3   Trials in advanced breast cancer have shown:
   (a) Docetaxel is more effective than paclitaxel in direct comparison
   (b) Docetaxel is more effective than doxoubicin
   (c) Paclitaxel is more effective than doxoubicin
   (d) No chemotherapy has an effect on overall survival
   (e) Combining taxoids and anthracyclines has a distinct survival gain for patients

4   Pre-operative chemotherapy:
   (a) Is the optimum way of treating most breast cancer
   (b) Should be confined to treating inoperable disease
   (c) Should be considered in the management of large tumours of the breast where the aim of treatment is to reduce the tumour volume making breast conservation possible
   (d) There is a clear advantage in randomised trials for pre-operative chemotherapy in terms of survival compared with standard treatment
   (e) Docetaxel has high activity in this setting

5   In studies with the antibody trastuzumab in advanced breast cancer, the following observations have been made:
   (a) It is a useful drug for all breast cancer
   (b) It should be confined to those tumours which overexpress the HER2 growth factor receptor
   (c) It is ineffective when used on its own
   (d) It has shown high activity in combination therapy with the taxoids
   (e) It is cardiotoxic

ANSWERS

1a True	2a True	3a False	4a False	5a False
b False	b False	b True	b False	b True
c False	c True	c False	c True	c False
d False	d False	d False	d False	d True
e True	e True	e False	e True	e True

Respiratory medicine and chest disease

Evolution or revolution: the treatment of airway inflammation

John Costello

□ INTRODUCTION

The airway is an interface with the environment and therefore subject to a number of pro-inflammatory stimuli. These include infections causing acute laryngo-tracheobronchitis, airborne allergens and irritants such as cigarette smoke and pollution. Asthma and chronic obstructive pulmonary disease (COPD) are the commonest causes of chronic airway inflammation and the mechanisms of inflammation are relevant when considering treatment.

There is now much evidence that airway inflammation plays an important part in asthma. Information from necropsies on patients with fatal asthma, airway biopsy studies and the presence of pro-inflammatory mediators, cytokines and chemokines in bronchoalveolar lavage fluid demonstrate a complex inflammatory cascade that initiates and sustains clinical asthma [1]. In particular, the immunoglobulin (Ig) E-mediated response to inhaled allergens in atopic asthma is fundamental to this process in which mast cells and eosinophils also play a central role. Bronchoconstrictor substances, such as histamine and leukotrienes (LTs), are released from the mast cells in acute asthma. This may be followed 4–6 hours later by a late asthmatic reaction mediated by cytokines and chemokines from resident mast cells, macrophages, epithelial cells and recruited lymphocytes and eosinophils.

□ AIRWAY INFLAMMATION

The role of the eosinophil in asthma

Current knowledge of airway inflammation in asthma points to a central role for the eosinophil (Fig. 1) [2]. The inflammatory cascade is initiated by the inhalation of antigens which stimulate mast cells and T helper (Th) 2 lymphocytes to produce histamine, LTs and cytokines. In particular, the Th2 lymphocyte secretes interleukin (IL)-4, granulocyte-macrophage colony stimulating factor (GM-CSF) and IL-5. IL-5 stimulates terminal differentiation of eosinophils by the bone marrow. The eosinophils are then taken up in the circulation and, following migration to the lung and interaction with selectins, adhere to the endothelium through the binding of integrins to adhesion molecules. The eosinophils transmigrate into the airway under the influence of chemokines and cytokines such as RANTES (regulated on activation, T cell expressed and secreted) eotaxin, monocyte chemotactic protein-1

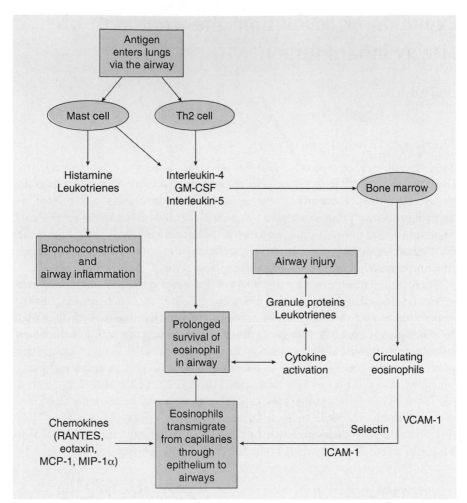

Fig. 1 Allergic inflammation in the airways and the role of eosinophils (GM-CSF = granulocyte-macrophage colony stimulating factor; ICAM = intercellular adhesion molecule; MCP = monocyte chemotactic protein; MIP = macrophage inflammatory protein; Th = T helper; VCAM = vascular cell adhesion molecule) [2].

and macrophage inflammatory protein-α. Their survival is prolonged by IL-5 and GM-CSF. When activated, inflammatory mediators are released from the eosinophil, including LTs and major basic protein (MBP), which may damage airway tissue. There is therefore a mechanism for a sustained inflammatory response to allergic stimuli.

In patients with asthma, airway eosinophilia is regulated by CD4+ T cells, mainly Th2. Th2 lymphocytes are important in allergic responses and host defence against parasites, whereas Th1 lymphocytes produce interferon γ and IL-2 which regulate defences against viral and bacterial infections. The presence of IL-12 at antigen presentation is critical to Th1 differentiation, and might therefore be of therapeutic value in shifting immune responses down this pathway and away from the Th2 phenotype. In animal models, either blocking IL-5 or administering IL-12 can inhibit airway inflammation and hyperresponsiveness.

The production of eosinophils in the bone marrow is regulated by IL-3, IL-5 and GM-CSF. Since IL-5 induces terminal differentiation of the eosinophils, particular attention has been directed to antagonism of its action as a possible mode of therapy.

Chronic obstructive pulmonary disease

The inflammatory cascade in COPD follows exposure of the airway to cigarette smoke and other irritants which interact with macrophages and epithelial cells in the airway (Fig. 2) [3]. There is consequent release of neutrophil chemotactic factors including IL-8 and LTB4. Proteases that break down connective tissue are released from the neutrophils and macrophages and mucus hypersecretion is stimulated. Cytotoxic T cells (CD8+ lymphocytes) are also involved in the lung damage. This mechanism therefore is largely neutrophil based.

There is some overlap between the inflammatory processes in asthma and COPD. Eosinophils may be found in the airway wall in acute exacerbations of the latter, while in acute episodes of asthma, particularly those associated with infection, the neutrophil may play an important role. In these circumstances, the pathological hallmarks of asthma and COPD may be blurred.

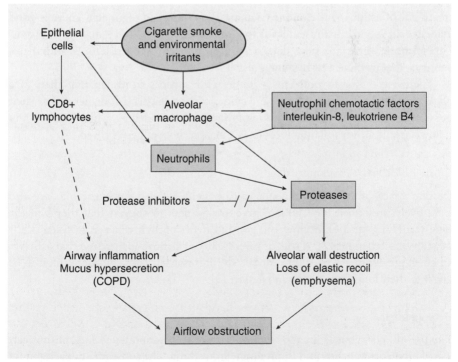

Fig. 2 Inflammatory mechanisms in chronic obstructive pulmonary disease (COPD) [3].

☐ TREATMENT OF AIRWAY INFLAMMATION

The treatment of airway inflammation has been laid out in a number of national and international guidelines [4,5]. Historically, the drug treatment of COPD tended to follow developments for asthma. Evolving understanding of the different mechanisms of inflammation may in future allow the conditions to be targeted with more specificity. The following agents have been demonstrated to have anti-inflammatory actions and are listed in current asthma and COPD guidelines:

- ☐ corticosteroids
- ☐ beta-agonists
- ☐ theophylline
- ☐ LT antagonists
- ☐ cromones
- ☐ (immunotherapy).

The last two will not be discussed further.

Corticosteroids

Asthma

Corticosteroids are the most widely used and potent anti-inflammatory drugs for the treatment of airway disease. Inhaled corticosteroids are now the cornerstone of treatment of asthma, either alone or as part of combined regimens. There is good evidence that regular treatment leads to fewer exacerbations and reduced symptoms. Furthermore, there are now data on interactions of corticosteroids with beta-agonists, theophylline and LT antagonists (see below).

There are, however, problems with inhaled corticosteroids, in that there is a plateau on the dose-response curve and evidence for side effects at higher doses. Their possible beneficial effect on prevention of the airway remodelling, which is thought to follow chronic airway inflammation in asthma, has not yet been proven [6].

Chronic obstructive pulmonary disease

Despite a lack of definitive evidence as to benefit, inhaled corticosteroids are also extensively prescribed for COPD. There are no data to suggest that they halt the long-term lung function decline, but good evidence of their value given systemically in acute exacerbations [7]. A trial of reversibility of airflow obstruction that achieves an effect greater than 15% with systemic steroids is essential if consideration is to be given to their long-term use by inhalation [3].

Beta-agonists

The use of beta-agonists for the relief of airflow obstruction dates back to the early use of inhaled adrenaline and isoprenaline for asthma. The subsequent development of the saligenins with more beta-2 specificity, such as salbutamol, and the resorcinols, such as terbutaline, led to their current position as the most widely prescribed drugs for the relief of airflow obstruction. In the last 10 years the arrival of the long-acting beta-agonists such as salmeterol, with a long lipophilic tail, and formoterol, have led not only to a further increase in prescribing for regular use but also to a developing interest in the possible anti-inflammatory actions of these drugs alone or in combination [8].

This has happened on the background of a debate in the early 1990s about the possible deleterious effects of regular inhaled short-acting beta-agonists. However, the clinical benefit of regular inhaled long-acting beta-agonists was defined by a study from Greening and Ind [9]. Addition of a long-acting beta-agonist, salmeterol, gave better asthma control than increasing the dose of inhaled corticosteroid in a group of 427 patients whose asthma was poorly controlled on low-dose inhaled corticosteroids. The findings were confirmed in a subsequent study [10].

The 'add on' form of therapy is now in widespread use in clinical practice. The model of adding on a different drug to low-dose inhaled corticosteroid, rather than increasing the dose of the latter, has been developed with other agents. With beta-agonists themselves, there is growing evidence that the clinical interaction between them and corticosteroids and beta-agonists has a molecular basis. The inactive steroid receptor is primed by the long-acting beta-agonist, so less inhaled corticosteroid may therefore be required for activation, resulting in increased anti-inflammatory activity [8].

Despite all the positive evidence for their benefits, some doubts remain concerning the long-term safety of regular inhaled beta-agonists, particularly in the short-acting formulations. Because beta-agonists are racemic molecules, and the 'S' enantiomer – which contributes nothing to bronchodilatation and may augment airway inflammation – is stereoselectively metabolised more slowly that the 'R' enantiomer, it has been hypothesised that the use of a single 'R' enantiomer might be preferable. To this end, 'R' salbutamol is now available in nebulised form in the US [11].

Theophylline

Theophylline, a 1,3-dimethylxanthine, has long been known to be a bronchodilator when given systemically and has been available as a treatment for airway disease for about 60 years. Use of theophylline began to fall away in the 1970s because of its irritant properties in the stomach and competition from the newly arrived beta-2-agonists. However, controlled-release formulations became available which sustained interest, and new data on anti-inflammatory actions of theophylline started to emerge in the early 1990s. In particular, theophylline was reported to have important inhibitory effects on the late asthmatic response [12]. As with the beta-agonists, an 'add on' effect of theophylline to low-dose inhaled corticosteroids was demonstrated to be more beneficial than increasing the dose of the latter [13].

Mechanism of action of theophylline

The mechanism of action of theophylline has been thought partly to reside in its role as a non-specific inhibitor of the phosphodiesterase (PD) family of enzymes.

Inhibition of PDE4 is known to increase cyclic AMP levels in mast cells, eosinophils, macrophages and neutrophils. Specific PD inhibition as a route into inhibiting inflammation in the airway was investigated, leading to the development of PDE4 inhibitors such as CP80633, CDP840 and SB207499 (Ariflo) [14].

However, theophylline is a weak PD inhibitor and other mechanisms for its action continue to be investigated. There is now a novel approach to understanding the anti-inflammatory actions of theophylline through its molecular mechanism. Theophylline has been shown in a series of careful studies to be recruited to the histone deacetylase complex which inhibits inflammatory gene transcription in the cell. This mechanism could explain the synergistic clinical data with inhaled corticosteroid [15].

Leukotriene antagonists

LTs are formed by the action of 5-lipoxygenase (5-LO) and 5-LO activating protein (FLAP) on arachidonic acid to form LTA4, which is in turn metabolised to LTB4 or the cysteinyl-LTs (LTC4, LTD4 and LTE4) (Fig. 3). LTB4 is a powerful chemotactic agent, whereas the cysteinyl-LTs cause bronchoconstriction and increase mucus secretion, airway wall oedema, eosinophilia and bronchial hyperreactivity. Clearly, these actions are of interest in the pathogenesis of asthma and COPD. In particular, LTB4 inhibition might reduce airway inflammation in COPD. Studies of these issues are being pursued.

The role of the cysteinyl-LTs has generated most pharmacological interest. Specific cysteinyl-LT receptor antagonists such as montelukast, zafirlukast and pranlukast are now available for clinical use in asthma. Data show that they give good control of symptoms, inhibit exercise-induced asthma, and are safe when given

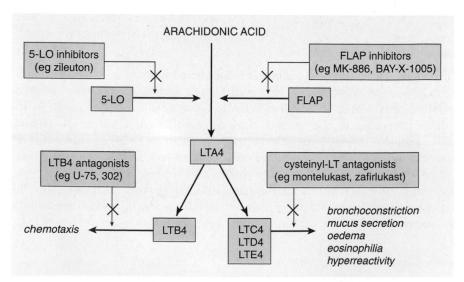

Fig. 3 The 5-lipoxygenase (5-LO) pathway showing the metabolism of arachidonic acid to leukotriene (LT) B4 and the cysteinyl-LTs (LTC4, LTD4 and LTE4) (FLAP = 5-LO activating protein).

by the oral route [16]. Additive effects to inhaled corticosteroids have also been demonstrated [17].

The leukotriene C4 synthase gene

One intriguing clinical observation with these agents is that they are effective in up to 70% of asthmatics, of whom about half will show major symptomatic improvement. It has been suggested that the ability to respond may be genetically determined, based on a polymorphism in the human LTC4 synthase gene. This gene is carried by 76% of patients with aspirin-induced asthma [18] compared with 42% of non-asthmatics and aspirin-tolerant asthmatics. The carriers also have higher levels of mRNA for LTC4 in eosinophils and an increased capacity of eosinophils to synthesise cysteinyl-LTs. Synthesis of LTC4 by calcium ionophore-stimulated blood eosinophils from normal subjects with variant genotypes in the presence of indomethacin is greater than from those with the 'wild type' LTC4 synthase genotype. Individuals who carry the variant genotype may respond better to the oral LTC4 receptor antagonist zafirlukast. If these studies are borne out by further evidence, it would be an important advance in treatment for patients with asthma.

Novel agents

Several novel treatments for airway inflammation are now under investigation (Table 1) or close to launch for clinical use.

Monoclonal antibodies

A monoclonal antibody to IgE (RhuMoAb-E25) given intravenously [19] inhibited the early and late asthmatic responses in a group of atopic asthmatics by 37% and 62%, respectively, but was inactive on either response when given in aerosolised form [20]. A further study in 317 subjects with moderate to severe asthma over

Table 1 Novel treatments for airway inflammation.

Asthma	COPD
• PDE4 inhibitors	• PDE4 inhibitors
• Monoclonal antibodies to IgE, IL-5	• Monoclonal antibodies to IL-8, TNFα, adhesion molecules
• IL-12	• Antioxidants (glutathione analogue)
• Antagonists of CD4+, TNFα, adhesion molecules, CTLA-4	• Tachykinin antagonists
	• Opioids
	• NκB inhibitors
	• IL-10

COPD = chronic obstructive pulmonary disease; CTLA = cytotoxic T lymphocyte antigen; Ig = immunoglobulin; IL = interleukin; PD = phosphodiesterase; TNF = tumour necrosis factor.

20 weeks had a significant effect on symptoms and led to a reduction of corticosteroid use [21]. Although this was linked to a 95% decrease in serum IgE, the clinical responses were only moderate. Further multicentre studies are awaited.

Cytokines

Several investigations into the role of cytokines are in progress. Two recently published studies have both mechanistic and therapeutic implications:

1   A study of the effect of recombinant human IL-12 on eosinophils, airway hyperresponsiveness and the late asthmatic response demonstrated that IL-12 given subcutaneously lowers the number of blood and sputum eosinophils, but without significant effects on airway hyperresponsiveness or the late asthmatic reaction [22].

2   A parallel study of the effects of intravenous administration of an IL-5 monoclonal antibody on eosinophils, airway hyperresponsiveness and the late asthmatic response also showed a marked decrease in blood eosinophils for up to 16 weeks and sputum eosinophils for up to four weeks, but again there was no effect on the late asthmatic response or airway hyperresponsiveness [23].

These approaches, on the one hand augmenting IL-12 and, on the other, blocking IL-5, are potential novel approaches to the treatment of asthma. Although there was a marked effect on eosinophil numbers, the lack of effect on both airway hyperresponsiveness and the late asthmatic reaction questions at a fundamental level the role of eosinophils in asthma. However, asthma is a complex disease, and it remains to be seen whether neutralising or augmenting a single cytokine is significant or will provide clinical benefit to patients.

☐ CONCLUSIONS

The approach to the treatment of airway inflammation is based on the evolution of current treatments and their combination in therapeutically useful regimens. Knowledge of the basic mechanisms of airway inflammation and the action of anti-inflammatory drugs in the airway is contributing to advances in therapeutics. Novel treatments, in particular those directed at specific mediators or cytokines, may not be beneficial as 'stand alone' therapies but possibly only when incorporated in multidrug targeted treatment regimens.

REFERENCES

1   Busse WW, Lemanske RF Jr. Asthma. Review. *N Engl J Med* 2001; **344**: 350–62.
2   Sanderson CJ. Interleukin-5, eosinophils, and disease. Review. *Blood* 1992; **79**: 3101–9.
3   Barnes PJ. Chronic obstructive pulmonary disease. Review. *N Engl J Med* 2000; **343**: 269–80.

4   British Thoracic Society Guidelines for the Management of Chronic Obstructive Pulmonary Disease. *Thorax* 1997; 52(Suppl 5).

5   National Heart, Lung and Blood Institute. Asthma management and prevention: a practical guide for public health officials and health care professionals. Publication No. 96-3659A. Bethesda, MD: National Institutes of Health, 1995.

6   Bousqet J, Jeffrey PK, Busse WW, Johnson M, Vignola AM. Asthma. From bronchoconstriction to airways inflammation and remodeling. Review. *Am J Resp Crit Care Med* 2000; 161: 1720–45.

7   Banner AS. Emerging role of corticosteroids in chronic obstructive pulmonary disease. *Lancet* 1999; 354: 440–1.

8   Taylor DR, Hancox RJ. Interaction between corticosteroids and beta agonists. Review. *Thorax* 2000; 55: 595–602.

9   Greening AP, Ind DW, Northfield M, Shaw G. Added salmeterol versus higher-dose corticosteroid in asthma patients with symptoms on existing inhaled corticosteroid. Allen & Hanburys Limited UK Study Group. *Lancet* 1994; 344: 219–24.

10   Pauwels RA, Löfdahl CG, Postma DS, Tattersfield AE, *et al.* Effect of inhaled formoterol and budesonide on exacerbations of asthma. Formoterol and Corticosteroids Establishing Therapy (FACET) International Study Group. *N Engl J Med* 1997; 337: 1405–11.

11   Handley D. The asthma-like pharmacology and toxicology of (S)-isomers of beta agonists. Review. *J Allergy Clin Immunol* 1999; 104: S569–76.

12   Sullivan P, Bekir S, Jaffar Z, Page C, *et al.* Anti-inflammatory effects of low-dose theophylline in atopic asthma. *Lancet* 1994; 343: 1006–8.

13   Evans DJ, Taylor DA, Zetterstrom O, Cheung KF, *et al.* A comparison of low-dose inhaled budesonide plus theophylline and high-dose inhaled budesonide for moderate asthma. *N Engl J Med* 1997; 337: 1412–8.

14   Torphy TJ, Barnette MS, Underwood DC, Griswold DE, *et al.* Ariflo (SB207499), a second generation phosphodiesterase 4 inhibitor for the treatment of asthma and COPD: from concept to clinic. Review. *Pulm Pharmacol Ther* 1999; 12: 131–5.

15   Ito K, Lim S, Caramori G, Chung KF, *et al.* A novel molecular mechanism for theophylline – induction of histone deacetylase activity (in press).

16   Sampson A, Holgate S. Leukotriene modifiers in the treatment of asthma. Look promising across the board of asthma severity. *Br Med J* 1998; 316: 1257–8.

17   Laviolette M, Malmstrom K, Lu S, Chervinsky P, *et al.* Montelukast added to inhaled beclomethasone in treatment of asthma. Montelukast/Beclomethasone Additivity Group. *Am J Resp Crit Care Med* 1999; 160: 1862–8.

18   Sanak M, Simon H, Szczeklik A. Leukotriene C4 synthase promoter polymorphism and risk of aspirin-induced asthma. *Lancet* 1997; 350: 1599–600.

19   Fahy JV, Fleming HE, Wong HH, Liu JT, *et al.* The effect of an anti-IgE monoclonal antibody on the early- and late-phase responses to allergen inhalation in asthmatic subjects. *Am J Resp Crit Care Med* 1997; 155: 1828–34.

20   Fahy JV, Cockcroft DW, Boulet LP, Wong HH, *et al.* Effect of aerosolized anti-IgE (E25) on airway responses to inhaled allergen in asthmatic subjects. *Am J Resp Crit Care Med* 1999; 160: 1023–7.

21   Milgrom H, Fick RB Jr, Su JQ, Reimann JD, *et al..* Treatment of allergic asthma with monoclonal anti-IgE antibody. *N Engl J Med* 1999; 341: 1966–73.

22   Bryan SA, O'Connor BJ, Matti S, Leckie MJ, *et al.* Effects of recombinant human interleukin-12 on eosinophils, airway hyper-responsiveness and the late asthmatic response. *Lancet* 2000; 356: 2149–53.

23   Leckie MJ, ten Brinke A, Khan J, Diamant Z, *et al.* Effects of an interleukin-5 blocking monoclonal antibody on eosinophils airway hyper-responsiveness, and the late asthmatic response. *Lancet* 2000; 356: 2144–8.

□ SELF ASSESSMENT QUESTIONS

1   Airway inflammation:
   (a) Is identical in chronic bronchitis and asthma
   (b) Is associated with bronchial hyperresponsiveness in asthma
   (c) Is driven by T helper 1 lymphocytes in asthma
   (d) Is characteristic of the late asthmatic reaction
   (e) Cysteinyl leukotrienes (LTs) play an important part in the late asthmatic reaction

2   In chronic obstructive pulmonary disease (COPD):
   (a) Inhaled irritants interact with macrophages and epithelial cells
   (b) Eosinophils may be found in the airway wall in acute exacerbations
   (c) Proteases from macrophages protect connective tissue
   (d) Loss of lung elastic recoil causes airflow obstruction in emphysema

3   Corticosteroids for the treatment of airway inflammation:
   (a) May have beneficial interaction with theophylline
   (b) When inhaled regularly reduce long-term function decline in COPD
   (c) Have proven benefit in preventing airway remodelling in asthma
   (d) Are useful in the treatment of exacerbations in COPD
   (e) When regularly inhaled reduce the number of exacerbations of asthma

4   Cysteinyl LT antagonists for the treatment of asthma:
   (a) Are beneficial to some extent in all asthmatics
   (b) Are given by the inhaled route
   (c) May specifically help aspirin-sensitive asthmatics
   (d) The response to treatment may be genetically determined
   (e) Inhibit exercise-induced asthma

5   The following may be useful in the treatment of asthma:
   (a) Monoclonal antibody to immunoglobulin E
   (b) Recombinant human interleukin-12
   (c) Phosphodiesterase 4 inhibitors

ANSWERS

1a False	2a True	3a True	4a False	5a True
b True	b True	b False	b False	b False
c False	c False	c False	c True	c True
d True	d True	d True	d True	
e True		e True	e True	

Lung transplantation

Paul Corris

□ INTRODUCTION

The modern era for lung transplantation began in 1981 when Bruce Reitz and colleagues from Stanford University introduced combined heart and lung transplantation (HLT) for patients with pulmonary vascular disease [1]. Indications for HLT were subsequently widened to include various pulmonary conditions [2]. Survival rates were good and in marked contrast to results obtained for single lung transplantation (SLT) over the preceding 25 years [3]. The success of HLT was based on reliable healing of the tracheal anastomosis compared with the bronchial anastomotic breakdown frequently seen following SLT. This reliable healing reflected a good blood supply to the proximal donor trachea via donor coronary artery/bronchial artery anastomoses, in contrast to the lack of blood supplied to the proximal donor bronchus following SLT. The lack of success with SLT was also based both on poor selection of potential recipients, some of whom were septic and had multi-organ failure, and on the apparently insuperable problems of rejection and infections.

It was realised, however, that many patients undergoing HLT received a new heart unnecessarily. In 1986, after a period of research, the Toronto Group reported success with SLT in patients with fibrosing lung disease [4]. Important potential factors were:

- □ careful patient selection

- □ restoration of a viable blood supply to the bronchial anastomosis by wrapping it with a pedicle of greater omentum

- □ the introduction of cyclosporin A as the principal immunosuppressant.

It has subsequently been shown that the bronchial anastomosis does not require a wrap of omentum for reliable healing and no centres now perform this procedure. Some centres experimented with direct revascularisation of donor bronchial artery to ensure good blood supply to the donor bronchus but this practice has also been abandoned.

In 1988, the double lung transplant operation (DLT) was introduced by Patterson et al [5]. This procedure used an en bloc transplantation of both lungs with a tracheal anastomosis. It was accompanied by much more frequent problems with airway healing than with the HLT operation [6]. In addition, the operation was, if anything, more complex than HLT, and the extensive mediastinal dissection frequently led to denervation of the recipient's native heart. Bleeding was at least as great a problem as with HLT and by 1989 the procedure as originally described had been largely abandoned. Noirclerc [7] provided the solution to the problem of airway healing by performing two separate bronchial anastomoses – because, as in SLT, the donor bronchus is better vascularised initially if the anastomosis is close to the lung parenchyma.

This concept was further developed by Pasque *et al* [8] with the bilateral sequential lung transplant (BSLT). As its name implies, two separate lungs are implanted with separate hilar anastomoses (each of bronchus, pulmonary artery and left atrial cuff). The heart and mediastinum are left largely undisturbed. The incision is a transverse bilateral thoracotomy, dividing the sternum horizontally. In contrast to HLT, both SLT and BSLT do not in general require cardiopulmonary bypass with associated anticoagulation.

A final development comprises the use of living lobar transplantation involving the implantation of two lobes from two living donors. This procedure is suitable only for children or small adults, and will not impact greatly on transplantation for chronic obstructive pulmonary disease (COPD).

☐ EVOLUTION OF LUNG TRANSPLANTATION IN CHRONIC OBSTRUCTIVE PULMONARY DISEASE

It was originally believed that patients with end-stage COPD were not suitable for SLT. Objections to SLT for emphysema arose because of perceived problems with the native lung which would be ventilated during a period of positive-pressure ventilation, leading to air trapping, subsequent mediastinal shift and compression of the transplanted lung. Perfusion would be directed towards the transplanted lung because of expected lower pulmonary vascular resistance, so ventilation perfusion V̇/Q imbalance would result.

These considerations proved to be more than only theoretical. Experience in the early 1970s demonstrated that severe ventilation perfusion imbalance and hyperinflation of the native lung did occur [9,10]. Therefore, patients with emphysema, including those with inherited alpha1-antitrypsin deficiency, were initially treated with combined HLT. The successful results in patients with alpha1-antitrypsin deficiency showed that such patients could undergo transplant procedures and retain normal lung function in the first 12–18 months without replacement therapy. The shortfall in donor heart lung blocks (ie combined heart and lung donation as a combined procedure for one recipient) led to the introduction of the *en bloc* DLT for emphysema but, as previously noted, this operation was associated with tracheal anastomotic complications in 50% of patients and quickly lost favour. Successful introduction of SLT for patients with fibrosing lung disease led to re-examination of this procedure for patients with emphysema because of the dramatic improvement in both donor lung preservation and surgical techniques since the early 1970s.

Following a preliminary report of successful SLT for emphysema by Mal *et al* [11] in France in 1989, the Washington Lung Transplant Group cautiously embarked on a programme of SLT in patients with emphysema and demonstrated the utility and safety of this procedure in carefully selected patients [8]. Although the mechanics of the native lung remain the same, improvements in patient selection, lung preservation and anaesthetic management have contributed to the success. Subsequent experience from other groups including our own has demonstrated the potential problem of residual infection in the native lung [12]. Moreover, most patients with large bilateral bullae may still show evidence of gross hyperinflation of the native lung in the early postoperative period after SLT. Thus, the BSLT transplantation was successfully applied to patients with emphysema who were not suitable for SLT.

There is now reasonable agreement about technical approaches to transplantation for COPD, in particular for emphysema with which experience is greatest:

☐ Patients with no evidence of large bilateral bullae are suitable for consideration for SLT.

☐ Patients with frequent pulmonary sepsis or marked bullous disease may be considered for HLT [13] or BSLT, with the latter increasingly used as the procedure of choice [14].

☐ INDICATIONS, CONSIDERATIONS AND CRITERIA FOR LUNG TRANSPLANTATION

Age

The shortfall in suitable donor organs has led to an upper age limit of 55–60 years for transplantation of heart and lungs or both lungs alone, and an upper age limit of 65 years for transplantation of single lung. The higher age limit for the latter reflects the increased availability of suitable single lungs.

Disease-specific guidelines

Transplantation is usually considered for a patient when estimated life expectancy is less than 18 months. However, it is inherently difficult to predict the survival in many patients with advanced obstructive disease. It is now recognised that patients with COPD may experience improved functional capacity following transplantation, but not necessarily improved survival. The International Society of Heart and Lung Transplantation (ISHLT) guidelines on referral of patients with COPD are as follows (Table 1):

☐ FEV_1 less than 25% predicted, without reversibility, *and/or*

☐ PaO_2 below 7.3 kPa, *and/or*

☐ elevated pulmonary artery pressure, with progressive deterioration such as cor pulmonale

☐ preference should be given to patients with elevated $PaCO_2$ with progressive deterioration who require long-term oxygen therapy as they have the poorest prognosis [15,16].

Table 1 Guidelines for transplant referral.

• FEV$_1$ <25% predicted
• Maximum medical treatment
• Capacity for rehabilitation
• Hypercapnia
• Pulmonary hypertension
• Unacceptable quality of life

Nutritional state

Many patients reaching the end stage of chronic pulmonary disease suffer from cachexia and malnutrition [17]. All transplant recipients lose weight in the first week following transplantation, and the presence of severe pre-operative nutritional deficiency leads to an inability to withstand the rigours of the postoperative period, increasing susceptibility to infection and poor wound healing. Obesity, on the other hand, increases surgical risk, predisposing to atelectasis and impairing postoperative mobility which is essential following lung transplantation. Ideally, recipients should weigh within 15 kg of their ideal body weight. There is an increased mortality in adult patients whose body weight is less than 40 kg. The early unsuccessful transplant recipients were all bed-bound. The majority of transplant centres now require that recipients are capable of self-care and able to participate in gentle exercise rehabilitation to maintain muscle bulk and physical fitness.

Infection

Localised sepsis pre-operatively may lead to severe systemic infection postoperatively because of the need for immunosuppressive therapy. Extrapulmonary sepsis therefore mitigates against successful transplantation. Patients with recurrent or persistent pulmonary infection are not suitable for SLT. Oral hygiene is important, and all patients should have any dental sepsis eradicated pre-operatively.

The presence of subpleural aspergilloma is a contraindication to any form of lung transplant. Removal of the lung containing an aspergilloma is likely to result in seeding of the pleural space with aspergillus, leading to fungal empyema. Removal of the contralateral lung for SLT leaves the aspergilloma *in situ*, and subsequent immunosuppression will inevitably lead to disseminated aspergillus infection.

Previous surgery

If there are pleural scars or adhesions, there is a risk of life-threatening haemorrhage when the native lungs are removed. There is a gradation of risk from scarring due to previous open lung biopsy via a limited thoracotomy to previous total pleurectomy. This is regarded as a contraindication for HLT. The risks of prior surgery have important consequences for the management of pneumothorax in potential recipients with emphysema. If pleurodesis is required, surgeons should be advised to perform limited anterior pleurodesis. The use of the anti-fibrinolytic aprotinin during transplant surgery reduces bleeding in patients who have undergone previous thoracotomy [18], and the recent development of BSLT via a transverse bilateral thoracotomy allows the surgeon much better access to the pleural space than is afforded by a sternotomy. In this regard, BSLT has advantages over the original HLT.

Systemic corticosteroids

Although early lung transplant programmes insisted on patients being weaned from corticosteroids, this proved difficult in practice, particularly in patients with COPD. Data from Newcastle show that bronchial anastomoses are at no greater risk in patients receiving up to 20 mg of prednisolone a day than in those not taking prednisolone [19], provided that there is no evidence of steroid-induced thinning of the skin, osteoporosis or myopathy.

Osteoporosis

Patients with COPD who are being considered for transplantation may already have been treated with corticosteroids for many years. Moreover, their intrinsic disease leads to markedly decreased physical activity. These factors, together with age and hormonal deficiencies, frequently result in a substantial loss of bone mineral density (BMD). Immunosuppressive agents post-transplantation, such as corticosteroids and cyclosporin, accelerate loss of bone mineral. Accordingly, patients who have severe osteoporosis or those with a history of compression fractures in the pretransplant period are at high risk for the recurrence of fractures postoperatively. Symptomatic osteoporosis is now regarded as a contraindication for transplant referral until therapy (usually with bisphosphonates) improves their BMD.

Cardiac disease

Ideally, patients with COPD under consideration for SLT or BSLT should have sufficient preservation of right ventricular function to allow single lung anaesthesia, obviating the need for cardiopulmonary bypass. The right ventricle has a great capacity to show improved function after successful surgery when pulmonary vascular resistance falls to normal. The Toronto Group has successfully performed an SLT in a patient with a right ventricular ejection fraction (RVEF) of only 12%, although the mean RVEFs of a series of patients they reported were 31% and 38% for SLT and DLT candidates, respectively [16]. Our group has shown that pulmonary vascular resistance, pulmonary artery pressure and right ventricular performance have returned to normal following SLT for pulmonary fibrosis even when markedly abnormal pre-operatively [20]. The presence of cor pulmonale complicating COPD is not a contraindication for successful SLT.

Psychological factors

No procedure in medicine provides more stress for recipients and family than lung transplantation. The process begins from the time of initial referral and lasts until postoperative rehabilitation is complete. Any potential recipient must be well motivated and want a lung transplant, be able to cope and have demonstrated a willingness to comply. A supportive family or circle of close friends is essential. Underlying psychiatric illness, abuse of alcohol or drugs (including cigarettes) are contraindications.

Presence of other major organ dysfunction

Good renal and hepatic function is essential, particularly in view of cyclosporin toxicity [21]. A creatinine clearance of over 50 ml/min is required and only minor abnormalities of liver function are acceptable. The latter is clearly important in patients with alpha1-antitrypsin deficiency who may have abnormalities of hepatic function as a result of their disease. The presence of portal hypertension would preclude consideration of lung transplantation. If well controlled, type 1 diabetes mellitus no longer rules out transplantation.

Volume reduction surgery

The successful introduction of lung volume reduction surgery (LVRS) may appear to have added an alternative surgical treatment option for patients under consideration for lung transplantation. In practice, however, patients deemed suitable for LVRS represent a different subgroup. The criteria for LVRS continue to evolve, but it is clear that all patients should have:

☐ ceased smoking

☐ a marked disability, despite completing a comprehensive pulmonary rehabilitation programme

☐ considerable airflow obstruction (FEV_1 <35% predicted)

☐ marked thoracic hyperinflation.

Importantly, the lungs should show sufficient heterogeneity in the distribution of emphysema to provide the surgeon with target areas of non-functioning volume occupying lung which is amenable to surgical resection. In general, patients with severe hypoxaemia, hypercapnia or pulmonary hypertension are not suitable. Patients with alpha1-antitrypsin deficiency have demonstrated a rapid decline following LVRS which is now considered a contraindication to the procedure in most surgical units.

LVRS and lung transplantation need not be considered as mutually exclusive procedures. There is now clear evidence that successful lung transplantation can be performed following LVRS in patients whose lung function and quality of life deteriorate, after apparent benefit, to the level at which poor prognostic features develop.

Lung transplantation: an exercise in quality rather than quantity?

Two published studies suggest that lung transplantation does not in general confer a survival benefit in patients with end-stage emphysema at two years of follow-up. In the first study, Hosenpud *et al* [22] analysed data from the Joint United Network for Organ Sharing/ISHLT Thoracic Registry to clarify the survival benefit of lung transplantation in patients with cystic fibrosis (CF), idiopathic pulmonary fibrosis and emphysema. Using a time-dependent, non-proportional hazard analysis, assessment of the risk of mortality after transplantation relative to that in patients on the waiting list suggested a survival benefit following lung transplantation for patients with CF and idiopathic pulmonary fibrosis. By contrast, in patients with emphysema the mortality rate on the waiting list was low, so survival following transplantation did not exceed waiting list survival during the two-year follow-up.

Some caution is needed over the interpretation of these findings, first, because the data came from many centres prior to publication of international guidelines, so participating centres were unlikely to have a uniform listing policy for all patients. Moreover, some centres employed a policy of listing patients at an early stage in the development of severe lung dysfunction, given the long waiting time for lung transplantation – which clearly biased the analysis towards waiting list survival. The data included selectively reported experience in the USA, where waiting time is the most important determinant of organ allocation, which clearly encourages larger transplant centres to list patients early.

The Dutch Lung Transplant Group has also published data demonstrating no difference in survival in patients with emphysema whether transplanted or remaining on the waiting list, although this study was underpowered to derive a clear conclusion. It is important to note that the conclusions were based on group mean data. Clearly, individual patients with emphysema who are hypoxaemic, hypercapnic, underweight, with pulmonary hypertension and a history of previous intubation for an episode of severe type II respiratory failure have a different prognosis from that of disabled but stable patients.

Matching donor to recipient

Donor matching is based on ABO compatibility and size by calculating the predicted total lung capacity (TLC) of both donor and recipient using height, age and sex. There is no direct measurement of donor lung TLC. In those patients with COPD who have much greater lung capacity than predicted, it is preferable to give larger lungs than calculated in this way, particularly if it will be an SLT. The size discrepancy between the transplanted lung and hemithorax commonly prevents sealing of any parenchymal leak which, if present, may lead to pneumothoraces persisting for several days. The chest wall remains compliant and, in practice, is observed to change shape in the first few days after transplantation.

A screening lymphocytotoxic cross-match using recipient serum and a banked pool of lymphocytes is carried out in all potential recipients accepted for transplantation to exclude the presence of preformed antibodies. Direct cross-match with lymphocytes from a potential donor is carried out prospectively only when this screening test is positive. Wherever possible, donor and recipient are matched for cytomegalovirus (CMV) status. If a CMV-negative recipient receives a CMV-positive organ, serious CMV infection can ensue. Most centres use prophylactic oral ganciclovir 1 g tds for the first three months. This approach prevents CMV disease when immunosuppression is highest, and delays its onset until the host response aids recovery. Alternative strategies include the use of weekly testing for levels of antigenaemia by polymerase chain reaction and treating when levels rise.

Choice of operation (Table 2)

There are several reasons why SLT is an attractive option in patients with emphysema:

- ☐ the procedure is technically straightforward

- ☐ most recipients do not have pleural adhesions

- ☐ the functional results of SLT are acceptable, most patients achieving an FEV_1 of 50% predicted.

These improvements are not as dramatic as those achieved following BLT but there are no major differences in maximum exercise performance. A significant degree of limitation usually persists with both procedures with maximum oxygen consumption of 45–52% predicted. However, patients who remain free of obliterative bronchiolitis (OB) enjoy a normal lifestyle and a good quality of life. The obvious advantage of SLT over BLT is that the former procedure enables more transplantations to be conducted if both donor lungs are acceptable.

Critics of the SLT option are concerned about hyperinflation of the native lung and potential compression of the contralateral graft. Although volume reduction on the opposite side can be considered, the use of SLT may be best limited to those patients without bullous disease and older patients who may be less able to tolerate the more major bilateral procedure. There is evidence that quality of life and long-term survival is slightly better in bilateral recipients than in their unilateral counterparts. The preference is therefore to offer BLT to younger patients and those of large stature with significant bilateral bullous disease.

One further consideration in the choice of operation relates to the potential risk of native lung sepsis following SLT. As a consequence, patients with a history of recurrent infective exacerbations associated with continued sputum production are usually offered BLT. All patients considered for SLT undergo computed tomography

Table 2 Transplantation for chronic obstructive pulmonary disease.

Single lung	Bilateral lung
Best use of resource	Better lung function but not exercise performance
Less extensive surgery	Better survival at 3 years and quality of life long term
Patients >50 years	Patients <50 years or with bilateral bullae

(CT) scanning to ensure that there is no evidence of bilateral bronchiectasis, which would indicate the need for the bilateral lung procedure.

Finally, the choice between left or right SLT is based on a pre-operative perfusion scan. Where perfusion is equal, either right or left transplantation is carried out, but where the difference in perfusion is greater than 40% to the left or 60% to the right, the preference is to transplant the lung with the least functional contribution.

☐ POSTOPERATIVE COMPLICATIONS AND FOLLOW-UP

Immunosuppression and postoperative management

Most patients are extubated within 36 hours of surgery and then begin an active programme of mobilisation. Fluid intake is restricted in the early postoperative period, with diuresis encouraged to avoid accumulation of fluid in the lungs.

Prophylactic antibiotics in the form of flucloxacillin and metronidazole are given for the first five days. The donor lungs are lavaged, with samples sent to microbiology prior to implantation, so that appropriate antibiotics may be started early to cover 'donor acquired' pulmonary sepsis. At present, patients receive azathioprine, anti-thymocyte globulin, methylprednisolone and cyclosporin during the immediate postoperative period. Alternative therapy substituting azathioprine with mycophenolate mofetil or cyclosporin with tacrolimus is favoured by some centres. Anti-thymocyte globulin is stopped after three days and methylprednisolone substituted by oral prednisolone at a rapidly tailing dose to a maintenance dose of 0.1 mg/kg. If there is no evidence of lung rejection at six months, maintenance steroids may be withdrawn gradually.

Rejection episodes are treated with intravenous pulsed methylprednisolone 10 mg/kg for three days followed by augmented oral prednisolone for one month. Patients with recurrent acute rejection episodes of steroid resistant rejection are treated with anti-thymocyte globulin, photophoresis or methotrexate.

Assessment of graft function

Analysis of blood gases and examination of chest radiographs are used to monitor graft function over the first few postoperative days. Thereafter, chest radiographs are performed daily for approximately one week, and lung function is monitored by continuous oximetry, daily spirometry and regular measurement of lung volumes and diffusing capacity. Patients undergoing SLT for COPD undergo a ventilation perfusion scan in the first week to ensure good perfusion and ventilation to the newly transplanted lung. In patients with emphysema, there is both early preferential ventilation and perfusion to the transplanted lung – unlike the situation following SLT for pulmonary fibrosis when preferential ventilation appears to lag behind preferential perfusion by about three weeks [23].

The principal problem in the management of lung transplant recipients is that clinically it is impossible to separate opportunist lung infections from lung rejection. Both complications can present identical respiratory symptoms and identical respiratory physical signs. A chest radiograph is unhelpful since pulmonary infiltrates may be common to both, and in the early postoperative period may also occur as a result of reimplantation injury. Moreover, the chest radiograph may be entirely normal in patients experiencing acute rejection. This is particularly true after the first month following transplantation.

During most episodes of acute rejection and infection the FEV_1 and diffusing capacity show a sustained fall of greater than 10%. Thus, unlike other solid organ transplant patients, graft function following lung transplantation can be monitored with ease. Many transplant units teach recipients to monitor their own using hand-held battery spirometers.

A diagnosis of rejection is currently based on transbronchial biopsy using alligator forceps under radiological screening [24]. The principal morphological changes found in acute rejection are perivascular infiltrates which may extend into alveolar septa at the later stages of rejection. Additionally, bronchial tissue may also show evidence of lymphocytic infiltrate. It is our practice to carry out three or four biopsies from each lobe of one lung. Rejection may be patchy, and the use of multiple biopsies from multiple lobes affords a greater chance of positive diagnosis. Moreover, opportunist infection and rejection may coexist. In a series reported from Papworth Hospital just under 25% of the biopsies performed in the face of a deteriorating clinical condition or a reduction in lung function showed the presence of both infection and rejection. For this reason, bronchoalveolar lavage is routinely combined with transbronchial biopsy, with the lavage submitted for viral culture, monoclonal staining for pneumocystis, and routine culture for bacteria and fungi. The practice of routine surveillance transbronchial lung biopsies on all patients at one week, one, three, six and 12 months and annually remains controversial. However, it has been shown to identify unexpected mild rejection in up to 20% of cases.

□ RESULTS

With appropriate selection of patients, the results of HLT, SLT and BSLT are good [12–14,25]. Approximately 10–15% of recipients die in the first few weeks following transplantation, usually because of problems with poor lung preservation leading to diffuse alveolar damage, sepsis or both. The one-year survival for UK centres is 70–80%, with a three-year survival of 55–60%. The most important complications leading to death are opportunist infections and the development of OB. Current data suggest approximately 30% of patients surviving the peri-operative period will develop OB within five years of their transplant. In most cases, this leads to a progressive deterioration in lung function unresponsive to medical therapy and ultimate progression to respiratory failure, death or consideration of retransplantation after 6–12 months.

After SLT for COPD, the transplanted lung receives approximately 80% of total ventilation and perfusion over the first year. As would be predicted, the flow volume curve after SLT for emphysema shows a two-compartment pattern, the initial high flow originating from the transplanted lung and the subsequent 'tail' of low flow from the native lung. Lung function, CT and transbronchial lung biopsies have revealed normal results in patients up to five years after transplantation, indicating the potential for prolonged survival in patients who do not develop OB.

☐ LONG-TERM COMPLICATIONS

Obliterative bronchiolitis

OB may be defined physiologically by the development of progressive irreversible airflow obstruction unresponsive to augmented steroids [26]. Pathology shows obliteration of bronchioles, the lumens of which are filled by organising fibrin associated with fibroblasts and mononuclear cells. Immunohistology has revealed infiltration of the walls of the bronchioles by CD8 lymphocytes [27]. The small bronchioles are left as fibrous bands extending out to the pleura, with associated dilatation of the bronchiectasis of proximal airways. Vascular sclerosis affecting both pulmonary arteries and pulmonary veins may also be seen in conjunction with OB. Current evidence suggests that the development of OB is related to the frequency and severity of rejection occurring in the first 6–12 months following transplantation, the presence of persisting rejection after the first month probably being most important. More recent evidence has demonstrated a clear relation-ship between the presence of both lymphocytic bronchiolitis, which represents airway directed rejection, and organising pneumonia in the subsequent development of OB.

The disease usually results in progressive loss of function due to airflow obstruction over a 6–12 month period, leading to respiratory failure and death. However, a few patients appear to 'stabilise', with evidence of inactive OB on biopsy and attenuation of the loss in FEV_1. Some patients with OB have demonstrated a clinical response to increased immunosuppression [28]. In patients who are maintained on cyclosporin, a switch to tacrolimus or total lymphoid irradiation may stabilise lung function. Other approaches have included cyclophosphamide.

Continued research aims to identify those patients at risk of this most important complication at an early stage when augmented immunosuppression might be successful in preventing irreversible bronchiolar obliteration.

Lymphoproliferative disorders

The association between immunosuppression and lymphoproliferative disorders has been well recognised. The most common form affects the B cell lineage resulting in B cell non-Hodgkin's lymphoma. Such lymphomas are usually associated with the Epstein-Barr virus. Abnormal lymphatic tissue has been found within lung transplant parenchyma itself as well as in lymph nodes and spleen. The lymphoma usually responds to a reduction in the level of immunosuppression.

☐ DISEASE RECURRENCE

There is no evidence so far that patients with COPD, including those with alpha 1-antitrypsin deficiency and emphysema, develop recurrence of their original disease. All transplant centres regard the cessation of smoking as an absolute requirement for acceptance on the active waiting list. Thus, provided recipients do not take up smoking again, the potential risk of disease recurrence should be reduced.

☐ CONCLUSIONS

Lung transplantation now offers an effective therapy for patients with end-stage COPD. Debate remains as to which operation these patients, particularly those with emphysema, are most suited. In practice, well chosen recipients, without the presence of frequent pulmonary sepsis or bilateral bullae, appear to do well with SLT, while patients with these complications do as well with BSLT as with HLT.

The major problems currently facing lung transplantation are a shortfall in suitable donor organs compared with the number of potential recipients. For this reason, we do not advocate that patients on the active waiting list should be intubated for chronic ventilation.

In the early postoperative period, opportunist infection and graft rejection remain the major problems. In the long term, OB will affect approximately 30% of patients, leading to potential graft failure. Much current research is aimed at reducing this figure. Patients with COPD who have received lung transplants and remain free of this complication enjoy an excellent standard of life, with normal or near normal restoration of activity and good prospects of prolonged survival.

REFERENCES

1   Reitz BA, Wallwork JL, Hunt SA, Pennock JL, *et al.* Heart lung transplantation: successful therapy for patients with pulmonary vascular disease. *N Engl J Med* 1982; **306**: 557–64.

2   Penketh A, Higenbottam T, Hakim M, Wallwork J. Heart and lung transplantation in patients with end stage lung disease. *Br Med J* 1987; **295**: 311–4.

3   Wildevuur CR, Benfield JR. A review of 23 human lung transplantations by 20 surgeons. Review. *Ann Thorac Surg* 1970; **9**: 489–515.

4   Unilateral transplantation for pulmonary fibrosis. Toronto Lung Transplant Group. *N Engl J Med* 1986; **314**: 1140–5.

5   Patterson GA, Cooper JD, Goldman B, Weisel RD, *et al.* Technique of successful clinical double-lung transplantation. *Ann Thorac Surg* 1988; **45**: 626–33.

6   Patterson GA, Todd TR, Cooper JD, Pearson FG, *et al.* Airway complications after double lung transplantation. Toronto Lung Transplant Group. *J Thorac Cardiovasc Surg* 1990; **99**: 14–20; discussion 20–1.

7   Noirclerc MJ, Metras D, Vaillant A, Dumon JF, *et al.* Bilateral bronchial anastomosis in double lung and heart-lung transplantations. *Eur J Cardiothorac Surg* 1990; **4**: 314–7.

8   Pasque MK, Cooper JD, Kaiser LR, Haydock DA, *et al.* Improved technique for bilateral lung transplantation: rationale and initial clinical experience. *Ann Thorac Surg* 1990; **49**: 785–91.

9   Stevens PM, Johnson PC, Bell RL, Beall AC Jr, Jenkins DE. Regional ventilation and perfusion after lung transplantation in patients with emphysema. *N Engl J Med* 1970; **282**: 245–9.

10 Vanderhoeft RJ, Rocmans P, Nemry C, de Francquen P, *et al.* Left lung transplantation in a patient with emphysema. *Arch Surg* 1971; **103**: 505–9.

11 Mal H, Andreassian B, Pamela F, Duchatelle JP, *et al.* Unilateral lung transplantation in end-stage pulmonary emphysema. *Am Rev Respir Dis* 1989; **140**: 797–802.

12 Colquhoun IW, Gascoigne AD, Gould FK, Corris PA, Dark JH. Native pulmonary sepsis after single-lung transplantation. *Transplantation* 1991; **52**: 931–3.

13   Khaghani A, Banner N, Ozdogan E, Musumeci F, *et al.* Medium-term results of combined heart and lung transplantation for emphysema. *J Heart Lung Transplant* 1991; **10**: 15–21.

14   Kaiser LR, Pasque MK, Trulock EP, Low DE, *et al.* Bilateral sequential lung transplantation: the procedure of choice for double-lung replacement. *Ann Thorac Surg* 1991; **52**: 438–45; discussion 445–6.

15   ISHLT International Guidelines for Selection of Lung Transplant Candidates. *J Heart Lung Transplant* 1998; **17**: 703–9.

16   Morrison DL, Maurer JR, Grossman RF. Preoperative assessment for lung transplantation. *Clin Chest Med* 1990; **11**: 207–15.

17   Hunter AM, Carey MA, Larsh HW. The nutritional status of patients with chronic obstructive pulmonary disease. *Am Rev Respir Dis* 1981; **124**: 376–81.

18   Bidstrup BP, Royston D, Sapsford RN, Taylor KM. Reduction in blood loss and blood use after cardiopulmonary bypass with high dose aprotinin (Trasylol). *J Thorac Cardiovasc Surg* 1989; **97**: 364–72.

19   Colquhoun IW, Gascoigne AD, Au J, Corris PA, *et al.* Airway complications after pulmonary transplantation. *Ann Thorac Surg* 1994; **57**: 141–5.

20   Doig JC, Corris PA, Hilton CJ, Dark JH, Bexton RS. Effect of single lung transplantation on pulmonary hypertension in patients with end stage fibrosing lung disease. *Br Heart J* 1991; **66**: 431–4.

21   Bennett WM, Pulliam JP. Cyclosporine nephrotoxicity. *Ann Intern Med* 1983; **99**: 851–4.

22   Hosenpud JD, Bennett LE, Keck BM, Edwards EB, Novick R. Effect of diagnosis on survival benefit of lung transplantation for end-stage lung disease. *Lancet* 1998; **351**: 24–7.

23   McCleod AT, Stone TN, Hawkins T, Dark JH, Corris PA. Ventilation perfusion relationships after single lung transplantation for pulmonary fibrosis. *Am Rev Respir Dis* 1989; **139**: A265.

24   Higenbottam T, Stewart S, Penketh A, Wallwork J. Transbronchial lung biopsy for the diagnosis of rejection in heart-lung transplant recipients. *Transplantation* 1988; **46**: 532–9.

25   Yacoub M, Khaghani A, Theodoropoulos S, Tadjkarimi S, Banner N. Single-lung transplantation for obstructive airways disease. *Transplant Proc* 1991; **23**: 1213–4.

26   Scott JP, Higenbottam TW, Sharples C, Clelland CA, *et al.* Risk factors for obliterative bronchiolitis in heart-lung transplant recipients. *Transplantation* 1991; **51**: 813–7.

27   Milne DS, Gascoigne AD, Wilkes J, Sviland L, *et al.* The immunohistopathology of obliterative bronchiolitis following lung transplantation. *Transplantation* 1992; **54**: 748–50.

28   Glanville AR, Baldwin JC, Burke CM, Theodore J, Robin ED. Obliterative bronchiolitis after heart-lung transplantation: apparent arrest by augmented immunosuppression. *Ann Intern Med* 1987; **107**: 300–4.

☐ SELF ASSESSMENT QUESTIONS

1   Which of the following are true?

(a) Successful lung transplantation in patients with emphysema requires transplantation of heart and lungs

(b) Bilateral lung transplantation requires routine cardiopulmonary bypass

(c) Bilateral lung transplantation requires wrapping of the bronchial anastomoses for successful healing

(d) Patients with alpha 1-antitrypsin deficiency emphysema require replacement therapy after transplantation

2   Which of the following are true?

(a) The presence of pulmonary hypertension in patients with emphysema represents an adverse prognostic feature

(b) Patients with emphysema should be referred for transplantation when their FEV_1 has fallen to 40% predicted

(c) Hypercapnia represents an adverse prognostic sign in patients with chronic obstructive pulmonary disease (COPD)
(d) Low-dose oral corticosteroid therapy constitutes a contraindication for transplantation

3   Criteria in support of consideration of volume reduction surgery for emphysema include:
(a) Marked hyperinflation
(b) Homogeneous disease
(c) Alpha1-antitrypsin deficiency
(d) Pulmonary hypertension

4   Episodes of acute graft rejection post-lung transplantation may be characterised by:
(a) A fall in FEV_1 of more than 10%
(b) Hypertension on chest X-ray
(c) A perivascular neutrophil infiltration
(d) An unexplained fever

5   Long-term complications following lung transplantation for COPD include:
(a) Obliterative bronchiolitis
(b) B cell lymphoproliferative disease
(c) Recurrence of emphysema in alpha 1-antitrypsin deficient patients
(d) *Pneumocystis carinii* pneumonia

ANSWERS

1a False	2a True	3a True	4a True	5a True
b False	b False	b False	b False	b True
c False	c True	c False	c False	c False
d False	d False	d False	d True	d False

How to manage the adolescent with cystic fibrosis

Kevin Webb

□ INTRODUCTION

The adolescent years of the patient with cystic fibrosis (CF) evenly straddle childhood and adulthood. CF patients from the two Manchester paediatric centres are referred to the adult CF unit at the age of 16 years. At present, there are 240 CF patients in this unit, of whom 60 (25%) are adolescents.

CF is no longer a disease solely associated with childhood, and nearly all paediatric patients now reach adulthood due to the superb care of the paediatricians. Currently, mean survival is into the fourth decade of life and it is predicted that CF babies born today will survive into their fifth and sixth decades [1].

For the CF adolescent maturing into adulthood, aspirations and ambitions are the same as those of their healthy peers, but they still have the burden of a lethal lung disease for which there remains an unfulfilled promise of a cure with gene therapy.

Adolescence is a time of change for CF patients on an adult unit. They become responsible for their own self-care and wish to lead an independent life. Their disease may take second place to personal issues such as relationships, social life and developing a career. A decline in self-care can result in irreversible disease progression. It is crucial for the CF team to manage the medical and personal issues of the adolescent in a professional and sensitive manner. Getting the balance right can determine both quality of life and longevity for the CF adolescent.

□ TRANSITION FROM PAEDIATRIC TO ADULT CARE

There has been considerable debate – but few comparisons or structured guidelines – about the best way of transferring CF adolescents to adult care [2,3]. It is essential for the adult unit to receive from the paediatric unit as much medical and personal information as possible about the transferring patient. The medical information is often detailed in an annual review. Different members of the multidisciplinary team can also communicate information about their own areas of expertise to each other.

A detailed social history is crucial and sets the scene for potential difficulties for all aspects of care. The adolescent is assuming responsibility for self-care, and parents may be reluctant to concede what they have achieved in maintaining the health of their child. They are concerned (often correctly) that their child will neglect self-care, with an associated decline in health.

It is also fundamental that the adult CF team makes the new adolescent patient welcome. On the Manchester unit, it is considered that it usually takes at least a year for the patient and team to get to know each other. In order to familiarise the adolescent patient with the adult unit, each adolescent receives before transfer a comprehensive introductory package which describes the unit facilities, provides a contact card with staff phone numbers and a recent copy of the patient-led news bulletin. A website for the unit has recently been installed.

One of the difficult questions at the time of transfer is whether the terminally sick adolescent should be transferred to adult care – this maxim can also apply to the prepubertal adolescent who may be intimidated by the much more mature adult CF patients.

☐ MEDICAL CARE

Chest care

Medical care for all CF patients should be delivered from a CF centre [4]. Treatment is complex and onerous (Table 1). Nutrition and pulmonary function, the two main prognostic factors for clinical outcome, are better when care is provided by continuous multidisciplinary paediatric and adult CF centred care [4]. Unfortunately, the treatment delivered by the multidisciplinary team increases rather than lessens the burden of self-care for the maturing adolescent. The major component is directed at delaying progression of lung disease. Chronic infection with *Pseudomonas aeruginosa* is treated aggressively and admission to hospital for courses of intravenous antibiotics frequent. At home, the daily burden of self-care has increased enormously. It now invades sleep for those patients with severe disease awaiting transplantation: night-time self-care can include continuous oxygen, enteral feeding and non-invasive ventilation. At the same time, the adolescent is trying to lead a normal life!

Extrathoracic medical disease

The basic defect for CF is expressed in epithelial cells lining all ductal systems. As CF patients mature into adulthood, an increasing number of extrathoracic problems become manifest (Table 2). Liver disease may present with bleeding from varices. On

Table 1 Treatment of the chest for cystic fibrosis patients.

• Antibiotics:
  – oral
  – nebulised
  – intravenous
	• Vitamins

	• Exercise

• Nutrition:
  – nasogastric feeding
  – gastrostomy
	• Physiotherapy

	• Home intravenous antibiotics
	• Oxygen
• Pancreatic supplements	• Home non-invasive ventilation

Table 2 Extrathoracic problems.

• Diabetes mellitus	• Increased cancer risk:
• Liver disease (biliary cirrhosis)	– small bowel
• Low bone density	– pancreas
• Incontinence	– biliary tree
• Abdominal pain:	• Vasculitis of skin
– pancreatitis	• Joint problems
– renal stones	
– bowel obstruction	

the Manchester unit 5–6 new cases of diabetes are diagnosed each year, all of whom should be treated with insulin. Delay in diagnosis and treatment can result in respiratory and nutritional decline [5].

Recent clinical problems presenting in some adolescent CF patients are low bone density [6] and, in females, urinary incontinence [7]. Low bone density results in back pain and an increase in fractures of ribs and long bones. Rib fractures can cause severe chest pain and sputum retention and result in severe infective exacerbations. The sporting activities enjoyed by many CF adolescents also make them vulnerable to an increased fracture rate.

Urinary leakage is remarkably common in adolescent CF females. It can cause great social embarrassment; there is a reluctance to use expiratory manoeuvres such as coughing or to perform lung function tests. The cause of the incontinence is unknown, and most patients are too embarrassed to have investigations and thereby the potential for treatment is reduced.

☐ SOCIAL AND PERSONAL ISSUES FOR THE CYSTIC FIBROSIS ADOLESCENT

Awareness of mortality

CF patients are optimistic about their disease and often cope by being positive, sometimes denying to themselves the severity of their disease. This works well until they have to face reality. Adolescents new to the adult unit are confronted with significant numbers of adults with CF who are chronically unwell, some in need of a transplant. Approximately 8–12 patients die each year on a large adult CF unit. Some of the adolescents will have developed friendships with these terminally ill patients, and find themselves attending funerals with the sharpened awareness that they are likely to die of the same disease as their friends. Unsurprisingly, some adolescents find this situation difficult to handle. A clinical psychologist attached to the Manchester unit has provided enormous help with the fears and anxieties of the adolescent population.

Independence, peer pressure, bad behaviour and fast-lane life

Improved survival has given us 'generations' of CF patients. Many CF adults are in the 30s and 40s. Consequently, on arrival in the adult unit the impressionable adolescent suddenly becomes the youngest patient there. The adolescent is often struggling to gain independence from parental pressure and sensitivity is required by the multidisciplinary team to resolve this area of conflict. Older patients can corrupt the younger patients by suggesting they need not do as much self-care as suggested by the team and compliance with treatment can drop dramatically.

The adolescent patients may also be introduced to smoking and soft drugs by the charismatic older patients. Smoking cigarettes and marihuana is frequent amongst CF patients and a smoking cessation clinic for our patients has recently been started.

Adolescence is a time when anger and frustration are expressed. CF disrupts lifestyle and can make this situation much worse. This anger is often directed at parents and carers. Adolescents can be extremely abusive to nursing staff and, despite the professional approach and understanding of the team, the resultant stress can be difficult to cope with. Careful handling of specific behaviour problems may be required.

Some disruptive behaviour may simply spring from family neglect. An example of what may happen occurred some years ago when a recently transferred adolescent with alcoholic parents accused the staff of sexual harassment. She also stated that she had been raped by a male nurse at the referring paediatric hospital. Neither fact was correct, but an experienced CF social worker had carefully to defuse a potentially explosive situation.

CF adolescents often live life in the 'fast lane'. Their awareness of a limited future often pushes them to live life to the full socially and take risks. They choose sporting activities which have a risk attached, such as bunji jumping, parachuting and paragliding [8]. The mobility allowance means that adolescents with CF can pass a driving test a year earlier than other adolescents. Repeated car crashes and multiple speeding fines with excess points are common amongst them.

Fertility, sterility, pregnancy and safe sex

Some of the adolescents' greatest concerns at the time of transfer to an adult CF unit are issues about fertility and relationships.

Males

The majority of paediatricians inform their male CF adolescents that they are infertile prior to their transition to the adult unit. Most of them would like infertility discussed prior to their transfer. Nevertheless, a recent study found that 26% of males with CF learnt about their infertility only when they were over the age of 20 years [9]. It can be disastrous for the CF male to find out by chance that he is infertile. This issue needs addressing with great sensitivity, emphasising that new therapeutic technologies such as microepididymal aspiration can now be used to enable CF males to become biological fathers [10].

Females

Despite previous reports, CF females appear to be as fertile as their healthy peers. There have been 40 pregnancies on the Manchester adult CF unit. CF females have similar wishes for a family as their healthy peers and, despite advice, most of their pregnancies are either unplanned or conception takes place against medical advice. Poor nutrition and lung function can make pregnancy hazardous for both mother and child [11]. The CF adolescent will sometimes explain her desire for a child as wanting someone to be left behind after she has died.

Safe sex

CF adolescents are sexually active. It is important to provide sensitive advice about safe sex. Chlamydial infection (a cause of female infertility) is increasing, and vaginal candidiasis is frequent in CF females taking long-term antibiotics.

Education and employment

Despite their disease, CF adolescents achieve a high level of education, with the same number as their healthy peers going on to higher education [12].

Attaining employment can be difficult. In the UK, 50% of CF patients are in paid employment [12]. The CF patient also has the dilemma of whether or not to disclose their disease status. Good career advice is essential for 16–19 years olds when they are trying to organise their future. Getting it wrong can prejudice work prospects.

☐ CONCLUSIONS

Adolescents with CF have special needs and high expectations. They want the same quality of life as their healthy peers, but they have a lethal disease with which mean actuarial survival is only into the fourth decade of life. As described above, trying to cope with health and disease creates conflict and potential premature decline in health status. Managing the CF adolescent requires the expertise of a multidisciplinary team based upon hard won experience, sometimes with failure. Although failure does occur, it is a testimony to CF adolescents how many mature into adulthood living a remarkably normal life.

REFERENCES

1   Elborn JS, Shale DJ, Britton JR. Cystic fibrosis: current survival and population estimates to the year 2000. *Thorax* 1991; 46: 881–5.

2   Conway SP. Transition from paediatric to adult-orientated care for adolescents with cystic fibrosis. Review. *Disabil Rehabil* 1998; 20: 209–16.

3   Transition from paediatric to adult care. A guide for purchasers, providers and clinical teams. Bromley, Kent: Cystic Fibrosis Trust, 1997.

4   Mahadeva R, Webb K, Westerbeek RC, Carroll NR, Dodd ME. Clinical outcome in relation to care in centres specialising in cystic fibrosis: cross sectional study. *Br Med J* 1998; 316: 1771–5.

5   Milla CE, Warwick WJ, Moran A. Trends in pulmonary function in patients with cystic fibrosis correlate with the degree of glucose intolerance at baseline. *Am J Respir Crit Care Med* 2000; 162: 891–5.

6   Haworth CS, Selby PL, Webb AK, Dodd ME, *et al.* Low bone mineral density in adults with cystic fibrosis. *Thorax* 1999; 54: 961–7.

7   Orr A, McVean RJ, Webb AK, Dodd ME. Questionnaire survey of urinary incontinence in women with cystic fibrosis. *Br Med J* 2001; **322**: 1521.

8   Webb AK, Dodd ME. Exercise and sport in cystic fibrosis: benefits and risks. *Br J Sports Med* 1999; **33**: 77–8.

9   Fair A, Griffiths K, Osman LM. Attitudes to fertility issues among adults with cystic fibrosis in Scotland. The Collaborative Group of Scottish Adult CF Centres. *Thorax* 2000; **55**: 672–7.

10 Oates RD, Honig S, Berger MJ, Harris D. Microepididymal sperm aspiration (MESA): a new option for treatment of obstructive azoospermia associated with cystic fibrosis. *J Assist Reprod Genet* 1992; **9**: 36–40.

11 Edenborough FP, Stableforth DE, Webb AK, Mackenzie WE, Smith DL. Outcome of pregnancy in women with cystic fibrosis. *Thorax* 1995; **50**: 170–4.

12 Walters S. Association of CF adults (UK) survey: analysis and report 1995. Bromley, Kent: Cystic Fibrosis Trust, 1996.

☐ SELF ASSESSMENT QUESTIONS

1   Prognosis in cystic fibrosis (CF) is related to:
(a) Rate of growth
(b) Nutrition
(c) Liver disease
(d) Pulmonary function
(e) Intravenous antibiotic usage

2   Urinary leakage is:
(a) Commoner in older CF females
(b) Related to expiratory manoeuvres
(c) Due to the basic defect
(d) Easy to treat
(e) Found in men

3   Extrathoracic complications of CF include:
(a) Pulmonary vasculitis
(b) Low bone density
(c) Cancer of the small bowel
(d) Epilepsy
(e) Hepatocellular failure

4   With regard to fertility:
(a) Females are relatively infertile
(b) Males have normal sperm
(c) Is affected by candidiasis in females
(d) All children of CF parents will be carriers of the CF gene
(e) CF parents cannot adopt

5   Adolescents with CF:
(a) Should be transferred to an adult unit only after puberty
(b) Cope well by denying disease severity

(c) Improve self-care on an adult unit
(d) Are no different from other adolescents
(e) Do not smoke

ANSWERS

1a False	2a False	3a False	4a False	5a False
b True	b True	b True	b True	b True
c False	c False	c True	c False	c False
d True	d False	d False	d True	d True
e False	e False	e False	e True	e False

The Croonian Lecture

Hepato-canalicular cholestasis: its mechanisms, causes and consequences

Piotr Milkiewicz and Elwyn Elias

☐ BILE ACIDS: PHYSIOLOGY

Bile formation and secretion are important functions of the liver, permitting excretion of highly lipophilic endogenous and exogenous substances. Primary and secondary bile acids, cholesterol and the phospholipid, phosphatidyl choline, are the main constituents of bile [1]. The major primary bile acids in man, cholic and chenodeoxycholic acid, are synthesised from cholesterol exclusively in the liver. They are conjugated within hepatocytes with glycine or taurine and then secreted into the bile where, together with phospholipid and cholesterol, they form micelles. Conjugation with amino acids reduces passive bile acid reabsorption by diffusion from the biliary tree and jejunum, but permits their conservation by carrier-mediated active transport from the terminal ileum and their return to the liver in the portal vein, thus completing the enterohepatic circulation (Fig. 1).

Bile acids entering the colon undergo deconjugation (loss of glycine and taurine) and 7α-dehydroxylation by colonic bacteria. This process leads to the formation of deoxycholic acid from cholic acid and lithocholic acid from chenodeoxycholic acid, secondary bile acids which are more hydrophobic and toxic than primary bile acids. Deoxycholic acid has recently been linked with the pathogenesis of colonic cancer [2] and with gallstone formation in patients with acromegaly treated with octreotide [3]. Significant amounts of deoxycholic and lithocholic acids have been found in oesophageal aspirates of patients with Barrett's metaplasia, prompting speculation about their potential involvement in the pathogenesis of oesophageal carcinoma [4]. Lithocholic acid has well documented hepatotoxic and cholestatic properties.

Recent discoveries have greatly enhanced our understanding of the events involved in the transport of bile acids at the level of the hepatocyte. This has led to detailed characterisation of the pathogenesis of several cholestatic syndromes and has therapeutic implications [5].

At the level of the sinusoidal membrane of the hepatocyte, bile acids are avidly taken up by at least two different, recently characterised and cloned transporters. Both conjugated and unconjugated bile acids are chiefly taken up by a bile acid-specific, sodium-taurocholate cotransporting protein which is expressed only in the liver and is structurally similar to the intestinal bile acid transporter. A proportion of bile acids is also taken up by a family of multispecific, sodium-independent

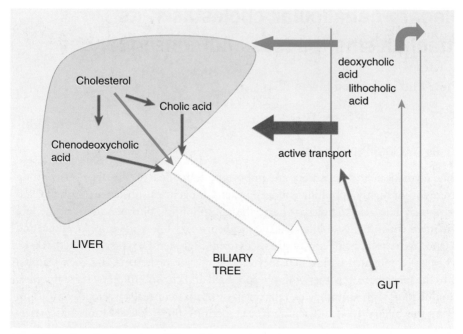

Fig. 1 Enterohepatic circulation of bile salts.

transporters called organic anion transporters. At the canalicular pole of the hepatocyte, bile acids are actively secreted into the bile against an enormous concentration gradient via two adenosine triphosphate-dependent transport systems. The bile salt export pump (BSEP) is responsible for the transport of non-metabolised bile acids, whereas multidrug resistant protein 2 (MRP2), formerly called multiorganic anion transporter, is involved in the canalicular excretion of a multiplicity of organic anions including sulphated and glucuronidated bile acids. Another canalicular transporter, not directly involved in the transport of bile acids but equally important in the pathogenesis of some cholestatic syndromes, is multidrug resistant protein 3 (MDR3). This is a phospholipid flippase, responsible for canalicular translocation of phosphatidylcholine from the inner to the outer leaflet of the canalicular membrane (see below). Hepatocyte transporters are shown schematically in Fig. 2 and demonstrated in human liver sections in Fig. 3.

☐ CHOLESTASIS

Cholestasis arises as a result of disruption of bile formation or flow. The focus of this chapter is canalicular cholestasis which, by definition, occurs at the level of the hepatocyte. The mechanisms of ductal (obstructive) cholestasis will not be discussed. Canalicular cholestasis can be induced by several factors (listed in Table 1), including inborn defects of hepatocyte transporters or bile acid metabolism, drugs and total parenteral nutrition. Cholestasis is usually associated with several clinical symptoms, the most common being:

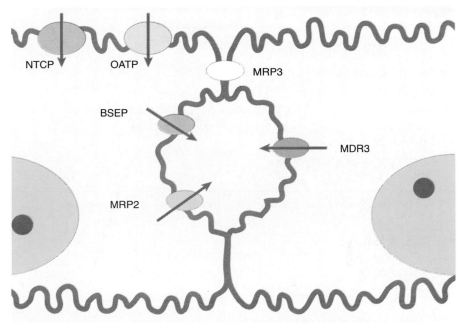

Fig. 2 Part of two adjacent hepatocytes which combine to form a bile canaliculus of 1 μm diameter are shown. Bile constituents are taken up from plasma by sodium-taurocholate cotransporting protein (NTCP) or organic anion transporter (OATP) and secreted into bile by transporters located within the canalicular membrane. Hereditary deficiency of these transporters is involved in the pathogenesis of inherited cholestatic syndromes (BSEP = bile salt export pump; MDR3 = multidrug resistant protein 3; MRP2 and 3 = multidrug resistant protein 2 and 3).

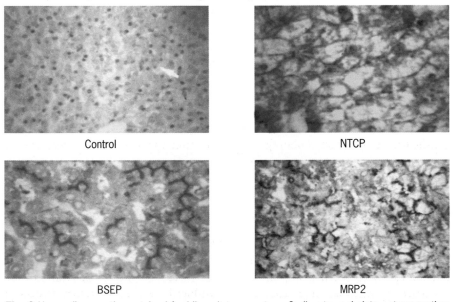

Fig. 3 Human liver sections stained for bile salt transporters. Sodium-taurocholate cotransporting protein (NTCP) can be seen within the sinusoidal and basolateral surface of the hepatocyte. Bile salt export pump (BSEP) and multidrug resistant protein 2 (MRP2) are confined to the bile canalicular membrane.

Table 1 Causes of intrahepatic cholestasis.

• Sex steroids
• Sepsis
• Total parenteral nutrition
• Drugs
• Alcohol
• Viral hepatitis
• Defects in bile acid synthesis
• Deficiency of canalicular transporters
• (PFIC 1, 2, 3, RFIC)

PFIC = progressive familial intrahepatic cholestasis; RFIC = recurrent familial intrahepatic cholestasis.

☐   pruritus

☐   steatorrhoea

☐   the consequences of malabsorption of fat-soluble vitamins, and

☐   hepatic osteodystrophy [6].

Pruritus

One of the most devastating symptoms of cholestasis is pruritus. If severe and intractable despite all available therapies, it may in itself be a sufficient indication for liver transplantation. Perhaps surprisingly, the intensity of pruritus does not correlate with plasma levels of bile acids. Recent work suggests that endogenous opioid peptides may exert a pruritogenic effect. This hypothesis has been supported by clinical studies demonstrating the pruritus-ameliorating effect of the opioid receptor antagonists, naloxone and naltrexone.

Steatorrhoea and malabsorption of fat-soluble vitamins

Decreased secretion of bile acids into the intestine, with consequent impairment of emulsification of dietary fat, leads to steatorrhoea. Bile acids are essential for absorption of fat-soluble vitamins. Their deficiency in patients with chronic cholestasis produces night blindness (vitamin A), osteomalacia (vitamin D) and coagulopathy (vitamin K).

Hepatic osteodystrophy

The aetiology of bone pathology in cholestasis is complex. It is not a simple consequence of osteomalacia due to vitamin D malabsorption, hypocalcaemia and secondary hyperparathyroidism. In most patients, hepatic osteodystrophy manifests with reduced bone formation and increased resorption leading to osteoporosis. A painful osteoarthropathy may also occur in some patients. All patients with chronic cholestasis are recommended to take supplementary vitamin D 800 iu and calcium 1 g daily. Bone mineral densitometry should be monitored and osteoporosis treated with bisphosphonates and hormonal replacement therapy as appropriate.

☐ HEREDITARY CHOLESTATIC SYNDROMES

Dysfunction of hepatocyte transporters

Recent characterisation and cloning of several transporters localised to the basolateral and canalicular membrane of the hepatocyte have clarified the aetiology of several inherited cholestatic syndromes.

Dubin-Johnson syndrome

In Dubin-Johnson syndrome there is a benign conjugated hyperbilirubinaemia, with autosomal recessive inheritance. Scleral icterus is often first noticed in teenagers or pregnant women. In the former, it is presumably because of competition for canalicular secretion between bilirubin diglucuronide and the pubertal surge of various conjugated sex hormone metabolites, while in pregnancy the high levels of sex hormones may be responsible. Retention of pigments within the hepatocyte typically makes the liver biopsy sample black. With the exception of serum bilirubin, routine liver function tests and serum bile acid levels are usually normal and life expectancy is not affected. The disease is the consequence of mutations in the *MRP2* gene, resulting in a scarcity of MRP2 protein in the canalicular membrane of the hepatocyte and impaired biliary secretion of various multicharged organic anions including bilirubin glucuronides [7]. Although the pigmented liver reflects permanent retention of some biliary waste within the liver, most compounds that would normally be excreted in bile are able to reflux into the bloodstream and are excreted in excess in urine. The diagnostic findings involving coproporphyrin I and III probably reflect this adaptation. In Dubin-Johnson syndrome the total 24-hour urinary excretion of coproporphyrin I and III is the same as in normal subjects, but the ratio of isomers III:I, normally 3:1 or 4:1, is inverted. The symptoms of Dubin-Johnson syndrome are benign because MRP2 is not involved in the transport of primary conjugated bile acids, so bile salt-dependent bile flow is not affected.

Progressive familial intrahepatic cholestasis type 1

An autosomal recessive disorder, progressive familial intrahepatic cholestasis type 1 (PFIC1), is also known as Byler's disease after Joseph Byler, a founder member of an Amish kindred in Pennsylvania, whose marriage to his first cousin led to generations of individuals with severe progressive intrahepatic cholestasis. The symptoms start in early infancy and manifest with recurrent episodes of intrahepatic cholestasis, diarrhoea, pancreatitis, pruritus and growth retardation. Routine liver function tests show marked elevation of alkaline phosphatase and bile acids in serum, with normal or only slightly increased γ-glutamyltransferase (γGT). The genetic defect was mapped to the FIC1 locus localised on chromosome 18q21-q22 [8]. In humans FIC1 is expressed in the pancreas, small intestine, urinary bladder and prostate. Although cholestasis is the most pronounced symptom of Byler's disease, the precise relation between the FIC1 locus and disruption of bile flow has not yet been elucidated.

Recurrent familial intrahepatic cholestasis

Now called recurrent familial intrahepatic cholestasis (RFIC), this syndrome was formerly called benign recurrent intrahepatic cholestasis. RFIC seems a more appropriate name because 'benign' does not reflect the severity of cholestatic symptoms during each attack. During their lifetime sufferers may experience a large number of episodes of jaundice, pruritus and steatorrhoea, each lasting several months. By definition, RFIC does not progress to chronic liver disease and cirrhosis, and there are long asymptomatic intervals between episodes. Serum bile acid levels are commonly increased before the first symptoms of cholestasis occur and, as in PFIC1, serum γGT is normal. Both PFIC1 and RFIC are associated with mutations of the same *FIC1* gene. PFIC1 and RFIC therefore represent cholestatic syndromes with widely different phenotypic expression arising from different mutations in a single gene [5].

Progressive familial intrahepatic cholestasis type 2

The genetic defect responsible for PFIC2 has been mapped to chromosome locus 2q24 which codes for BSEP, localised to the canalicular membrane of the hepatocyte [9]. Although PFIC2 shares several clinical and biochemical features with PFIC1, the disease progresses more rapidly, usually without significant periods of remission. Unlike PFIC1, PFIC2 commonly begins as non-specific giant cell hepatitis and histological sections may demonstrate more advanced inflammatory changes. Extrahepatic manifestations such as pancreatitis or diarrhoea, encountered in PFIC1, are not features of PFIC2.

Progressive familial intrahepatic cholestasis type 3

PFIC3 is associated with mutations of the *MDR3* gene located to chromosome 7q21 which codes for a flippase. This concentrates a specific phospholipid, phosphatidyl-choline (also known as lecithin), into the lumenal-facing leaflet of the bilaminar canalicular membrane whence it enters bile [10]. Mixed micelles formed by phospholipids and bile salts are able to solubilise cholesterol and protect the canalicular membrane and biliary epithelial cells from being damaged by the detergent bile salts. In PFIC3, lack of biliary phospholipid due to MDR3 malfunction leads to bile acid-induced damage of hepatocytes and cholangiocytes. In contrast to PFIC1 and PFIC2, serum γGT levels are high in PFIC3 and liver histology shows features of ductular proliferation and portal and periportal fibrosis, progressing to cirrhosis.

☐ POTENTIAL DYSFUNCTION OF HEPATOCYTE TRANSPORTERS

Obstetric cholestasis

Obstetric cholestasis (OC) (intrahepatic cholestasis of pregnancy) usually manifests in the second or third trimester of pregnancy with pruritus, most pronounced in the palms and soles. Serum bile acid concentrations are almost always elevated, with alanine aminotransferase the next most sensitive diagnostic test. Jaundice is relatively uncommon, complicating the most severe and prolonged episodes. OC is associated with increased risk of stillbirth, and it is recommended that pregnancy should not be allowed to continue beyond the 37th week of gestation. The symptoms classically disappear within 1–2 days after delivery.

Historically, OC has been attributed to the cholestatic effect of sex hormones, many of which have profoundly cholestatic properties, most notably 17β-oestradiol glucuronide. However, recent findings show that OC occurs more commonly in mothers of patients with PFIC or RFIC, which suggests that mothers heterozygous for mutations of genes coding for transporter proteins are predisposed to OC. In the family of an infant with PFIC3, maternally and paternally related women who were heterozygous for the MDR3 mutation had suffered from OC [11]. In another patient with OC and elevated γGT, but no family history of PFIC, a single amino acid substitution disrupted transporter trafficking to the membrane of transfected cells [12].

In the light of these findings, it is reasonable to speculate that mild malfunction of canalicular transporters leads to clinical symptoms of cholestasis when the transporter's capacity to excrete substrates is exceeded, which may occur with the high levels of sex hormones produced in pregnancy.

☐ TREATMENT OF CHOLESTASIS

Several agents used in the treatment of cholestasis are listed in Table 2. Two compounds, ursodeoxycholic acid (UDC) and S-adenosyl-L-methionine (SAMe), the subject of our recent research work, will be described in more detail.

Ursodeoxycholic acid

UDC is probably the most commonly prescribed drug in cholestatic disorders. It is a dihydroxy bile acid, traditionally derived from polar bear bile and used for many centuries in Chinese medicine. Several mechanisms have been postulated to account for its hepatoprotective properties, including:

☐ depletion of more toxic endogenous bile salts by feedback inhibition of *de novo* hepatic synthesis of bile acids and competitive inhibition of their absorption by gut

☐ its choleretic (enhancing bile flow) or immunomodulatory effects, and

☐ hepatocyte membrane protection.

Piotr Milkiewicz and Elwyn Elias

Table 2 Agents (established and experimental) used in the treatment of cholestasis-induced pruritus.

Agent	Mode of action	Clinical comment
Established		
Cholestyramine	Sequestration of bile acids and other organic anions in the intestine	Most effective when taken with breakfast. Separate by hours from administration of thyroxine, ursodeoxycholic acid, vitamin D, etc
Ursodeoxycholic acid	Replacement of toxic endogenous bile acids, stimulation of apical (canalicular) exocytosis by activation of protein kinase C	Safe, rarely may cause diarrhoea
Rifampicin	Speculative effects on pruritogen include: • induction of P450 to produce its urinary metabolite • inhibition of its formation by altering intestinal bacteria	Causes hepatitis, rarely requiring drug withdrawal
Antihistamines	Sedative effect	May cause confusion and psychomotor impairment
Naloxone/Naltrexone	Antagonisation of excess opioidergic tone associated with pruritus	Danger of opioid withdrawal symptoms can be countered by low escalating dose
Experimental		
Ondansetrone	Specific 5-hydroxytryptamine antagonist	
Propofol	Unknown	
S-adenosyl-L-methionine	Increased sulphation and methylation of potential pruritogen	Poor bioavailability when taken orally

It has been proposed that UDC or its taurine conjugated derivative (TUDC) may enhance the secretory potential of the liver in cholestasis by stimulation of a signalling network within the hepatocyte, leading to activation of calcium-dependent protein kinase C [13]. TUDC has recently been demonstrated to protect against cholestasis-induced disruption of the pericanalicular cytoskeleton and dispersal of canalicular transporters away from the canalicular membrane (Figs. 4 and 5 [14]. UDC has been shown to relieve the symptoms of cholestasis in several diseases, including primary biliary cirrhosis, OC, cystic fibrosis and in a proportion of patients with inherited cholestatic syndromes [13].

S-adenosyl-L-methionine

SAMe is a major methyl donor in mammalian cells and also an intermediate metabolite in the synthesis of cysteine and glutathione. Transmethylation with

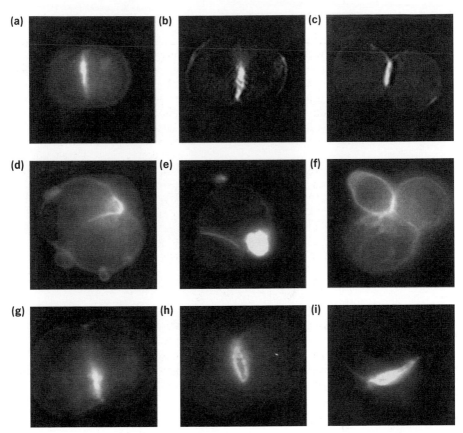

Fig. 4 Microphotographs showing intracellular distribution of F-actin in hepatocyte couplets: **(a)–(c)** controls; **(d)–(f)** treated with taurolithocholate (TLC); **(g)–(i)** treated with TLC and tauroursodeoxycholate (TUDCA). Filamentous actin is normally concentrated in the pericanalicular pole of the hepatocyte. TUDCA protects against disruption of the cytoskeletal structures introduced by TLC (reproduced, with permission, from [14]).

SAMe is one of the preferred mechanisms used by hepatocytes to detoxify a variety of substances [15]. Liver glutathione, derived from SAMe through the trans-sulphuration route, plays an important role in the maintenance of the normal redox potential. Chronic liver disease leads to an acquired deficiency of the enzyme SAMe synthetase, with subsequent impairment of detoxifying processes. In a recent double-blind, placebo-controlled trial SAMe was shown to be beneficial in patients with chronic, alcohol-induced liver disease [16]. Our experimental data show that SAMe protects and reverses cholestasis induced by cholestatic bile salts. When SAMe and TUDC are given simultaneously, their effectiveness in ameliorating cholestasis is additive [17].

These findings have led us to postulate that SAMe, as a precursor of sulphate, may facilitate sulphation of hydrophobic bile salts, thus decreasing their toxicity and precipitating their removal from the hepatocyte (Fig. 6). This hypothesis has been supported by subsequent experiments, clearly showing that the protective effect of

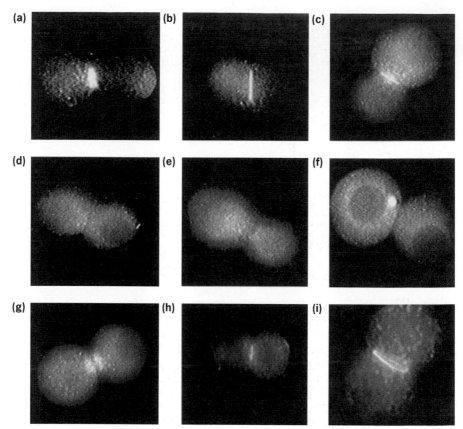

Fig. 5 Microphotographs showing canalicular localisation of multidrug resistant protein 2 (MRP2). Taurolithocholate (TLC)-treated hepatocyte couplets show dispersal and a diffuse, scattered pattern of MRP2 compared with controls. Tauroursodeoxycholate (TUDCA) partially protects against these changes: **(a)–(c)** controls; **(d)–(f)** treated with TLC; **(g)–(i)** treated with TLC and TUDCA (reproduced, with permission, from [14]).

SAMe is inhibited by addition of dehydroepiandrosterone, a competitive substrate for the sulphotransferase involved in sulphation of bile acids and sex hormones [18]. The possible clinical application of these findings has yet to be validated.

Acknowledgements

We wish to thank Professor Roger Coleman, Dr Charles Mills and Dr Marcelo Roma for their contribution to our research on intrahepatic cholestasis.

REFERENCES

1   Sherlock S, Dooley J. *Diseases of the liver and biliary system*, 10th edn. Oxford: Blackwell Science, 1993: 17.

2   Qiao D, Stratagouleas ED, Martinez JD. Activation and role of mitogen-activated protein kinases in deoxycholic acid-induced apoptosis. *Carcinogenesis* 2001; 22: 35–41.

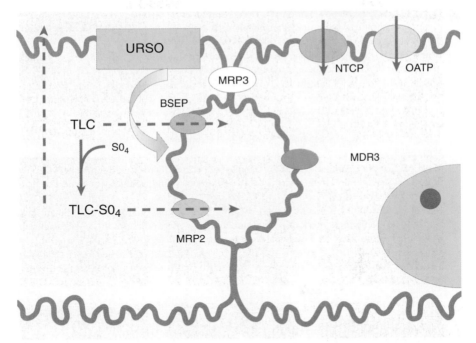

Fig. 6 Schematic representation of the mechanisms potentially involved in an additive effect of S-adenosyl-L-methionine and ursodeoxycholate (URSO) in taurolithocholate (TLC)-induced cholestasis. Sulphation of TLC (TLC-SO₄) makes it a suitable substrate for multidrug resistant protein 2 (MRP2) secretion into bile. It can be excreted in urine as well as bile because it is more hydrophilic than TLC. URSO increases recruitment of transporters (bile salt export pump (BESP) and MRP2) to the canalicular membrane (MDR3 = multidrug resistant protein 3; MRP3 = multidrug resistant protein 3; NTCP = sodium-taurocholate cotransporting protein; OATP = organic anion transporter).

3   Dowling RH. Review: pathogenesis of gallstones. *Aliment Pharmacol Ther* 2000; 14(Suppl 2): 39–47.

4   Jankowski JA, Harrison RF, Perry I, Balkwill F, Tselepis C. Barrett's metaplasia. *Lancet* 2000; **356**: 2079–85.

5   Jansen PLM, Muller M. The molecular genetics of familial intrahepatic cholestasis. Review. *Gut* 2000; **47**: 1–5.

6   Sherlock S, Dooley J. *Diseases of the liver and biliary system*, 10th edn. Oxford: Blackwell Science, 1993: 214.

7   Paulusma CC, Kool M, Bosma PJ, Scheffer GL, *et al.* A mutation in the human canalicular multispecific organic anion transporter gene causes the Dubin-Johnson syndrome. *Hepatology* 1997; **25**: 1539–42.

8   Bull LN, van-Eijk MJ, Pawlikowska L, De Young JA, *et al.* A gene encoding a P-type ATPase mutated in two forms of hereditary cholestasis. *Nat Genet* 1998; **18**: 219–24.

9   Strautnieks SS, Bull LN, Knisely AS, Kocoshis SA, *et al.* A gene encoding a liver-specific ABC transporter is mutated in progressive familial intrahepatic cholestasis. *Nat Genet* 1998; **20**: 233–8.

10 de Vree JM, Jacquemin E, Sturm E, Cresteil D, *et al.* Mutations in the MDR3 gene cause progressive familial intrahepatic cholestasis. *Proc Natl Acad Sci USA* 1998; **95**: 282–7.

11 Jacquemin E, Cresteil D, Manouvrier S, Boute O, Hadchouel M. Heterozygous non-sense mutation of the MDR3 gene in familial intrahepatic cholestasis of pregnancy. *Lancet* 1999; **353**: 210–1.

12   Dixon PH, Weerasekera N, Linton KJ, Donaldson O, *et al.* Heterozygous MDR3 missense mutation associated with intrahepatic cholestasis of pregnancy: evidence for a defect in protein trafficking. *Hum Mol Genet* 2000; **9**: 1209–17.

13   Beuers U, Boyer JL, Paumgartner G. Ursodeoxycholic acid in cholestasis: potential mechanisms of action and therapeutic applications. Review. *Hepatology* 1998; **28**: 1449–53.

14   Milkiewicz P, Roma MG, Mills CO, Coleman R, *et al.* Tauroursodeoxycholate (TUDCA) protects against redistribution of multidrug resistant protein 2 (Mrp2) and disruption of F-actin caused by taurolithocholate (TLC). A study in isolated rat hepatocyte couplets. *Hepatology* 1999; **30**: 461A.

15   Lieber CS. Role of S-adenosyl-L-methionine in the treatment of liver diseases. *J Hepatol* 1999; **30**: 1155–9.

16   Mato JM, Camara J, Fernandez de Paz J, Caballeria L, *et al.* S-adenosylmethionine in alcoholic liver cirrhosis: a randomized, placebo-controlled, double-blind, multicenter clinical trial. *J Hepatol* 1999; **30**: 1081–9.

17   Milkiewicz P, Mills CO, Roma MG, Ahmed-Choudhury JA, *et al.* Tauroursodeoxycholate and S-adenosyl-L-methionine exert an additive ameliorating effect on taurolithocholate-induced cholestasis: a study in isolated rat hepatocyte couplets. *Hepatology* 1999; **29**: 471–6.

18   Milkiewicz P, Roma MG, Cardenas R, Mills CO, *et al.* Effect of tauroursodeoxycholate and S-adenosyl-L-methionine on 17beta-estradiol glucuronide-induced cholestasis. *J Hepatol* 2001; **34**: 184–91.

□ SELF ASSESSMENT QUESTIONS

1   Deoxycholic acid:
   (a) Is hydrophilic and non-cholestatic
   (b) May stimulate proliferation of the colorectal epithelium
   (c) Is protective in cholestatic liver disorders
   (d) Has been linked with gallstone disease in patients with acromegaly
   (e) May be involved in the pathogenesis of oesophageal carcinoma

2   In inherited cholestatic syndromes:
   (a) Progressive familial intrahepatic cholestasis (PFIC) type 1 (formerly called Byler's disease) is a benign syndrome with normal life expectancy
   (b) Genetic mutation of bile salt export pump gene has been found in patients with PFIC3 syndrome
   (c) Ursodeoxycholate (URSO) is a recommended treatment in PFIC2 syndrome
   (d) FIC1 locus mutation has been found in both PFIC1 and recurrent familial intrahepatic cholestasis syndrome
   (e) Dubin-Johnson syndrome rapidly progresses and requires liver transplantation in early childhood

3   In cholestasis:
   (a) Intensity of pruritus correlates with the serum level of bile salts
   (b) Steatorrhoea is a recognised symptom
   (c) Malabsorption of vitamin D may lead to night blindness
   (d) Osteomalacia is a result of malabsorption of vitamin D
   (e) Coagulopathy may be treated with vitamin K

4 In obstetric cholestasis:
   (a) Symptoms classically manifest in the first trimester of pregnancy
   (b) Jaundice is present in almost all patients
   (c) There is increased risk of stillbirth
   (d) Symptoms resolve in the mother 2–3 months after delivery
   (e) In some patients the disease may be related to heterozygosity for multidrug resistant protein 3 (MDR3) mutation

5 In pruritus related with cholestasis:
   (a) Propofol is the drug of choice
   (b) URSO may work via activation of protein kinase C cascade
   (c) Rifampicin may cause symptomatic relief by induction of P450
   (d) Activation of opiate receptor by endogenous pruritogens is considered to play a role
   (e) Treatment with cholestyramine relieves symptoms in a significant proportion of patients

ANSWERS

1a	False	2a	False	3a	False	4a	False	5a	False
b	True	b	False	b	True	b	False	b	True
c	False	c	False	c	False	c	True	c	True
d	True	d	True	d	True	d	False	d	True
e	True	e	False	e	True	e	True	e	True